krausnet

ADVANCES IN STROKE THERAPY

Advances in Stroke Therapy

Editor

F. Clifford Rose, F.R.C.P.
Chairman
Department of Neurology
Charing Cross Hospital
London, England

Raven Press ■ New York

Raven Press, 1140 Avenue of the Americas, New York, New York 10036

Great care has been taken to maintain the accuracy of the information contained in the volume. However, Raven Press cannot be held responsible for errors or for any consequences arising from the use of the information contained herein.

Library of Congress Cataloging in Publication Data
Main entry under title:

Advances in stroke therapy.

Includes bibliographical references and index.
1. Cerebrovascular disease—Treatment.
2. Cerebrovascular disease—Patients—Rehabilitation. I. Rose, F. Clifford (Frank Clifford)
[DNLM: 1. Cerebrovascular disorders—Therapy.
2. Tomography, Emission computed. 3. Cerebrovascular disorders—Prevention and control. WL 355
A244]
RC388.5.A35   616.8'1   82–47508
ISBN 0–89004–847–9   AACR2

Opening Address

The Medical Society of London has been in the forefront of the movement to combine all branches of medicine. From its foundation in 1773, the principle of Fellowship was first an equal partnership between the physician, the surgeon, and the family practitioner, and now includes many others. The annual Mansell Bequest Symposium has been a fine example of the Society's early principles. In each of the symposia, the speakers have been drawn from all branches of our profession.

The other great ideal of our founder, John Coakley Lettsom, was to foster association with colleagues overseas. He was an American by birth, and overseas members of the profession have been welcome at our Society since those very early days. The Mansell Bequest Symposium has continued that great tradition, inviting speakers every year from many parts of the world.

The Medical Society of London has been pleased and honoured to act as host for this symposium, the publication of which provides a permanent record of the very high quality these meetings have achieved.

Ewart M. Jepson, President
Medical Society of London

Preface

Stroke is the third most common medical cause of death, after cancer and coronary disease. It is also one of the major causes of chronic disability. For these reasons, any approach that will lighten the lot of the patient, the load on his relatives, and the burden on the community will be greatly welcomed.

The first part of this volume is concerned with basic aspects, while the second part reevaluates techniques for diagnosis and management, with particular attention given to the use of positron emission tomography. The section on treatment of acute stroke reveals that we do not yet have any really effective cure, and indicates that the following section on the prevention of stroke must be regarded as a crucial topic. The following sections review some of the problems of surgery, the scientific basis of remedial therapy, whether stroke units are effective, and the management of the stroke patient in the community and outside the hospital service.

Taken together these considerations give us an update on what can be done for stroke, the great medical challenge of the 1980s.

This volume will be of interest to neurologists, rehabilitation physicians and allied personnel, and all general physicians involved in the management of stroke.

F. Clifford Rose

Contents

Contributors

A. J. Akhtar
Department of Geriatric Medicine
Royal Victoria Hospital, and
Department of Geriatric Medicine
University of Edinburgh
Edinburgh, United Kingdom

N. R. Ambler
The Royal Victoria Hospital
Dover, Kent
United Kingdom

H. J. M. Barnett
Department of Clinical Neurological
  Sciences
University of Western Ontario
London, Ontario, Canada

J. C. Baron
Service Hospitalier Frèdèric Joliot
Hôpital d'Orsay
Orsay, France

A. M. Bidabe
Department of Neuroradiology
Unité de Pathologie Vasculaire Cérébrale
University of Bordeaux
Bordeaux, France

P. W. Blower
Department of Rheumatology and
  Rehabilitation
Greenwich District Hospital
Greenwich, London
United Kingdom

B. Boneu
Service de Neurologie—CHU
Toulouse Purpan
Toulouse, France

M.-G. Bousser
Clinique des Maladies du Système
  Nerveux
Hôpital de la Salpêtrière
Paris, France

R. Busto
Department of Neurology
University of Miami School of Medicine
Miami, Florida

J. M. Caillé
Department of Neurology
Unité de Pathologie Vasculaire Cérébrale
University of Bordeaux
Bordeaux, France

R. Capildeo
Department of Neurology
Charing Cross Hospital
London, United Kingdom

J. P. Cassel
Department of Neurosurgery
Unité de Pathologie Vasculaire Cérébrale
University of Bordeaux
Bordeaux, France

P. Castaigne
Hôpital de la Salpêtrière
Paris, France

P.-L. Chin
Department of Geriatric Medicine
Cumberland Infirmary
Carlisle, United Kingdom

M. Clanet
Service de Neurologie—CHU
Toulouse Purpan
Toulouse, France

F. Cohadon
Departments of Neurosurgery and
  Experimental Medicine
University of Bordeaux
Bordeaux, France

D. Comar
Service Hospitalier Frédéric Joliot
Hôpital d'Orsay
Orsay, France

L. de Coninck
Unité de Pathologie Vasculaire Cérébrale
University of Bordeaux
Bordeaux, France

B. M. Coull
Comprehensive Stroke Center of Oregon
Oregon Health Sciences University
Portland, Oregon

J. F. Dartigues
Department of Statistics, Epidemiology
  and Computer Science
University of Bordeaux
Bordeaux, France

J. David
Service de Neurologie—CHU
Toulouse Purpan
Toulouse, France

S. Dunbar
Department of Physiotherapy and
  Occupational Therapy
Royal Victoria Hospital
Edinburgh, United Kingdom

H. H. G. Eastcott
St. Mary's Hospital
London, United Kingdom

V. Eaton Griffith
St. Martin's
Grimm's Hill
Great Missenden
Bucks, United Kingdom

W. S. Fields
Department of Neurology
University of Texas Medical School
Houston, Texas

P. Floras
Department of Neuroradiology
Unité de Pathologie Vasculaire Cérébrale
University of Bordeaux
Bordeaux, France

R. S. J. Frackowiak
Department of Neurology
Hammersmith Hospital
London, United Kingdom

W. M. Garraway
Department of Medical Statistics and
  Epidemiology
Mayo Clinic
Rochester, Minnesota

M. Gawel
Department of Neurology
Charing Cross Hospital
London, United Kingdom

R. M. Greenhalgh
Professorial Department of Surgery
Charing Cross Hospital Medical School
London, United Kingdom

B. Guiraud-Chaumeil
Service de Neurologie—CHU
Toulouse Purpan
Toulouse, France

S. Haberman
Department of Actuarial Sciences
The City University
London, United Kingdom

M. Height
Stroke Unit
Royal Victoria Hospital
Edinburgh, United Kingdom

P. Y. Henry
Department of Neurology
University of Bordeaux
Bordeaux, France

S. Hepinstall
Department of Medicine
University Hospital
Queen's Medical Centre
Nottingham, United Kingdom

R. D. Illingworth
Department of Neurosurgery
Charing Cross Hospital
London, United Kingdom

M. Irving
Cumberland Infirmary
Carlisle, United Kingdom

P. Loiseau
Department of Neurology
University of Bordeaux
Bordeaux, France

B. Isaacs
Department of Geriatric Medicine
University of Birmingham
Birmingham, United Kingdom

A. Lowenthal
Department of Neurology
Independent University of Antwerp
Wilrîjk, Belgium

E. W. Jones
Department of Medicine
University Hospital
Queen's Medical Centre
Nottingham, United Kingdom

E. McGuirk
Department of Speech Therapy
University Hospital
Nottingham, United Kingdom

C. Kellershohn
Service Hospitalier Frédéric Joliot
Hôpital d'Orsay
Orsay, France

J. Marquardsen
Department of Neurology
Aalborg Hospital
Aalborg, Denmark

K. Kogure
Department of Neurology
University of Miami School of Medicine
Miami, Florida

J. Marshall
Institute of Neurology
National Hospital for Nervous Diseases
London, United Kingdom

D. A. Lane
Department of Haematology
Charing Cross Hospital
London, United Kingdom

T. W. Meade
Epidemiology and Medical Care Unit
Northwick Park Hospital
Harrow, Middlesex
United Kingdom

R. Langton-Hewer
Frenchay Hospital
Bristol, United Kingdom

J. R. A. Mitchell
Department of Medicine
University Hospital
Queen's Medical Centre   ·
Nottingham, United Kingdom

D. Laplane
Hôpital de la Salpêtrière
Paris, France

L. Mitchell
Stroke Unit and Department of Geriatric
*   Medicine*
Royal Victoria Hospital
Belfast, United Kingdom

N. J. Legg
Department of Neurology
Hammersmith Hospital
London, United Kingdom

N. B. Lincoln
Department of Health Care of the Elderly
Sherwood Hospital
Nottingham, United Kingdom

G. P. Mulley
Department of Health Care of the Elderly
Sherwood Hospital
Nottingham, United Kingdom

J. M. Orgogozo
Department of Neurology
Unité de Pathologie Vasculaire Cérébrale
University of Bordeaux
Bordeaux, France

J. J. Péré
Department of Neurology
Unité de Pathologie Vasculaire Cérébrale
University of Bordeaux
Bordeaux, France

A. Rascol
Service de Neurologie—CHU
Toulouse Purpan
Toulouse, France

F. Clifford Rose
Department of Neurology
Charing Cross Hospital
London, United Kingdom

A. Rosie
Cumberland Infirmary
Carlisle, United Kingdom

R. W. R. Russell
Department of Neurology
St. Thomas's Hospital
London, United Kingdom

P. Scheinberg
Department of Neurology
University of Miami School of Medicine
Miami, Florida

R. Smith
Cumberland Infirmary
Carlisle, United Kingdom

T. J. Steiner
Department of Neurology
Charing Cross Hospital
London, United Kingdom

R. S. Stevens
Stroke Rehabilitation Centre
Royal Victoria Hospital
Dover, Kent, United Kingdom

L. Symon
Institute of Neurology
National Hospital
London, United Kingdom

P. M. Taylor
Department of Medicine
University Hospital
Queen's Medical Centre
Nottingham, United Kingdom

D. J. Thomas
St. Mary's Hospital
London, United Kingdom

D. T. Wade
Department of Neurology
Frenchay Hospital
Bristol, United Kingdom

J. P. H. Wade
Department of Neurology
St. Thomas's Hospital
London, United Kingdom

C. Warlow
Department of Clinical Neurology
Radcliffe Infirmary
Oxford, United Kingdom

J. P. Whisnant
Department of Neurology
Mayo Clinic and Medical School
Rochester, Minnesota

R. J. S. Wise
Department of Neurology
Hammersmith Hospital
London, United Kingdom

F. M. Yatsu
Department of Neurology
Comprehensive Stroke Center of Oregon
Oregon Health Sciences University
Portland, Oregon

ADVANCES IN STROKE THERAPY

Advances in Stroke Therapy, edited by
F. C. Rose. Raven Press, New York © 1982.

Mechanisms of Brain Swelling due to Ischemia

Peritz Scheinberg, K. Kogure, and R. Busto

Department of Neurology, University of Miami School of Medicine, Miami, Florida

The onset of brain ischemia is accomplished by an explosion of physiological and biochemical events, of which the relationships to each other and their roles in the development of infarction are still inadequately understood. This chapter focuses on only one of these events, brain swelling. There is little doubt that the increase in brain water that occurs in ischemia is of clinical importance; it is equally true that our ability to treat brain ischemia is dependent upon an understanding of its biological mechanisms. Clinicians are aware that stroke occasionally may be accompanied by sufficient edema to cause intercompartmental herniation and death. Increased brain water may be harmful in less dramatic ways, i.e., capillary compression impairing reperfusion and damage to the metabolic machinery of the cell itself.

The studies described here were performed in rats and have been reported in detail elsewhere (4), to which the reader interested in detailed methodology is referred. Cerebral ischemia, produced experimentally by arterial embolization, causes an almost immediate increase in brain water (5), cytoxic edema being caused by faulty energy metabolism that impairs the Na^+ extrusion pump. The severity of the edema is determined by at least two factors other than depressed energy metabolism, namely the hydrostatic pressure difference between the intravascular serum and the center of the ischemic zone and increased tissue osmolality.

The importance of a pressure differential in moving water from serum to ischemic brain is illustrated by the observation that brain ischemia caused by decapitation is accompanied by a rapid decrease in energy metabolism, but no increase in brain water. Similarly, ischemia induced by the Brierley-Pulsinelli technique, in which essentially all blood flow to the brain ceases, is accompanied by an insignificant increase in brain water (6). On the contrary, induced hypertension significantly increases the efflux of water into the brain 5 minutes after embolization in ischemic areas adjacent to tissue that is still being perfused. The situation is similar in brain that is reperfused after temporary ischemia; there is an increase in brain water that had not existed during ischemia.

Studies by others have shown that the increase in tissue osmolality that occurs in ischemia contributes to reperfusion tissue edema. Hossman and colleagues (2) demonstrated a decrease in extracellular space and increased tissue osmolality during ischemia, denoting a shift of water from the extracellular to the intracellular com-

1

partment. The increase in tissue osmolality cannot be accounted for solely by increased Na^+ and K^+ ions; ideogenic osmoles, possibly intermediates of anaerobic glycolysis, and conformational changes in protein molecules may also contribute.

Prenecrotic ischemic brain edema is ordinarily not accompanied by extravasation of large protein molecules into the brain, and is, therefore, termed cytotoxic. We have confirmed the observations of many observers (1,3), that prove a correlation between increased perfusion pressure and macromolecule extravasation into ischemic tissue. In addition, our studies have demonstrated that this breach in the blood–brain barrier is accompanied by increased edema and increased Na^+ concentration in all areas of the ischemic hemisphere.

The significance of these biologic events in clinical terms may be not yet certain, although there no longer can be any doubt that the level of arterial pressure plays an important role in the severity of ischemic brain edema. In the experiments reported here, there was a significantly greater mortality rate in the rats made briefly hypertensive during induced ischemia than in those that remained normotensive after ischemia.

REFERENCES

1. Hossman, K. A., and Olsson, Y. (1977): Influence of ischemia on the passage of protein tracers across capillaries in certain blood-brain injuries. *Acta Neuropathol.*, 18:113.
2. Hossman, K. A., and Tagaki, S. (1976): Osmolality of brain in cerebral ischemia. *Exp. Neurol.*, 51:124.
3. Johansson, B., and Linder, L. E. (1974): Blood brain barrier dysfunction in acute arterial hypertension induced by clamping of the thoracic aorta. *Acta Neurol. Scand.*, 50:360.
4. Kogure, K., Busto, R., and Scheinberg, P. (1981): The role of hydrostatic pressure in brain edema. *Ann. Neurol.*, 9:273–282.
5. Kogure, K., Busto, R., Scheinberg, P., et al. (1974): Energy metabolites and water content in rat brain during the early stage of development of cerebral infarction. *Brain*, 97:103.
6. Pulsinelli, W. A., and Brierley, J. B. (1979): A new model of bilateral hemispheric ischemia in the unanesthetized rat. *Stroke*, 10:267.

Advances in Stroke Therapy, edited by
F. C. Rose. Raven Press, New York © 1982.

Pathophysiology of Brain Ischaemia: Recent Experimental Results and Early Clinical Correlations

Lindsay Symon

Department of Neurological Surgery, Institute of Neurology, National Hospital, Queen Square, London, England

In another symposium two years ago (18), I reviewed some studies of experimental cerebral infarction. At that time, it was already clear that thresholds of blood flow existed in the experimental primate brain whereby electrical function could be shown to fail at a blood flow level of around 16 ml/100 g/min (7), a flow threshold higher than and clearly separate from a lower level of ischaemia that evoked failure of the membrane ionic pump, as evidenced by potassium efflux into the extracelluar space (4). The level of blood flow necessary to produce permanent infarction, no doubt time-related (16,19), was at a similar level. It was clear also that there was a spatial separation between brain rendered nonfunctional by a degree of ischaemia adequate to abolish electrical activity, and a true infarct in which there was potassium release and subsequent disruption of cellular structure. These two concepts, the evidence of separate thresholds of ischaemia for failure of function of the tissue and for structural disruption, and the evidence of a separate area of brain which though not functioning, is not infarcted, and which we have called the "ischaemic penumbra" (3), have challenged our management of clinical stroke. The clinical implication is that restoration of a modest amount of flow in the penumbra would result in restoration of electrical function and considerable improvement in clinical function, as far as the patient was concerned.

This chapter presents an update on laboratory experimental work concerned with thresholds of ionic movement and their modification, with such clinical correlation as has been possible to make in the relatively uncontrolled circumstances of patient management.

FURTHER STUDIES ON THE FLOW THRESHOLD FOR MEMBRANE FUNCTION

Much experimental evidence has established a flow threshold for the failure of energy metabolism (2) and, in particular, the maintenance of the ionic pumping mechanisms of cell membranes as indicated by the movement of potassium from the intracellular to the extracellular space. It is interesting to note that when the

3

flow threshold of electrical failure was first described (7), it was far from clear how electrical failure related to disruption of the energy state, ionic transport, or ionic homeostasis. Our initial working hypothesis was that failure of the electrical response would be associated with the influx of cellular potassium and subsequent membrane depolarization. We have, however, clearly established that extracellular potassium concentration in the cortex remains normal, or only slightly transiently elevated at flow levels where electrical function has already ceased (4). Astrup et al. (2) have further shown, in experiments with bicuculline-induced continuous generalized seizures in the rat, that hypotension induced during seizures will abolish the seizure activity before massive efflux of potassium into the extracelluar space. Further metabolic studies (17) have shown that at levels of blood flow associated with electrical failure, the tissue has almost normal concentration of ATP and only slightly reduced phosphocreatine concentration. Astrup and colleagues have further observed that the rate of clearance of potassium in the interictal periods was gradually reduced before electrical signs of ischaemia appeared, and our own work on clearance of transient flux of potassium into the extracellular space has again confirmed that what is presumably a cell-mediated clearance mechanism from the extracellular space, is impaired at blood flow levels higher than those associated with electrical failure. As far as actual membrane permeability is concerned, however, it is clear that extracellular levels of potassium remain low until blood flow falls to the region of 10 ml/100 g/min; there is then a sharp efflux of potassium into the extracellular space, which, if maintained for periods of longer than 1 hr, is associated with failure of reversibility of potassium movement as well as substantial failure of the evoked response to recover on reperfusion (6,8).

More recent work has used triple-barrelled, ion-sensitive microelectrodes (10): one barrel measuring extracellular potassium as before, one reference barrel as before, and one barrel containing a calcium ion exchanger, so that it is possible to measure extracellular calcium activity and extracellular potassium activity at the same point simultaneously. Using these electrodes, the baseline activity for potassium has been confirmed as 3.9 ± 0.8 mM K_e, and baseline calcium as 0.31 ± 0.10 mM Ca_e (mean $\pm$ SD). As blood flow approached the critical level of 10 ml/100 g/min, there was a major change in extracellular ionic activity. The threshold blood flows for potassium and calcium cannot be separated statistically, but the events are not simultaneous, potassium always moved first (11). (Fig. 1). Interestingly, the fall in the extracellular calcium level could be related to the attainment of a critical level of extracellular potassium activity. The extracellular calcium always fell after K_e rose to an average value of 13.4 ± 3.8 mM. The delay between the initial rise in potassium and the initial fall in calcium levels was related to blood flow: the lower the blood flow the shorter the delay. The potassium level could rise to between 10 and 20 mM before the calcium was effected. The average minimum value of calcium reached in dense ischaemia was 0.28 ± 0.7 mM. Where spontaneous ionic activity was recorded, the potassium level began to rise before the calcium level fell, and the K_e value attained before the movement of calcium

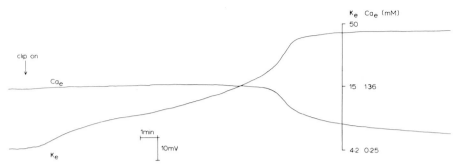

FIG. 1. Continuous traces of extracellular and calcium ionic activity from the opercular cortex of a baboon under chloralose anaesthesia. At the time of middle cerebral clip, an initial blood flow level of approximately 9 ml/100 g/min was obtained in the region of the electrode, falling with an induced hypotension to a flow of approximately 3 ml/100 g/min at the end of the trace. With this fall in flow, efflux in potassium into the extracellular space occurred and as potassium rose above 13–15μl, a disappearance of calcium ionic activity from the extracellular space was recorded.

was again 10.5 ± 3.0 mM, not significantly different from the potassium level associated with calcium movement in ischaemia.

These experiments have suggested that depolarization-induced membrane permeability changes are the cause of calcium and potassium movement in ischaemia, ions travelling down their concentration gradients, as a result of changes in the energy relationships of tissue consequent upon ischaemia. The increase of extracellular potassium is due to a progressive overload of potassium clearance mechanisms with increased leakage of intracellular potassium. The question of whether extracellular calcium movement is critically related to the extracellular potassium concentration, or whether it is dependent upon specific energy failure, cannot be answered at this time. However, the final Ca_e found in densely ischaemic tissue, with the local CBF of around 6 ml/100 g/min, is 0.28 mM, indicating that calcium activity in the intra- and extracellular compartments is in equilibrium.

The significance of the demonstration of calcium movement in ischaemia has been highlighted by Hass (12), who has recently suggested a hypothesis for the molecular mechanisms of cellular damage in ischaemia. Raised intracellular calcium activity stimulates breakdown of the phosphatidylinositol pool, with serious consequences for neurotransmitter metabolism during reperfusion. Raised intracellular calcium activity also stimulates phospholipase activity, releasing free fatty acids. A major member of this group is arachidonic acid, the precursor of prostaglandins and other related substances believed to have further deleterious effects upon ischaemic cerebral tissue.

EVIDENCE OF RECOVERABILITY OF ISCHAEMIC TISSUE

The concept of amelioration of neurological signs by reperfusion of the penumbra is an attractive one. There is now a certain amount of data available, relating the degree of depression of blood flow and tissue pO_2 in experimental ischaemia to the possibility of electrical recovery in the affected cortex (6). Depression of local tissue blood flow below 10 ml/100 g/min or of tissue pO_2 below 10% of the control level of oxygen tension over a period of 16 to 55 min, is associated with failure of electrical potentials to return. Comparable experiments in which similar occlusion times were associated with local tissue blood flow near the threshold of electrical failure, and tissue pO_2 of not less than 50% control values, have shown that recovery of electrical potential of 80 to 100% of control was possible. Lengthening the period of ischaemia beyond 50 min provided the observed flow and oxygen levels remained above critical values, made no significant difference in potential for recovery in the tissue. From the differences in threshold flow for failure of the ionic pumps and electrical potential, we would have predicted that ionic movement would be more resistant in time to ischaemia than electrical function. Parallel experiments measuring extracellular potassium movement (8) showed that reperfusion of tissue subjected to flows below 15 ml/100 g/min for an average of 136 min showed evidence of partial or complete recovery of extracellular potassium to control levels in all animals. This occurred in two phases in the exponential fashion. The more rapid portion of potassium clearance was significantly correlated with postocclusion flow and with the length of time during occlusion that flow was below an arbitrary threshold of 10 ml/100 g/min. In four of these experiments, although the potassium level returned to normal, evoked response remained substantially impaired, having regained less than 50% of control after 100 min. In the remainder, there was evidence of delayed recovery of the evoked response to almost normal. This is again evidenced from the pattern and type of course of recovery in that normalization of ionic pumping mechanisms may occur more readily than electrical function following reperfusion after ischaemia, while in a densely ischaemic lesion, a persistently elevated level of potassium is the norm.

Experimental studies of induced transient elevations of potassium (5) have been used to assess the efficiency of clearance mechanisms in the cortex. The clearance of potassium is usually at a rate roughly proportional to blood flow. However, such potassium clearance shows some impairment of function at a fairly high level of blood flow above the threshold for electrical failure, and there is a progressive failure of clearance until flows of approximately 6 ml/100 g/min, when potassium clearance in the cortex apparently ceases.

CORRELATIVE HUMAN STUDIES

Attempts to correlate levels of blood flow with loss of function or death of tissue in human circumstances are much less easy. This is in part because the measurement of human cerebral blood flow is less precise than the techniques available in animals, and in part because both blood flow measurement and electrical analysis, being of necessity noninvasive, are less specific to particular tissues. Measurement of tissue extracellular concentrations is of course impossible, and since one is largely dependent upon the vagaries of human pathology, repetitive analysis of exactly similar circumstances is difficult.

Our attempts have concentrated upon the analysis of blood flow and electrical function in the closely observed circumstances of subarachnoid haemorrhage. Here, particularly following surgery and clipping of aneurysms, transient disturbances of the cerebral circulation, which are usually dignified by the term vasospasm (1), have enabled us to make repeated observations of perfusion and electrical activity in the pre- and postoperative period. We have been concerned with the place and degree of induced hypotension during the operative management of intracranial aneurysms in view of the demonstration in 1972 by Heilbrun et al. (13) of widespread loss of autoregulation in hemispheres recently affected by subarachnoid haemorrhage. We have employed induced hypertension to increase perfusion in the postoperative period, and have been able to make a number of observations on electrical activity associated with blood flow and neurological status during this technique. Repeated measurements of regional cerebral blood flow have been made by the xenon inhalational technique (15), and there is suggestive evidence relating regional cerebral blood flow to ischaemic complications. It appears that the development of a hyperaemic phase following surgery for intracranial aneurysms is associated with a more favourable postoperative course than persistence of low flow or unchanged blood flow in the postoperative period.

Some support for this clinical observation has been leant by the observations of Jakubowski, Bell, and Symon in baboons (*unpublished data*). Our electrical studies have employed the use of central conduction time (CCT) (14,21), a measurement of the passage of a somatosensory evoked response elicited by median nerve stimulation between two electrodes, one over the C_2 level (N_{14}), and one signifying the arrival of this postsynaptic volley at the contralateral cortex (N_{20}). This value represents conduction in the central pathways only, and is independent of peripheral nerve or spinal cord tracts. It is a remarkably constant measurement, values of 5.6 ± 0.4 msec having been obtained in control circumstances and in a group of 13 subarachnoid haemorrhage cases without evident aneurysm. We have now studied over 70 patients with angiographic evidence of intracranial aneurysm and have related ischaemic events to the electrical activity. Thus, we have found that there is a significantly longer CCT ($p = 0.01$) in patients who fall into the Hunt and Hess grade 4 in the affected hemisphere than in normal patients. We have found also that preoperative values of central conduction time more than 2 standard deviations (SD) from our norm are significantly associated with a higher proportion of complications than in patients showing CCT in the affected hemisphere within 2 SD of the norm (20). Differences in CCT between the two hemispheres also has been found to be helpful. The mean and standard deviations for the normal population of this interhemispheric difference has been found to be 0.22 ± 0.15 msec, and a difference of greater than 0.6 msec (2 SD) between mean CCT, has been considered suggestive of abnormality in the admission or preoperative period. In individual cases also, the development of postoperative hemiparesis has been associated with prolongation of the conduction time in the affected hemisphere with conduction time usually being a more sensitive measurement, becoming prolonged before the development of neurological signs, and remaining prolonged after apparent clinical resolution (Fig. 2).

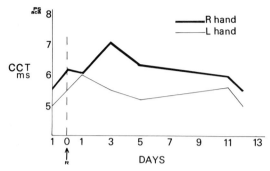

FIG. 2. CCT measurements from right and left hands (*left and right* hemispheres) of a patient with subarachnoid haemorrhage operated on at the sixth postbleed day. The operation was on the right hemisphere, and significant prolongation of left hemispheric conduction time was recorded on the third postoperative day, the patient developing a mild right hemiparesis between the second and third days. Conduction times in the right hemisphere (recorded from left hand stimulation) remained normal throughout. The patient made an uninterrupted recovery thereafter.

Evidence of a threshold relationship between blood flow and neuronal function has been obtained in instances in which a transient hemiparesis has been reversed by elevation of the systemic blood pressure, taking into account the loss of autoregulation in ischaemic hemispheres, as demonstrated by Heilbrun et al. (13) in man, and by Hargadine (9) in the baboon. Reversal of neurological progression has been achieved by the induction of hypertension raising measured blood flow and appropriately shortening CCT.

Measurements of electrical activity also have been shown to have some prognostic value. In addition to the clearly disadvantageous situation of a CCT in the affected hemisphere more than 2 SD from the norm in the preoperative period and correlating well with poor grades of preoperative case, significant prolongation of the conduction time at 5 days and 2 weeks has been associated in a significant proportion of cases with a poor neurological recovery at 2 months.

PREOPERATIVE RECORDING

Recording of conduction time in a number of cases during the induction of hypotension at surgery has shown the capacity of the technique to monitor the development of significant ischaemia during operation. Figure 3 shows the preoperative and postoperative findings in a giant terminal carotid aneurysm which, under normothermia and at normal blood pressure, had the terminal carotid, proximal anterior cerebral, and proximal middle cerebral arteries occluded with temporary clips for periods of 7 min and 30 sec. Prolongation of the conduction time was considerable but, in the postoperative period, although initially for approximately 20 min following recovery from anaesthesia there was a dense paresis of the upper limb, thereafter was complete resolution to normal within 1 hr and restoration of full function without neurological defect. The measurement of conduction time and its correlation with blood flow measurement, preferably by tech-

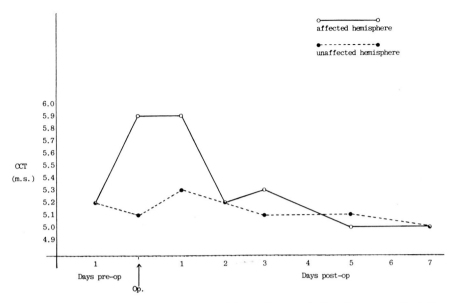

FIG. 3. CCT recorded from the left (affected) hemisphere to right median nerve stimulation, and in the contralateral hemisphere in a patient following temporary occlusion of the internal carotid, middle cerebral, and anterior cerebral vessels during excision of a giant aneurysm. The patient had a distinct hemiparesis that resolved within one-half hr, but central conduction time grossly elevated during surgery, remained significantly prolonged to the second postoperative day. The patient made a full and uninterrupted recovery.

niques more specific than the present externally collimated measurement of xenon, is being pursued in our attempts to set limits of safety for the functional and structural survival of human tissue during ischaemia.

REFERENCES

1. Allcock, J. M., and Drake, C. G. (1965): Ruptured intracranial aneurysms—the rate of arterial spasm. *J. Neurosurg.*, 22:21–69.
2. Astrup, J., Blennow, G., and Nilsson, B. (1979): Effects of reduced cerebral blood flow or EEG pattern, cerebral extracellular potassium and energy metabolism in the rat cortex during bicucculine-induced seizures. *Brain Res.*, 117:115–126.
3. Astrup, J., Siesjo, B. K., and Symon, L. (1982): Thresholds of cerebral ischaemia—the ischaemic penumbra. *Stroke (in press)*.
4. Astrup, J., Symon, L., Branston, N. M., and Lassen, N. (1977): Cortical evoked potential and extracellular K^+ and H^+ at critical levels of brain ischaemia. *Stroke*, 8:51–57.
5. Branston, N. M., Strong, A. J., and Symon, L. (1982): Kinetics of resolution of transient increases in extracellular potassium activity: relationships to regional blood flow in primate cerebral cortex. *(In preparation.)*
6. Branston, N. M., Symon, L., and Crockard, H. A. (1976): Recovery of the cortical evoked response following temporary middle cerebral artery occlusion in baboons: Relation to local blood flow and pO2. *Stroke*, 7:151–157.
7. Branston, N. M., Symon, L., Crockard, H. A., and Pasztor, E. (1974): Relationship between cortical evoked potential, blood flow and local cortical blood flow following acute middle cerebral artery occlusion in the baboon. *Exp. Neurol.*, 45:195–208.
8. Branston, N. M., Symon, L., and Strong, A. J. (1978): Reversibility of ischaemically induced changes in extracellular potassium in primate cortex. *J. Neurol. Sci.*, 37:37–49.

9. Hargadine, J. R., Branston, N. M., and Symon, L. (1980): Central conduction time in primate brain ischaemia—a study in baboons. *Stroke*, 6:637–642.
10. Harris, R. J., and Symon, L. (1981): A double ion-sensitive micro-electrode for extracerebral cortical measurement. *J. Physiol. (Lond.)*, 312:3P.
11. Harris, R. J., Symon, L., Branston, N. M., and Bayhan, M. (1982): Changes in extracellular calcium activity in cerebral ischaemia. *J. Cerebral Blood Flow Metabol, (in press)*.
12. Hass, W. K. (1981): Beyond cerebral blood flow, metabolism and ischaemic thresholds; examination of the role of calcium in the initiation of cerebral infarction. In: Cerebrovascular Disease III, edited by J. S. Meyer, H. Lechner, M. Reivich, E. O. Ott, and A. Arinibar, pp. 3–17. Excerpta Medica, Amsterdam.
13. Heilbrun, N. P., Olesen, J., and Lassen, N. A. (1972): Regional cerebral blood flow studies in subarachnoid haemorrhage. *J. Neurosurgery*, 37:36–44.
14. Hume, A. L., and Cant, B. R. (1978): Conduction time in central somatosensory pathways in man. *Electroencephalogr. Clin. Neurophysiol.*, 45:361–375.
15. Merory, J., Thomas, D. J., Humphrey, P. R. D., Du Boulay, G. H., Marshall, J., Ross Russell, R. W., Symon, L., and Zilkha, E. (1980): Cerebral blood flow after surgery for recent subarachnoid haemorrhage. *J. Neurol. Neurosurg. Psychiat.*, 43:(3)214–221.
16. Morawetz, R., De Girolami, B., Ojeman, R. G., Marcoux, F. W., and Cromwell, R. M. (1978): Cerebral blood flow determined by hydrogen clearance during middle artery occlusion in unanaesthetised monkeys. *Stroke*, 9:143–149.
17. Siesjo, B. K., and Plum, F. (1973): Pathophysiology of anoxic brain damage. In: *Biology of Brain Dysfunction, Vol. 1*, edited by G. E. Gaul, pp. 319–372. Plenum Press, London.
18. Symon, L. (1979): Experimental cerebral infarction. In: *Progress in Stroke Research*, edited by R. M. Greenhalgh and F. C. Rose, pp. 79–89. Pitman Medical, England.
19. Symon, L., and Brierley, J. (1975): Morphological changes in cerebral blood vessels in chronic ischemic infarction flow correlation obtained by the hydrogen clearance method. In: *The Cerebral Vessel Wall*, edited by J. Cervos-Navarro, and F. Matakas, pp. 165–174. Raven Press, New York.
20. Symon, L., Cone, J., Hargadine, J. R., Wang, A. D. J., and Watson, A. (1981): Central conduction time as a functional monitor in brain ischaemia. *J. Cerebral Blood Flow*, 1:(1)S243–S246.
21. Symon, L., Hargadine, J., Zawirski, M., and Branston, N. M. (1979): Central conduction time as an index of ischaemia in subarachnoid haemorrhage. *J. Neurol. Sci.*, 44:95–103.

Advances in Stroke Therapy, edited by
F. C. Rose. Raven Press, New York © 1982.

Cerebral Blood Flow

John Marshall

Institute of Neurology, National Hospital for Nervous Diseases, Queen Square, London, England

CEREBRAL BLOOD FLOW AND METABOLISM

The brain comprises about 2% of body weight, yet takes 20% of cardiac output. This reflects the high metabolic demands of this extremely sophisticated organ. Since reliable measurement of the cerebral blood flow (CBF) in man became possible through the introduction of the nitrous oxide clearance technique by Kety and Schmidt (13), it has been known that there is a close link between CBF and metabolism. A condition such as myxoedema in which cerebral metabolism is reduced is associated with low CBF (21) whereas hyperthyroidism is accompanied by a high CBF (20,22).

CEREBRAL BLOOD FLOW AND MENTAL ACTIVITY

There are generalized and relatively gross disturbances of cerebral metabolism. The fine coupling that exists between CBF and metabolism has been demonstrated exquisitely by Scandinavian workers. They have shown, for example, that movements of the hand are associated with a focal increase of CBF in the appropriate area of the motor cortex (17); even more exciting is their demonstration of focal increases in CBF in association with speech and with various forms of mental activity (10,11,18,19).

AUTOREGULATION

The importance of CBF for metabolism is reflected in the mechanism of autoregulation that enables CBF to be maintained at a constant level (as required by current metabolic demands) over a wide range of blood pressures. In the past, it was all too readily assumed that a fall in pressure is accompanied by a fall in flow, and phenomena such as transient ischaemic attacks (TIAs) were attributed to this (3). Subsequent work established that it is uncommon for a TIA to be caused by a fall in blood pressure (12), autoregulation maintaining CBF down to a mean arterial pressure of approximately 60 mm Hg. TIAs are commonly the result of emboli (7).

HYPERTENSION AND CBF

Hypertension has an important effect upon autoregulation, raising the level of pressure below which autoregulation fails (23). It is this phenomenon that probably led to the mistaken conclusion that blood flow and pressure are linearly related. While it is essential to lower an elevated blood pressure because of the effect it has on cerebral, cardiac, and renal morbidity and upon mortality, this must be done gradually. There is evidence that the point below which autoregulation fails can be restored to the normal level over time.

BLOOD FLOW AND STENOSIS

Another activity about which false assumptions were made regarding blood flow is stenosis of large arteries, particularly of the internal carotid. Once it was realized that carotid stenosis was frequently associated with TIAs and cerebral infarction, the conclusion was drawn that it was due to a reduction of flow through the stenosis. Measurement of blood flow in man showed this not to be the case (2). The lumen of a vessel must be reduced by about 90% before there is a significant effect on flow. Stenoses of this degree occur but are uncommon. Most stenoses are of lesser degree and do not impair flow. The reason for their removal is because they provide a source of emboli (7).

CBF AND DEMENTIA

Similar confusion has arisen about the relationship of CBF to dementia. Reduction of CBF in dementia has been well established (5,14,15). Because dementia is sometimes associated with vascular disease, the assumption was sometimes made that low CBF was the cause of the dementia. That this is not so has been demonstrated by the fact that raising the pCO_2 increases CBF in these cases though not as much as in normal subjects (26). CBF is low not because the vessels are incapable of supplying more blood but because there is not the metabolic demand for it from a brain containing many small infarcts. That metabolic demand is the main determinant of CBF is further attested by Alzheimer's dementia, in which there is no vascular disease, yet CBF is low (8).

While there can be no doubt that reduced metabolic demand is the main determinant of low CBF in multi-infarct dementia, there is evidence that there may be a degree of primary reduction in blood flow. Studies of patients with asymptomatic cerebrovascular disease have shown low CBF, normal $CMRO_2$, and increased arteriovenous oxygen difference. The increased extraction of oxygen indicates that the blood supply was not adequate to the metabolic demands of the brain.

The conclusion must be that some reduction in CBF may play a role in the production of vascular dementia. The main determinant of the low CBF in established cases is certainly the reduced metabolic demand, but this may not be the whole story. Reduced CBF may be partly causal in the early stages of dementia.

CBF AND VISCOSITY

Emphasis so far has been laid on the close relationship between CBF and metabolism, the latter being the main determinant of the former. Recent work however has shown that rheological aspects of CBF cannot be ignored (9,24,25). Increased blood viscosity found in various forms of polycythaemia is associated with low CBF. So important is this aspect that it is the subject of a separate chapter. For present purposes, it is important to stress that while metabolic demand is the main determinant of CBF, viscosity also plays a part. The significance of this observation is that viscosity can be altered readily by the simple process of haemodilution; hence, it has therapeutic implications and potential.

CBF AND STROKE

The various aspects of CBF discussed thus far finally lead to consideration of CBF and stroke. As with TIAs, reduction in CBF is an infrequent cause of stroke. This may occur in cardiac arrest or during a profound fall in blood pressure to a level far below the lower limit of autoregulation, as may occur in massive haemorrhage. In such circumstances, 'watershed' infarcts occur at the site of the anastomoses between anterior, middle, and posterior cerebral arteries.

Most frequently, a stroke is caused by infarct resulting from occlusion of an artery, most commonly by embolism, less frequently by thrombosis *in situ*. There is an immediate, profound reduction in CBF in the infarcted territory and a widespread reduction of lesser degree that may extend to the opposite cerebral hemisphere (4). Diaschisis is the explanation of the widespread depression of CBF, any cerebral lesion affecting function to some extent throughout the brain.

The profound reduction in CBF at the site of infarct may not last; collateral supply from adjacent vascular territories may restore flow. This may prove to be excessive, giving rise to the phenomenon that has been described as luxury perfusion (16). This represents an uncoupling of the close link that normally exists between CBF and metabolism, the uncoupling being the result of damage to the vessels and their receptors during the initial period of ischaemia.

Luxury perfusion is not a constant feature of infarcts, moreover, it may not be established immediately. The place of measures to improve flow in the early stages of an infarct must therefore be considered. Here the influence of viscosity on flow is important. Changes such as aggregation of red blood cells associated with infarction may cause increased viscosity, thus impeding the local restoration of flow. How important the no-reflow phenomenon described in experimental infarction is in animals (1) in the clinical situation is uncertain, but haemodilution and maintenance of perfusion pressure were two factors associated with reduction in the frequency of the occurrence of this phenomenon. Clinical experience with haemodilution after cerebral infarction certainly suggests that it reduces morbidity and mortality (6).

CONCLUSION

While there can be no doubt that the main determinant of CBF is the metabolic demands of the brain and that reduction in flow usually reflects a reduction in demand, blood flow cannot be considered solely in those terms. Factors such as viscosity influence flow irrespective of metabolic demands. Such factors are commonly overridden by the metabolic factor, but this is not always so. There are situations in which haemodynamic and rheological factors are important; they may be more susceptible to therapeutic intervention than metabolic factors. For this reason, it would be unwise to ignore blood flow in its own right in the approach to the therapy of cerebrovascular disease.

REFERENCES

1. Ames III, A., Wright, R. L., Kowada, M., Thurston, J. M., and Majno, G. (1968): Cerebral ischaemia II. The no-reflow phenomenon. *Am. J. Pathol.*, 52:437–453.
2. Brice, J. G., Dowsett, D. J., and Lowe, R. D. (1964): The effect of constriction on carotid blood-flow and pressure gradient. *Lancet*, i:84–85.
3. Denny-Brown, D. (1960): Recurrent cerebrovascular episodes. *A.M.A. Arch. Neurol. Psychiat.*, 2:194–210.
4. Fieschi, C., Agnoli, A., Battistini, N., Bozzao, L., and Prencipe, M. (1968): Derangement of regional cerebral blood flow and of its regulatory mechanisms in acute cerebrovascular lesions. *Neurology (Minneap.)*, 18:1166–1179.
5. Freyhan, F. A., Woodford, R. B., and Kety, S. S. (1951): Cerebral blood flow and metabolism in psychoses of senility. *J. Nerv. Ment. Dis.*, 113:449–456.
6. Gottstein, U., Sedlymeyer, I., and Heuss, A. (1976): Treatment of acute cerebral ischaemia with low-molecular dextran. Results of a retrospective study. *Dtsc. Med. Wochenschr.*, 101:223–227.
7. Gunning, A. J., Pickering, G. W., Robb-Smith, A. H. T., and Ross Russell, R. (1964): Mural thrombosis of the internal carotid artery and subsequent embolism. *Q. J. Med.*, 33:155–195.
8. Hachinski, V. C., Iliff, L. D., Zilkha, E., Du Boulay, G. H., McAllister, V. L., Marshall, J., Ross Russell, R. W., and Symon, L. (1975): Cerebral blood flow in dementia. *Arch. Neurol.*, 32:632–637.
9. Humphrey, P. R. D., Du Boulay, G. H., Marshall, J., Pearson, T. C., Ross Russell, R. W., Symon, L., Wetherley-Mein, G., and Zilkha, E. (1979): Cerebral blood-flow and viscosity in relative polycythaemia. *Lancet*, ii:873–877.
10. Ingvar, D. H., and Risberg, J. (1967): Increase of regional cerebral blood flow during mental effort in normals and in patients with focal brain disorders. *Exp. Brain Res.*, 3:195–211.
11. Ingvar, D. H., and Schwartz, M. S. (1974): Blood flow patterns induced in the dominant hemisphere by speech and reading. *Brain*, 97:273–288.
12. Kendall, R. E., and Marshall, J. (1963): Role of hypertension in the genesis of transient focal cerebral ischaemic attacks. *Br. Med. J.*, 2:344–348.
13. Kety, S. S., and Schmidt, C. F. (1945): The determination of cerebral blood flow in man by the use of nitrous oxide in low concentrations. *Am. J. Physiol.*, 143:53–66.
14. Lassen, N. A., Munck, O., and Tottey, E. R. (1957): Mental function and cerebral oxygen consumption in organic dementia. *Arch. Neurol. Psychiatr.*, 77:126–133.
15. Lassen, N. A., Feinberg, I., and Lane, M. H. (1960): Bilateral studies of cerebral oxygen uptake in young and aged normal subjects and in patients with organic dementia. *J. Clin. Invest.*, 39:491–500.
16. Lassen, N. A. (1966): The luxury-perfusion syndrome and its possible relation to acute metabolic acidosis localised within the brain. *Lancet*, ii:1113–1115.
17. Olesen, J. (1971): Contralateral focal increase of cerebral blood flow in man during arm work. *Brain*, 94:635–646.
18. Risberg, J., and Ingvar, D. H. (1973): A study of regional cerebral blood flow changes during psychological testing in a group of neurologically normal subjects. *Brain*, 96:737–753.

19. Risberg, J., Halsey, J. H., Wills, E. L., and Wilson, E. M. (1975): Hemispheric specialization in normal man studied by bilateral measurements of the regional cerebral blood flow. *Brain*, 98:511–524.
20. Scheinberg, P. (1950): Cerebral circulation and metabolism in hyperthyroidism. *J. Clin. Invest.*, 29:1010–1012.
21. Scheinberg, P., Stead, E. A., Brannon, E. S., and Warren, J. V. (1950): Correlative observations on cerebral metabolism and cardiac output in myxedema. *J. Clin. Invest.*, 29:1139–1146.
22. Sokoloff, L., Wechsler, R. L., Balls, K., Mangold, R., and Kety, S. S. (1950): The blood flow and O_2 consumption of the human brain in hyperthyroidism. *Am. J. Med. Sci.*, 219:465.
23. Strandgaard, S., Olesen, J., Skinhøj, E., and Lassen, N. A. (1973): Autoregulation of brain circulation in severe arterial hypertension. *Br. Med. J.*, 1:507–510.
24. Thomas, D. J., du Boulay, G. H., Marshall, J., Pearson, T. C., Ross Russell, R. W., Symon, L., Wetherley-Mein, G., and Zilkha, E. (1977): Cerebral blood-flow in polycythaemia. *Lancet*, ii:161–163.
25. Thomas, D. J., du Boulay, G. H., Marshall, J., Pearson, T. C., Ross Russell, R. W. Symon, L. Wetherley-Mein, G., and Zilkha, E. (1977): Effect of haematocrit on cerebral blood-flow in man. *Lancet*, ii:941–943.
26. Yamamoto, M., Meyer, J. S. Sakai, F., and Yamaguchi, F. (1980): Aging and cerebral vasodilator responses to hypercarbia. Responses in normal aging and in persons with risk factors for stroke. *Arch. Neurol.*, 37:489–496.

Advances in Stroke Therapy, edited by
F. C. Rose. Raven Press, New York © 1982.

Polycythaemia and Stroke

R. W. Ross Russell and J. P. H. Wade

Department of Neurology, St. Thomas' Hospital, London, England

It has been known for a long time that patients with primary proliferative poly-cythaemia (PPP) suffer a high incidence of vascular thrombosis (2), particularly in the brain. More recently, it has been demonstrated that the frequency of cerebral ischaemic attacks correlates with the height of the haematocrit (Hct) (6). Epidemiological studies also suggest an increased incidence of cerebral infarction in those who have high Hct within the normal range but do not have PPP (5). A remarkable clinicopathological study from Japan has also shown a striking relationship between cerebral infarction at autopsy and raised Hct during life (9).

The relationship between viscosity and the rate of flow through tubes was first defined by Poiseuille, but the laws governing blood flow *in vivo* are more complicated, since blood viscosity varies at different points in the circulation, being greatest under conditions of slow flow (low shear). The modern types of viscometer can measure blood viscosity over a range of shear rates *in vitro*, but it is uncertain what shear rates apply in the resistance vessels of the circulation. By varying the constituents of blood and plasma, it has been shown that the proportion of red cells to plasma (Hct) is the major factor determining whole blood viscosity (1). The question to be asked is whether the high incidence of vascular occlusion seen in polycythaemia is due to increased blood viscosity.

The first point to be examined is the relationship between cerebral blood flow (CBF) and viscosity. Since an increase in viscosity raises peripheral vascular resistance, it might be expected to reduce CBF unless there is some compensatory mechanism such as an increase in vessel calibre. This compensation proves to be incomplete, since there is an inverse relationship between CBF and Hct in patients with PPP, and since CBF increases after venesection (7). It is of interest to examine the relationship between CBF and Hct over the normal range of haemoglobin as well as in the pathological states of anaemia and polycythaemia. Results show that the lower the haemoglobin the higher the flow and vice versa (4,8). These findings are consistent with the idea that viscosity might be critical in governing CBF, but there is another possible explanation. Since the arterial oxygen content (proportional to the amount of haemoglobin and its oxygen saturation) of polycythaemic blood is increased and the oxygen content of anaemic blood decreased, it is also possible that CBF is regulated by the capacity of blood to deliver oxygen to the brain. In fact, as close a relationship can be plotted between oxygen content and CBF as between Hct or viscosity and CBF.

Some further light on the relative importance of these two factors can be gained by studying the reactivity of the cerebral circulation to CO_2, a powerful vasodilating agent. If viscosity were restricting CBF in patients with PPP, then it might be expected that the resistance vessels would be widely dilated in an attempt to maintain normal flow. Consequently, the capacity for further dilation to other agents such as CO_2 would be impaired. We therefore examined CO_2 reactivity in patients with PPP before and after venesection (11). The expected increase in flow occurred after venesection but there was no significant difference in reactivity. Although viscosity was high, the vascular bed was not fully dilated suggesting that CBF was low for other reasons. Evidence implicating oxygen carriage as an important factor in determining CBF has come from two further studies. Wade et al. (12), examining patients with high oxygen affinity haemoglobinopathy and Gottstein (3), studying patients with cyanotic heart disease, found high CBF values in spite of elevated viscosity. Clearly viscosity is not the limiting factor when there is a chronic hypoxic stimulus tending to increase CBF. If the effects of viscosity can be overruled in this way, it seems unlikely that it is the factor responsible for regulating CBF throughout the normal range of haemoglobin or in anaemic states.

When the Hct level is grossly elevated, the situation may be different. Oxygen carriage to the brain is defined as CBF $\times$ arterial oxygen content. This is constant throughout a wide range of Hct values, but certain discrepancies arise when patients with very high Hct levels are studied. For instance, if patients with PPP are venesected and oxygen carriage is measured before and after, a significant increase is found indicating that more oxygen is carried to the brain at lower Hct levels than at high (10). It is possible that viscosity is a factor here, and similar results have been found for other tissues, such as in the leg (14). Does this mean that the brains of patients with PPP are in a state of mild oxygen starvation and that the efficient coupling of flow and metabolism has been disrupted? To answer this, we need to measure $CMRO_2$ in polycythaemic patients before and after venesection. Our studies here are not complete, but preliminary results in only three patients show no change in $CMRO_2$, and the steady values for jugular venous oxygen tension give no indication of tissue hypoxia in untreated patients. It seems that although CBF is increased by venesection, the brain does not make use of the additional oxygen carriage.

These findings may be summarised as follows:

a) CBF is inversely related to Hct and also to oxygen content of arterial blood.

b) Throughout the physiological range of Hct and in anaemic patients, an efficient mechanism exists to ensure a constant delivery of oxygen to the brain. Viscosity seems unlikely as a controlling factor at this level.

c) At high levels of Hct, probably because of increased viscosity, this mechanism is less efficient and less oxygen is carried to the brain.

d) There is usually sufficient reserve in the system to ensure that although oxygen carriage is reduced, the supply is sufficient for metabolic requirements and there is no evidence of tissue hypoxia.

Does the brain or other organ actually work better when its circulation is increased irrespective of the oxygen content of the blood? There is some evidence, though not very strong, that this is so. Willison (13) showed subjective improvement on tests of mental alertness in a group of patients with high Hct after venesection, suggesting either that metabolism had improved or that venesection was having some nonspecific alerting effect. Measurements of this kind are extremely important but notoriously difficult and are subject to influences such as training, observer bias, and suggestion. More observations are certainly needed but there is an indication that, in some parts of the circulation, a reduction in Hct may actually improve organ function particularly if arterial disease is superimposed.

To return to the question posed at the beginning—why do patients with high haematocrit suffer cerebral vascular occlusion? We have indicated that this is unlikely to be due to a state of chronic cerebral hypoxia as a result of increased viscosity. However slow flow itself may be thrombogenic by favouring the build up of platelet aggregations, the accumulation of coagulation factors, and by decreasing the mechanical dispersion of microthrombi. These factors may be especially important in diseased vessels or in states of quantitative or qualitative platelet abnormality. Though the mechanisms are still obscure, there seem good grounds for intermittently reducing the Hct of patients suffering from TIA who have Hct greater than 0.5 and in whom the polycythaemia is not secondary to pulmonary or cardiac disease. There is already evidence that such treatment is beneficial in patients with PPP (6).

A critical piece of information is still needed to complete the puzzle—do patients with high flow and high Hct have a thrombotic tendency? If not (and this seems likely), then the answer is that it is retarded flow and not raised viscosity that is the critical factor.

ACKNOWLEDGMENTS

We acknowledge the National Hospital, Queen Square and St. Thomas' Hospital, London in collaboration with J. Marshall, G. H. Du Boulay, L. Symon, D. J. Thomas, P. Humphrey, T. C. Pearson, and G. Wetherley-Mein. Research supported by the Medical Research Council and by the Special Trustees to St. Thomas' Hospital.

REFERENCES

1. Begg, T. B., and Hearns, J. B. (1966): Components in blood viscosity: the relative contribution of haematocrit, plasma fibrinogen and other proteins. *Clin. Sci.*, 31:87–93.
2. Chievitz, E., and Thiede, T. (1962): Complications and causes of death in polycythaemia vera. *Acta Med. Scand.*, 172:513–523.
3. Gottstein, U., Bersnmeier, A., and Blömer, H. (1957): Der hirnkreislauf bei ange borenen herzfelhern mit zyanose. *Verh. Dtsch Ges. Kreislaufforsch.*, 23:290–296.
4. Humphrey, P. R. D., Marshall, J., Ross Russell, R. W., Wetherley-Mein, G., Du Boulay, G. H., Pearson, T. C., Symon, L., and Zilkha, E. (1979): Cerebral blood flow and viscosity in relative polycythaemia. *Lancet*, ii:873–876.
5. Kannel, W. B., Gordon, T., Wolf, P. A., and McNamara, P. (1972): Hemoglobin and the risk of cerebral infarction. *Stroke*, 3:409–420.

6. Pearson, T. C., and Wetherley-Mein, G. (1978): Vascular occlusive episodes and venous hae-matocrit in primary proliferative polycythaemia. *Lancet*, ii:1219–1222.

7. Thomas, D. J., Marshall, J., Ross Russell, R. W., Wetherley-Mein, G., Du Boulay, G. H., Pearson, T. C., Symon, L. and Zilkha, E. (1977): Cerebral blood flow in polycythaemia. *Lancet*, ii:161–164.

8. Thomas, D. J., Marshall, J., Ross Russell, R. W. Wetherley-Mein, G., Du Boulay, G. H., Pearson, T. C., Symon, L., and Zilkha, E. (1977): Effect of haematocrit on cerebral blood flow in man. *Lancet*, ii:941–943.

9. Tohgi, H., Yamanouchi, H., Murakami, M., and Kameyama, M. (1978): Importance of hematocrit as a risk factor in cerebral infarction. *Stroke*, 9:369–374.

10. Wade, J. P. H. (1980): MD Thesis, Cambridge University

11. Wade, J. P. H. (1981): Reactivity of the cerebrovascular bed to carbon dioxide in patients with primary high haematocrit before and after venesection. *Acta Neurol. Scand.*, 63:306–314.

12. Wade, J. P. H., Du Boulay, G. H., Marshall, J., Pearson, T. C., Ross Russell, R. W., Shirley, J. A., Symon, L., Wetherley-Mein, G., and Zilkha, E. (1980): Cerebral blood flow in subjects with a high oxygen affinity haemoglobin variant. *Acta Neurol. Scand.*, 61:210–215.

13. Willison, J. R., Thomas, D. J., Du Boulay, G. H., Marshall, J., Paul, E. A., Pearson, T. C., Ross Russell, R. W., Symon, L., and Wetherley-Mein, G. (1980): Effect of haematocrit on alertness. *Lancet*, i:846–848.

14. Yates, C. J. P., Andrews, V., Berent, A., and Dormandy, J. A. (1979): Increase in leg blood flow by normovolaemic haemodilution in intermittent claudication. *Lancet*, i:166–168.

Advances in Stroke Therapy, edited by
F. C. Rose. Raven Press, New York © 1982.

Investigative Aspects of Acute Stroke

D. J. Thomas

St. Mary's Hospital, London, England

The purpose of investigating acute stroke is to supplement the clinical history and examination in order to increase the accuracy of diagnosis, such that the management of the patient may be improved and a clearer prognosis provided. There are several important questions that require answers:

Has the patient had a stroke at all, or is the hemiparesis due to a cerebral tumour, multiple sclerosis, a Todd's paresis, or a traumatic haematoma?
Has the patient had a haemorrhage, an infarct, or a haemorrhagic infarct?
What is the site and size of the lesion?
Which arterial territory is likely to have been involved?
If an infarct, did it result from a local arterial occlusion, or was an embolus arising from the heart or major vessels responsible? Are further emboli probable? Is there evidence of a thrombotic tendency?
If a haemorrhage, was it subarachnoid or intracerebral? Is there evidence of longstanding hypertension? Is there a haemorrhagic tendency?
Are there any other abnormalities? Have there been previous infarcts, perhaps bilaterally? Is there significant ventricular dilatation or cortical atrophy?
Are there signs of complications, e.g., cerebral oedema, ventricular compression, or shift?
Is there evidence of reduced cerebral blood flow, loss of linkage between flow and metabolism?
Is there anything in the patient's general condition that might influence the intracerebral problem adversely, e.g., severe hypertension, recent myocardial infarct, cardiac failure, or a haematological disturbance?
What investigations may be helpful for monitoring progress and for measuring the response to treatment?

The investigative techniques that are available should be considered in the light of these questions. New methods need to be developed in order to answer them more precisely.

GENERAL ASSESSMENT

Haematological Tests

Is the patient anaemic or polycythaemic? Are the red cells normal? Is there a thrombocytosis or leucocytosis?

Anaemia is only rarely a factor in the pathogenesis of stroke and unless produced by recent acute blood loss, should not be corrected by blood transfusion (3). A high-normal or elevated haematocrit more likely is important, both aetiologically and rheologically. The possibility of dehydration must be excluded and corrected. A high platelet or white count with a haematocrit above 0.50 is suggestive of polycythaemia rubra vera. However, a case can be made for immediate haemodilution in acute stroke (2) in order to optimize CBF promptly and not wait for the results of red cell mass, plasma volume, leucocyte alkaline phosphatase, intravenous pyelogram, and erythropoietin levels.

Sedimentation rate is also valuable, not only because it may indicate certain aetiological factors like an arteritis or atrial myxoma, but because a high value may imply abnormal red cell—red cell aggregation. This is usually associated with an elevated plasma fibrinogen or globulins and both plasma and whole blood viscosity.

In cases of cerebral haemorrhage, if there is a history or any other signs of bleeding tendency, a defect of one of the common coagulation factors should be considered and if found, appropriate replacement therapy given.

Serological Tests

Serological tests to exclude syphilis are advisable.

Biochemical Tests

Blood glucose, urea, and electrolytes should be measured promptly. Urinary protein or glucose should be excluded. The plasma globulins and fibrinogen should be assayed especially if the ESR is high. If the globulins are very high as in some of the myelomas, plasmaphoresis may be considered (4). It is possible to reduce a high fibrinogen acutely with the venoms of certain vipers (1), but whether this is beneficial in acute stroke remains to be seen. With the knowledge of the haematocrit and fibrinogen and globulin levels, the routine measurement of whole blood viscosity is probably unnecessary. It is my policy to measure the "cardiac enzymes" in all patients with acute stroke in case there has been a recent myocardial infarct.

Electrocardiography

An electrocardiogram will not only give evidence of myocardial infarction, past or recent, but will also provide evidence of preexisting, sustained hypertension. It is clearly essentially in the diagnosis and monitoring of cardial arrhythmias.

X-RAY COMPUTERIZED TOMOGRAPHY

Computerized tomography (CT) is of such great value in assessing a patient who has suffered a sudden hemiparesis that one should not consider a research program on stroke or establishing an acute stroke unit without ready access to a CT scanner. Not only is it capable of providing precise anatomical information, but it also has potential for yielding valuable physiological information about blood flow, the blood–brain barrier, and cerebral oedema.

In many medical centres the best that has been possible so far is a single scan done at a random intervals after the ictus. Clinicians are sometimes disillusioned by an apparently normal scan in a patient with a dense hemiparesis. The usual explanation for this is that the scan was performed when the lesion was passing through a stage when it was isodense with the surrounding brain. In most cases, a further scan will illustrate the problem.

A CT scan will identify readily the small minority of patients with a sudden hemiparesis due to tumour rather than stroke. It will differentiate easily between a haemorrhage, an infarct, or a haemorrhagic infarct. The presence of the latter should always suggest the possibility of an embolism. If a haemorrhage is present, its size and position can be seen clearly. In a case where the history is obscure, the possibility of a subarachnoid haemorrhage may be inferred from the position of the bleed. A large superficial haematoma combined with signs of rising intracranial pressure may prompt beneficial neurosurgical evacuation.

The site and size of an infarct may be determined in most cases, and the arterial territory that has been involved may be deduced. Watershed territory infarction is clearly demonstrated, and may point to a hypotensive crisis as having been responsible. Involvement of clinically silent areas may be diagnosed, e.g.; the extension of a right hemisphere infarct into the frontal lobe may explain the patient's lack of motivation and poor response to rehabilitation. There may be signs of several other infarcts. If bilateral infarcts can be seen, then a proximal cause for the cerebral emboli, usually the heart, should be considered.

Intracranial complications of stroke also may be demonstrated. Ventricular size, position, and degree of shift can be determined. An assessment of the amount of cerebral oedema can be made.

The use of iodine-containing contrast material permits the integrity of the blood–brain barrier to be determined. Under normal circumstances, the contrast does not leak from the vessels into the cerebral substance. Using scanners with very fast scanning times, the rate of disappearance of the contrast can be measured from serial scans and estimates of regional cerebral blood flow obtained. Nonradioactive xenon is a potentially valuable contrast material. If its concentration in the inspired gas is high, it acts as an anaesthetic and may be of value with restless patients. It is a safe and rapidly cleared anaesthetic agent and would be used widely if it were not so expensive. It diffuses rapidly and freely over small distances and can give a useful assessment of the size and distribution of the area of hypoperfusion in and around the area of an infarct.

Other, unsuspected lesions may be demonstrated; there may be impressive cortical atrophy, ventricular dilatation, or evidence of an old infarct elsewhere. Last, the CT scan may be used for monitoring progress and response to treatment. After the oedema has cleared, a better assessment of the size and position of the infarct can be made and compared with the functional deficit.

NONINVASIVE TESTS

There is now little place for the use of electroencephalography, echoencephalography, and technetium brain scanning in acute stroke. Ultrasonic examination of the major neck vessels is more commonly considered in the management of transient ischaemic attacks. Combined with oculoplethysmography, it may provide evidence of a haemodynamically significant stenosis of the internal carotid artery but noninvasive assessment of the vertebral arteries is more difficult. Also, it is not possible as yet to differentiate between a very tight internal carotid stenosis and an occlusion, angiography being necessary if surgery is considered.

Unfortunately a simple noninvasive test for reliably detecting thrombus at the carotid bifurcation has yet to be developed. When it arrives it will be most useful as a guide to the use of thrombolytic and anticoagulant therapy.

Echocardiography may be a useful adjunct to cardiological assessment if a cardiac source for a cerebral embolism is possible and anticoagulation is being considered to prevent further, perhaps more damaging, emboli.

ANGIOGRAPHY

Apart from its use in cases of subarachnoid haemorrhage, early angiography after stroke has gone out of fashion. There are two main reasons for this. First, angiography is not without its hazards. If a general anaesthetic is necessary, the transient hypotension that may occur may be damaging. A large volume of contrast material may aggravate the degree of cerebral oedema and thrombi may be dislodged. Second, it is now appreciated that carotid surgery or extracranial–intracranial anastomosis in the acute phase are not helpful and especially in the case of the former, it may make the deficit more profound. Current policy is to consider angiography at two weeks, by which time cerebral autoregulation may have recovered, in patients in whom there is still a lot more to lose functionally and in whom a significant carotid stenosis is likely.

However, the present underutilization of cerebral angiography is likely to be a passing phase. To consider angiographic procedures to be simply diagnostic is probably too limited. The use of embolization techniques in the treatment of arteriovenous malformation and cerebral tumours is developing rapidly. It is possible that fine catheters may be used for the delivery of thrombolytic substances proximal to an arterial thrombus immediately after stroke. This may prove to be more valuable and less dangerous than their use intravenously.

MEASUREMENT OF CEREBRAL BLOOD FLOW AND METABOLISM

Measurement of cerebral blood-flow and metabolism already have been covered in some detail in the previous three chapters, but some general points may be in order. Normally, blood flow and metabolism are closely linked, but the use of positron-emitting isotopes and tomographic cameras have shown that in the early hours after stroke, areas of critical perfusion exist where there is an increased oxygen extraction ratio and flow is less than optimal for the metabolic demand. Later, certainly around the periphery of an infarct, the reverse seems to be the case. There appears to be luxury perfusion where flow has recovered but metabolic demand is low.

This technique is extremely expensive, requiring a cyclotron on site because the clinically useful positron-emitting isotopes are short-lived. A computerized tomographic camera and a large team of highly trained physicists, chemists and technicians are needed in addition to committed physicians. In most medical centres, the best that can be achieved is an assessment of blood flow without knowledge of whether there is critical or luxury perfusion in the penumbra of the stroke. Obviously, if the overall blood flow to the brain is low as in hyperviscosity, hypotension, or hypovolaemia, attempts must be made to improve it. However, it remains to be demonstrated whether it is preferable to treat critical perfusion by depressing metabolism or by increasing cerebral blood flow.

LUMBAR PUNCTURE

This is still indicated in cases of suspected subarachnoid haemorrhage but, in other forms of stroke, lumbar puncture is rarely necessary. With small lesions no abnormality may be found and with large lesions, it may be hazardous.

CONCLUSION

It is becoming clear that in order to attempt to improve stroke management, patients must be referred promptly within a few hours, before extensive, permanent damage has occurred. The establishment of stroke units should streamline patient assessment and investigation and thereby permit the use of the most appropriate treatment as early as possible. Without special units, committed to the assessment, investigation, and management of stroke, potentially useful forms of therapy will be given to heterogeneous groups with no overall gain and their benefit in certain subgroups may be missed.

REFERENCES

1. Bell, W. R. Pitney, W. R. and Goodwin, J. F. (1968): Therapeutic defibrination in the treatment of thrombotic disease. *Lancet*, i:490–493.
2. Gottstein, U., Seldmeyer, I., and Heuss, A. (1976): Treatment of acute cerebral ischemia with low molecular dextran. *Dtsch. Med. Wochenshr.*, 101:223–227.
3. Isbister, J. P., and Scurr, R. D. (1978): Blood transfusion therapy: components, indications, complications and controversies. *Anaesth. Intensive Care*, 6:297–309.
4. Preston, F. E., Cook, K. B., Foster, M. E., Winfield, D. A., and Lee, D. A. (1978): Myelomatosis and the hyperviscosity syndrome. *Br. J. Haematol.*, 38:517–530.

Advances in Stroke Therapy, edited by
F. C. Rose. Raven Press, New York © 1982.

Are Noninvasive Techniques of Value in Stroke Management?

William S. Fields

*Department of Neurology, University of Texas Medical School at Houston,
Houston, Texas 77030*

Because of the risks inherent in any invasive technique such as arteriography, physicians and surgeons are continually searching for methods of diagnosis of common and internal carotid artery lesions that employ noninvasive tests. Over the past 20 years, a large number of such tests have been developed, a fact that attests not only to the difficulty of finding a fully satisfactory one, but also to the technological advances that have augmented the number of potential avenues one may take to evaluate the anatomy as well as the physiology of the carotid arterial system (2,17).

Unfortunately, in spite of thousands of clinical examinations, arteriographic studies, and surgical interventions, there is still no full understanding of the epidemiology of carotid disease, the pathophysiology of occlusive changes, the natural history of extracranial carotid lesions, and the pathogenesis of ischemic insults distal to disease in the cervical carotid bifurcation. For these reasons, we do not really know which lesions are important enough for us to search for and act upon; for example, the identification of asymptomatic lesions may lead to surgical intervention that is not indicated. Furthermore, many clinicians remain skeptical about noninvasive diagnosis of carotid disease because hemodynamic tests cannot provide information about atheromatous plaques and tests designed to provide anatomic information cannot delineate many ulcerated lesions.

Other clinicians, both medical and surgical and particularly the latter, have great enthusiasm for noninvasive diagnosis of carotid disease as a means of identifying in many patients what they believe to be a treatable cause of stroke, and also for learning more about the characteristics of carotid lesions that may have some prognostic importance. Virtually everyone who has a laboratory for noninvasive carotid evaluation is asked frequently about the direction which the field is taking and the degree of success that has thus far been achieved. Perhaps the three questions most frequently asked are: a) Can arteriography be replaced by noninvasive diagnosis? b) Is noninvasive diagnosis really any good? c) Which is the most appropriate test to use? Most who ask the last question are interested in obtaining an instrument that will be simple to use as well as cost-effective.

Noninvasive testing may never replace conventional arteriography but it can be extremely important in determining which patients with suspected carotid lesions have sufficient evidence of disease, presumed to be related to their symptoms, to make arteriography imperative. Noninvasive testing also can be important in providing further insight into the natural history and pathophysiology of carotid disease. Although each person entering the field with a new instrument may feel that he has the most useful test, in general those who operate carotid evaluation laboratories find the use of a battery of tests to be the most effective method for noninvasive diagnosis (10).

The techniques for noninvasive diagnosis are most readily separated into those that are "direct" and those that are "indirect." Direct tests provide anatomic or physiologic information concerning the carotid artery itself. Those designated as indirect examine for hemodynamic changes in distal arterial beds such as those in the orbital and cerebral circulations.

Since the ophthalmic artery is the first major branch of the internal carotid, obstructive lesions at the cervical bifurcation may produce pressure and flow changes in the orbital branches of that artery and its periorbital ramifications. Indirect tests that measure changes in the orbital bed are the most common noninvasive techniques employed today. These include periorbital directional Doppler ultrasonography (13,14) and two types of oculoplethysmography (OPG). One method of OPG (Gee method) (7) determines systolic ophthalmic artery pressure, while the other (Kartchner and McRae method) (9) monitors the relative arrival time of the ocular pulse wave and is thereby related to flow. Recent attempts have been made to incorporate both techniques into a single instrument, but this effort thus far has been unsuccessful.

Before they become positive, indirect tests depend upon a hemodynamic change and for this reason will be negative in the presence of nonobstructing atheromatous lesions, especially those that are ulcerated. In addition, both types of indirect tests are not specific for the carotid artery because they monitor two major circulatory beds. For example, periorbital Doppler ultrasonography and OPG both examine the carotid via the ophthalmic artery and a positive test may signify an abnormality in either vessel. Although the number of abnormalities in the ophthalmic artery is small, nevertheless, abnormal directional Doppler studies may be due to ophthalmic rather than carotid lesions.

As already mentioned, direct tests monitor physiology and/or anatomy at the carotid bifurcation itself. Direct physiologic tests include bruit analysis and Doppler flow velocity determinations. The latter are important in respect to imaging systems.

The two most common methods of bruit analysis are both referred to as phonoangiography. One examines intensity/time relationships while the other measures intensity/frequency relationships. The former presents a display of the intensity of the bruit as a function of time (7) and the latter uses spectral analysis to describe the relationship of the intensity to the frequency of the bruit thereby assisting in the derivation of accurate numerical estimates of the residual diameter of the vascular lumen (6). The methods are quite different and are designated "direct bruit analysis" and "spectral bruit analysis" but, for either to be useful, a bruit must be present to be analyzed. In approximately 30% of patients with severe carotid lesions when there is a residual lumen of 2 mm or less, no bruit is audible. In addition, another 10% of patients, even though they have bruits, are unable to cooperate by holding their breath long enough to permit a satisfactory analysis of the bruit. Furthermore, neither type of bruit analysis can localize the lesion reliably.

Direct pathoanatomic tests provide an image of the bifurcation and may demonstrate atheromatous lesions including those that may not yet have produced a detectable hemodynamic change in the distal arterial bed. In addition, these tests also may provide further information as to whether an abnormality detected in an indirect test is a result of carotid artery disease. There are two distinct groups of imaging techniques suitable for the carotid artery. One is the high frequency B-scan system (1,8) and the other, continuous or pulse-wave Doppler devices (3,16), both of which employ ultrasonic waves. B-scanners record echos that are related to variations in the acoustical impedance of the tissues under observation. The Doppler systems, on the other hand, register frequency shifts that are related to velocity of flow. B-scan systems provide instantaneous imaging of the vessel wall in real-time so that it is seen while pulsating. Although the resolution of B-scan systems may be as high as 0.5 to 1 mm in one plane, at present, the principal diagnostic value of the method is in delineating extensive lesions which distort the sound wave. Accurate determination of the residual lumen is not always possible. Hopefully improvement in instrumentation will provide better resolution of images and more reliable information regarding ulceration even in the absence of severe occlusive disease.

Doppler systems construct a static image of the lumen over a period of 10 to 20 min as the examiner passes the probe transversely across serial segments of the moving column of blood. After the transverse dimensions and course of the vessel are imaged, the probe then can be moved longitudinally along the common and internal carotid arteries in order to detect any evidence of flow velocity changes that might indicate either stenosis or occlusion. Some researchers are of the opinion that with Doppler imaging systems, the audio information obtained is more useful diagnostically than the visual, and methods have been developed to enhance the audio value.

Virtually the same potential limitations are inherent in the B-scan and Doppler imaging systems as in the indirect hemodynamic measuring devices. Neither can predict consistently the presence of ulcerated plaques. Occasionally, however, after arteriography has been performed, one can retrospectively identify ulceration in the prearteriographic scan.

With the B-scan system, some lesions are not capable of being imaged because they are sonically translucent, i.e., they have the same acoustical impedance as the moving blood. A B-scan image of a vessel with such a lesion may demonstrate what appears to be a normal lumen. The Doppler system, however, would provide some indication of the lesion because of the changes in Doppler sounds produced by alterations in velocity of flow. Neither system can differentiate consistently a "subocclusive" lesion from complete occlusion of the carotid artery. The B-scan system can demonstrate very nicely chronically occluded fibrosed vessels but may produce an image of an acute occlusion that mimics that observed with severe stenosis. The Doppler system fails to resolve extremely slow flow velocities and is unable to image the lumen in the vessel that is either almost occluded or completely occluded.

In the opinion of most observers, potential exists for obtaining high resolution images and important hemodynamic information by developing a real time B-scan imager with a Doppler interface. Thus far, attempts to build such an instrument have not been applicable to clinical use.

Radionuclide imaging (scintigraphy) recently has been employed to detect the localization on arterial lesions of autologous platelets labeled with indium-111. This method has been tested over the cervical carotid bifurcation and the results compared with contrast arteriography. It appears to offer considerable promise for evaluating the pathophysiologic characteristics of atherosclerotic lesions in patients with extracranial cerebrovascular disease (4,5).

Another promising approach to noninvasive testing is in the early stages of investigation. This method, referred to as "computerized fluoroscopy" or "digital video angiography," requires the intravenous injection of a bolus of iodinated contrast material (11,12). Fluoroscopy is then performed over the neck and upper thorax in order to construct a real time image of the arteries. The information obtained is collected either in digital form or converted from analogue to digital form. It then is manipulated by the computer and a hard-copy obtained of the computer-enhanced image. The computations contain subtractions that enable a more satisfactory interpretation of the intravascular images. If this method proves capable of producing high resolution hard copy, it may soon replace other tests, both direct and indirect. Furthermore, it may permit identification of ulcerated nonobstructing plaques or fresh thrombi not visualized by direct methods currently in vogue. It even may serve ultimately as a substitute for conventional, invasive arteriographic procedures in specific situations such as serial studies to determine progression or regression of lesions. The latter would be applicable both in following atherosclerotic stenosis and intracranial arterial vasospasm seen in association with subarachnoid hemorrhage. The procedure is rapid and safe and can be performed on out-patients, but, it cannot be used on patients who are uncooperative since the subject must remain perfectly still and not swallow for 15 sec.

The criteria for the ideal noninvasive tests for carotid artery disease are listed in Table 1. It has been extremely difficult to assess the relative effectiveness of noninvasive methods by comparing results from different laboratories. Unfortunately, the methods of procedure as well as the methods for interpretation are not adequately standardized. One problem is that many laboratories do not report the results of an individual test but only an overall diagnostic impression from a battery of tests. Reports are not always provided of both false positives and false negatives and the findings for stenosis and occlusion are not invariably reported separately. Perhaps the most significant difficulty of all is the fact that the composition of patient populations vary. It may be true, for example, that patients under observation

TABLE 1. *Criteria for the ideal noninvasive tests for carotid artery disease*

Practicability
  Performed rapidly
  Performed by a skilled technician
  Useful in patients not completely cooperative
  Performed supine or sitting
  Performed at bedside or in laboratory
Safety
  No risk to local tissue
  No risk of systemic or neurologic complications
  No discomfort
Information obtainable
  Reproducible data of high sensitivity and specificity
  Both pathoanatomic and hemodynamic data
Expenditure
  Must be cost-effective

Adapted from Ackerman, ref. 2.

in the northwestern part of the United States versus the northeastern part of the United States versus Western Europe may be entirely different.

With respect to the direct tests, it has been difficult to assess the value of B-scan imaging systems because of continuing modifications in technology and data analysis. Published reports on the more widely used Doppler imaging system and its various modifications indicate an overall accuracy of somewhere between 85 and 90% in identifying major stenotic and occlusive lesions. Direct bruit analysis has proved to be far less effective than spectral bruit analysis.

For the most part, indirect tests would seem to provide adequate diagnostic information when a stenosis of 60 to 75% is present and become quite valuable when there is a stenosis of 85 to 90%. With subocclusive or complete occlusion, the true positive rate is somewhere between 90 and 95% with a false positive rate of 1 to 5%. Most investigators also agree that periorbital directional Doppler ultrasonography is less reliable than OPG in identifying stenosis of the internal carotid artery but, from the clinical point of view, the two techniques may complement each other, physiologically as well as diagnostically. One monitors the superficial orbital arterial bed and the other the deep orbital arterial bed and measurement of both will provide a check of one on the other, particularly in circumstances where the pattern of disease or the degree of patient cooperation may severely limit the application of one study. Other indirect tests of the orbital circulation are also in use, although most investigators tend to find them less reliable than those already mentioned.

Direct tests applied to the cervical carotid bifurcation are of considerable value since no indirect test can identify the location of a lesion in the carotid or ophthalmic system nor can it provide any information about atheromatous change in even moderately involved vessels. Indirect tests are required because a cervical carotid lesion may lie beyond the reach of an imaging system or may fail to produce a bruit suitable for analysis. Although most atheromatous lesions lie within a short distance of the carotid bifurcation, a highly placed distal extracranial lesion or stenosis within the carotid siphon may be detected only by the use of indirect methods. It is, therefore, extremely important to appreciate how both direct and indirect tests can complement each other physiologically. Effective, noninvasive diagnosis employs a battery of tests including indirect methods that monitor both superficial and deep beds of the orbital circulation and direct tests that monitor the region of the cervical carotid bifurcation.

The coordination of a battery of tests requires the establishment of a laboratory with a well-trained and dedicated technician supervised by a physician or surgeon who understands both the instrumentation and cerebral vascular disease. In general, noninvasive diagnosis should be used to determine which patient should have an arteriogram rather than to determine which one should not.

The selection of patients for noninvasive diagnostic study becomes a very important clinical consideration. At present, in many departments, patients with typical carotid transient ischemic attacks (TIAs), both monocular and hemispheric, are subjected immediately to arteriography since they will require arteriography irrespective of what the noninvasive tests might show.

Individuals who have either amaurosis fugax or carotid TIAs but in whom there are potential medical contraindications to arteriography first should have noninvasive tests. In this group, positive tests can assist in determining whether arteriography should be done in spite of the fact that the patient may be considered a "relatively high risk" individual.

Another large group referred for noninvasive studies includes persons with symptoms that are not clearly identifiable as TIAs. In such individuals, the results of the studies may tip the balance in favor of doing an arteriographic examination, but it must be emphasized that the laboratory tests, particularly in a patient population in which atherosclerosis is both common and widespread, should never be employed as a substitute for a careful clinical history.

In those persons who have had a recent stroke or minor deficits following a series of TIAs, noninvasive diagnostic techniques may reveal either suspected or completely unexpected carotid lesions. This revelation then may lead to an arteriographic study and subsequent surgery that may prevent a recurrent stroke. In many medical centers in the United States, patients with asymptomatic carotid bruits are subjected to noninvasive testing in the expectation of identifying surgically accessible lesions. Unfortunately, the natural history of asymptomatic lesions is entirely unknown and for this reason it is preferable to use noninvasive tests merely to provide a more precise manner by which to follow these patients for any evidence of progression of disease.

Noninvasive diagnostic testing can assist in the attainment of new knowledge regarding the natural history of carotid lesions by enabling us to follow patients who present with early hemodynamic change or with some direct evidence of an early atheroma. A small number of patients will show rapid progression from nonhemodynamic to rather severe hemodynamic changes over a short period of time while others will show no hemodynamic or B-scan imaging changes over a period of several years. With new instrumentation either currently under investigation or in the developmental stage, it may be possible to correlate more effectively noninvasive diagnostic results with clinical and arteriographic data that then could help to delineate the prognostic aspects of carotid lesions, provide further information concerning the pathophysiology of cerebral insults of carotid-middle cerebral disease, and enable us to appreciate the limitations of arteriography (15).

The field of noninvasive diagnosis in carotid lesions is, at the present time, in a state of considerable flux. The relative value of the various types of procedures must be clarified and this pertains to both the indirect and direct methods of examination. Hopefully what is learned during the course of the next several years will permit one to make judgments with respect to which direction to follow in planning treatment. It should be clearly understood that noninvasive diagnosis of carotid disease does not have, as yet, the capability for replacing conventional arteriography. However, it does provide important diagnostic information that may contribute to clinical decisions and to a better understanding of the natural history of extracranial vascular disease.

SUMMARY

Noninvasive diagnostic testing for vascular disease is now well established. New techniques and refinements of older ones are consistently being evaluated in order to assist in planning for both medical and surgical management. To date, no single technique has replaced invasive contrast arteriography, but this is the ultimate goal of noninvasive diagnosis.

REFERENCES

1. Ackerman, R. H., Pryor, D., and Taveras, J. (1978): Evaluation of a real-time ultrasound imaging system for the carotid artery. *Neurology*, 28:340 (abstr.).
2. Ackerman, R. H. (1979): A perspective on non-invasive diagnosis of carotid disease. *Neurology*, 29:615–622.
3. Blackwell, E., Merory, J., Toole, J. F., and McKinney, W. (1977): Doppler ultrasound scanning of the carotid bifurcation. *Arch. Neurol.*, 34:145–148.
4. Davis, H. H., Heaton, W. A., Siegel, B. A., Mathias, C. J., Joist, J. H., Sherman, L. A., and Welch, M. J. (1978): Scintigraphic detection of atherosclerotic lesions and venous thrombi in man by indium-111-labeled autologous platelets. *Lancet*, i:1185–1187.
5. Davis, H. H., II, Siegel, B. A., Sherman, L. A., Heaton, W. A., Naidich, T. P., Joist, J. H., and Welch, M. H. (1980): Scintigraphic detection of carotid atherosclerosis with indium-111-labeled autologous platelets. *Circulation*, 61:982–988.
6. Duncan, G. W., Gruber, J. O., Dewey, C. F., Myers, G. S., and Lees, R. S. (1975): Evaluation of carotid stenosis by phonoangiography. *N. Engl. J. Med.*, 293:1124–1128.
7. Gee, W., Oller, D. W., and Wylie, E. J. (1976): Non invasive diagnosis of carotid occlusion by ocular pneumoplethysmography. *Stroke*, 7:18–21.
8. Green, P. S., Taenzer, J. C., and Ramsey, S. D. (1977): *A Real-Time Ultrasonic Imaging System for Carotid Arteriography*. Stanford Research Institute Publication, Menlo Park, California.
9. Kartchner, M. M., and McRae, L. D. (1977): Non-invasive evaluation and management of the "asymptomatic" carotid bruit. *Surgery*, 82:840–847.
10. Keagy, B. A., Pharr, W. F., Thomas, D. D., and Bowes, D. E. (1980): Oculoplethysmography-phonoangiography: its value as a screening test in patients with suspected carotid artery stenosis. *Arch. Surg.*, 115:1199–1202.

11. Kruger, R. A., Mistretta, C. A., Houk, T. L., Riederer, S. J., Shaw, C. G., Goodsitt, M. M., Crummy, A. B., Zwiebel, W., Lancaster, J. C., Rowe, G. C., and Fleming, D. (1979): Computerized fluoroscopy in real-time for non-invasive visualization of the cardiovascular system. *Radiology*, 130:49–57.
12. Meaney, T. F., Weinstein, M. A., Buonocore, E., Pavlicek, W., Borkowski, G. P., Gallagher, G. H., Sufka, B., and MacIntyre, W. J. (1980): Digital substraction angiography of the human cardiovascular system. *AJR*, 135:1153–1160.
13. Moore, W. S., Bean, G., Burton, R., and Goldstone, J. (1977): The use of ophthalmosonometry in the diagnosis of carotid artery stenosis. *Surgery*, 82:107–115.
14. Muller, H. (1972): The diagnosis of internal carotid artery occlusion by directional Doppler sonography of the ophthalmic artery. *Neurology*, 22:816–823.
15. Sandok, B. A. (1978): Non-invasive techniques for diagnosis of carotid artery disease. *Stroke*, 9:427 (Editorial).
16. Spencer, M. P., Reid, J. M., David, D. L., and Paulson, P. S. (1974): Cervical carotid imaging with a continuous-wave Doppler flowmeter. *Stroke*, 5:145–154.
17. Toole, J. F., and Janeway, R. (1972): Diagnostic tests in cerebrovascular disorders. In: *Handbook of Clinical Neurology*, edited by P. J. Vinken, and G. W. Bruyn, pp. 216–223. Vol. 11, Elsevier North-Holland Publishing Co. Amsterdam.

Advances in Stroke Therapy, edited by
F. C. Rose. Raven Press, New York © 1982.

The Pathophysiology of Stroke Studied by Positron Emission Tomography

N. J. Legg, R. J. S. Wise, and R. S. J. Frackowiak

Department of Neurology, Hammersmith Hospital, London, England

The first event in a cerebral infarct is failure of blood supply, usually due to thrombosis or embolism. Tissue distal to this occlusion then becomes ischaemic, and may die. The extent of the ischaemia depends on whether the occlusion is proximal or distal, on the possibility of collateral supply, on perfusing pressure, on blood viscosity, and other factors. The occlusion itself may be temporary or permanent, as platelet thrombi in particular will break up and disperse, restoring patency of the vessel.

These variations in the circumstances surrounding an infarct are sufficient to explain why the pathophysiology of stroke is not a simple matter. In the presence of vascular stenosis, raising the blood pressure may improve perfusion to an is- chaemic area, but this manoeuvre would be risky in infarcts where vessels had themselves become fragile within the lesion and thus liable to haemorrhage. Fur- thermore, in the presence of ischaemia, cell metabolism gives rise to local acidosis and other changes that produce a loss of normal vascular autoregulation. This underlies the phenomenon of luxury perfusion (4) in which blood flow to the damaged area is in excess of normal. The original concept was based on an absolute increase in blood flow, as judged by the normal range and by flow in the rest of the brain, rather than on a relative increase, judged by the metabolic demands of the ischaemic area, and the measurements were made by the invasive technique of intracarotid xenon injection and measurement of clearance. In order to understand the processes that underly the evolution of an acute cerebral infarct, there is need for a noninvasive method that will disclose the nature of the circulatory disturbance in different patients. In particular we need to know which are exhibiting luxury perfusion and which have "critical" perfusion, since methods of treatment are likely to be different for the two categories.

Such a method is provided by positron emission tomographic scanning (PET) using oxygen 15. Steady-state oxygen scanning was established by Lenzi et al. (5,6) using a gamma camera, and was later adapted for tomographic analysis. The method and the results in normal subjects have been described fully by Frackowiak et al. (3). In summary, trace quantities of radioactive oxygen are inhaled either as the pure gas or as carbon dioxide. Scans performed during carbon dioxide inhalation provide a measurement of regional cerebral blood flow (CBF), and those obtained during oxygen inhalation can be used to provide a measurement of regional cerebral metabolic rate for oxygen ($CMRO_2$). The results are shown as tomographic slices of the head in the orbitomeatal plane, each 1.6 cm thick. The ratio between blood flow and oxygen metabolism, which can be envisaged as the ratio between oxygen supply and oxygen demand, is expressed as the oxygen extraction ratio (OER), and is relatively constant throughout the brain. A typical normal scan is shown in Fig. 1. The method used at the Hammersmith Hospital also generates precise quantitative data for all three variables (2).

Stroke patients show various changes from normal. The metabolic rate for oxygen is invariably low, and blood flow is usually low as well, but the ratio between the two is frequently abnormal, indicating that there is uncoupling of the normal close ratio between supply and demand. When blood flow is relatively greater than metabolic rate for oxygen, the oxygen extraction ratio is decreased; this represents luxury perfusion. When blood flow is relatively less than oxygen demand, the oxygen extraction ratio is high; and this indicates critical perfusion.

In luxury perfusion, the blood flow is always increased relative to oxygen demand, and sometimes it is increased in absolute terms as well (see Figs. 2 and 3). The prevalence of luxury perfusion is considerably higher than was thought on the basis of xenon studies, since the earlier method showed only absolute luxury perfusion, whereas the present one demonstrates relative luxury perfusion as well. Whether absolute or relative, the condition indicates a loss of control of arterial diameter;

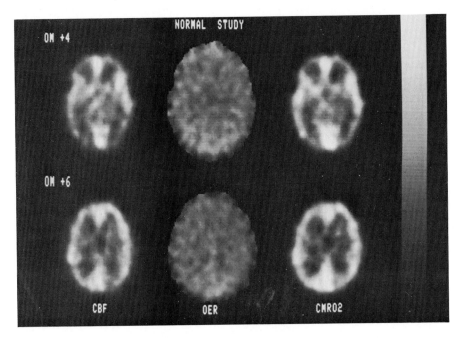

FIG. 1. Normal PET scans of the head in two planes, 2 and 4 cm above the orbitomeatal line. CBF and $CMRO_2$ are closely matched, and the OER is therefore even throughout the slices.

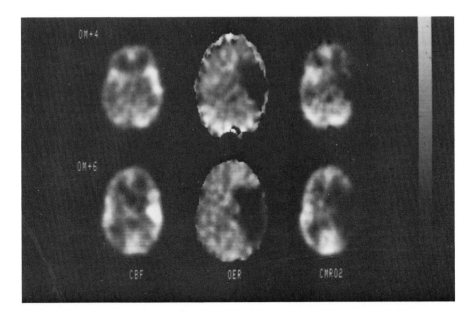

FIG. 2. Right hemisphere infarct showing absolute luxury perfusion. CMRO$_2$ is decreased, but CBF is increased above that in normal surrounding brain, and the OER is reduced.

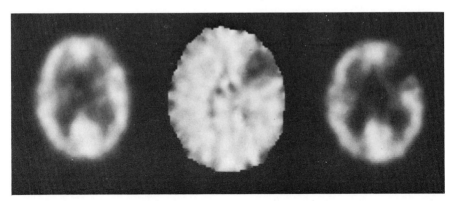

FIG. 3. Right frontal infarct showing relative luxury perfusion. Both CMRO$_2$ **(right)** and CBF **(left)** are decreased, but the decrement is relatively less in CBF than in CMRO$_2$, and the OER **(center)** is therefore reduced.

the dilatation is thought to be due to breakdown products from anoxic tissue. It seems unlikely on first principles that specific therapy is necessary or desirable in this situation since the blood supply is more than sufficient for the needs of the tissue that remains alive.

The opposite condition, of critical perfusion, appears an ideal one for treatment, for it indicates the presence of viable cells whose blood supply is at present inadequate; if the blood supply can be increased, recovery may still be possible.

Evidence that this is indeed the situation comes from observing the evolution of blood flow and metabolism in individual patients in whom critical perfusion is often seen to give way to luxury perfusion due to a decrease in metabolic rate for oxygen accompanied by an increase in blood supply, indicating that cells have died during the period of critical perfusion. An example is seen in Fig. 4. It therefore appears that treatment designed to increase blood flow during the period of critical perfusion might prevent the death of cells whose blood supply is temporarily compromised. It remains to be established in how many cases this situation is found, and for how long. Once cells have died and luxury perfusion has set in, it would be pointless to pursue treatment.

Evidence that critical perfusion can be modified is illustrated in the following case report (10).

> A 75-year-old woman suffered a left hemisphere cerebrovascular accident and was admitted to hospital. Her admission blood pressure was 180/100 and her neurological deficit, in the form of a right hemiparesis and dysphasia, was mild. She deteriorated over 24 hr, and the next day had a dense right hemiplegia and global aphasia. Three days after the onset of stroke, she was transferred to the Hammersmith Hospital. She was still hemiplegic and aphasic, her blood pressure was by then 150/70, and she was dehydrated. Previous outpatient records between 1976 and 1979 showed that her usual blood pressure was 170/90. An X-ray CT scan showed a large infarct in the left middle cerebral artery territory without

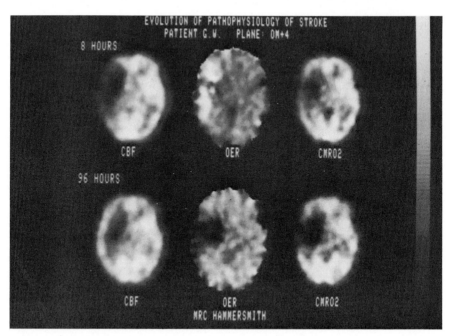

FIG. 4. Left hemisphere infarct showing critical perfusion at 8 hr and relative luxury perfusion at 36 hr. Between these two scans there has been both an increase in CBF and a decrease in $CMRO_2$.

evidence of haemorrhage. Subsequent noninvasive studies indicated that the left internal carotid artery was occluded.

A PET scan, performed three days after the onset of stroke, showed substantial reduction of both CBF and $CMRO_2$ in the area of the infarct. The OER was markedly increased in this area indicating critical perfusion. On the assumption that vascular autoregulation was abolished and that blood flow was therefore linearly dependent on the perfusion pressure, it was decided to raise her blood pressure by an infusion of angiotensin II. This was felt to be safe in view of the earlier records of a habitual blood pressure higher than the one she now showed. Her pressure was therefore raised to a level of between 190/90 and 200/100. A repeat ECAT scan 30 min later showed a marked increase in blood flow in the left temporal region and a decrease in the OER, showing that critical perfusion had been successfully reversed (Fig. 5).

The change in blood flow was examined quantitatively by taking the values for blood flow in strips of cortex around the edge of the left hemisphere from frontal through temporal to occipital lobes. These were taken to represent the flow in cortical grey matter, although contamination with a small amount of white matter and of subarachnoid space has to be assumed. Comparison of these values for scans taken both before and during angiotensin infusion showed that blood flow increased in the frontal region by nearly 80% and in the temporal region by nearly 90%. In the temporal region, this represented a recovery to about 80% of normal.

The angiotensin drip was maintained, and the patient was rescanned on the following day. The OER was still normal initially, but during the scan, angiotensin was discontinued and the blood pressure allowed to fall. When this happened,

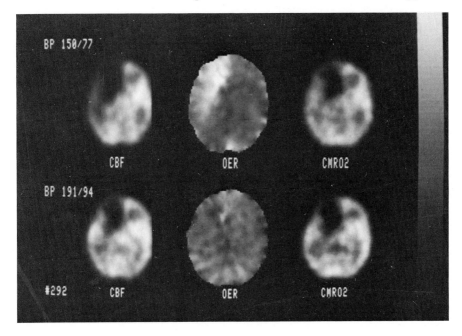

FIG. 5. Left frontotemporal infarct showing correction of critical perfusion by hypertensive therapy. At the higher blood pressure, CBF has increased and the OER has returned to normal.

critical perfusion reappeared. The angiotensin was again started, the blood pressure again rose, and again, the critical perfusion was abolished.

Unfortunately there was not clinical improvement in the patient during these manoeuvres, and quantitative estimates of the cortical $CMRO_2$, using the same analytical method as for CBF, showed no significant rise in metabolic rate in the area of the infarct. In other words, there was no tissue that showed an ability to increase its metabolism when blood flow was increased for 24 hr.

The measurements of blood flow in the frontal and temporal regions showed readings either below or only just above the threshold for irreversible ischaemia of neuronal tissue as described experimentally by Symon *(this volume)*, and therefore clinical improvement might not have been expected. It may be that at the relatively late stage three days after the stroke when the patient was first scanned, the residual metabolising tissue consisted only of nonneuronal cells. However, it has been shown in clinical studies that within a few hours of onset of cerebral ischaemia, the use of hypertensive agents can result in recovery of neurological function (7–9) and this patient might have responded, were treatment started earlier.

On first principles, one would expect this approach to be less helpful in occlusion of the middle cerebral artery than in cases like the present one, where failure of perfusion was due to a proximal block with inadequate collateral supply. In this patient, relative hypotension, contributed to by dehydration, may have been a factor in her deterioration.

The use of positron emission tomography makes it possible to study cerebral physiology in sufficient detail for changes in CBF and CMR to be observed on a regional basis and with quantitative data, which greatly extends our assessment and understanding of the underlying defects and the therapeutic responses following acute stroke. To establish the scope of feasibility of this and other methods of treatment, further cases need to be scanned in detail, with careful monitoring of the changes that can be induced by drugs that raise blood pressure, alter vascular reactivity, or suppress neuronal activity during ischaemia. Our preliminary results suggest that there may be a substantial proportion of stroke patients whose ultimate deficit could be reduced if the mechanisms of their ischaemic damage could be assessed and appropriately treated.

REFERENCES

1. Farhat, S. M., and Schneider, R. C. (1967): Observations on the effect of systemic blood pressure on intracranial circulation in patients with cerebrovascular insufficiency. *J. Neurosurg.*, 27:441–445.
2. Frackowiak, R. S. J., Lenzi, G. L., Jones, T., and Heather, J. D. (1980): Quantitative measurement of regional cerebral blood flow and oxygen metabolism in man using 15_0 and positron emission tomography. *J.C.A.T.*, 4:727–736.
3. Frackowiak, R. S. J., Jones, T., Lenzi, G. L., and Heather, J. D. (1980): Regional cerebral oxygen utilisation and blood flow in normal man using oxygen-15 and positron emission tomography. *Acta Neurol. Scand.*, 62:336–344.
4. Lassen, N. A. (1966): The luxury perfusion syndrome and its possible relation to acute metabolic acidosis localised within the brain. *Lancet*, ii:1113–1114.
5. Lenzi, G. L., Jones, T., McKenzie, C. G., Buckingham, P. D., Clark, J. C., and Moss, S. (1978): Study of regional cerebral metabolism and blood flow relationships in man using the method of

continuously inhaling oxygen-15 and oxygen-15 labelled carbon dioxide. *J. Neurol. Neurosurg. Psychiatr.*, 41:1–10.

6. Lenzi, G. L., Jones, T., McKenzie, C. G., and Moss, S. (1978): Non-invasive regional study of chronic cerebrovascular disorders using the oxygen-15 inhalation technique. *J. Neurol. Neurosurg. Psychiatr.*, 41:11–17.

7. Merory, J., Thomas, D. J., Humphrey, P. R. D., Du Boulay, G. H., Marshall, J., Ross Russell, R. W., Symon, L., and Zilkha, E. (1980): Cerebral blood flow after surgery for recent subarachnoid haemorrhage. *J. Neurol. Neurosurg. Psychiatr.*, 43:214–221.

8. Wise, G. R. (1970): Vasopressor-drug therapy for complications of cerebral arteriography. *New Engl. J. Med.*, 282:610–612.

9. Wise, G. R., Sutter, R., and Burkholder, J. (1972): The treatment of brain ischaemia with vasopressor drugs. *Stroke*, 3:135–140.

10. Wise, R. J. S., Frackowiak, R. S. J., Jones, T., Legg, N. J. (1981): Critical perfusion in acute stroke. *(in press).*

Advances in Stroke Therapy, edited by
F. C. Rose. Raven Press, New York © 1982.

Noninvasive Study of Cerebral Blood Flow and Oxygen Metabolism with Positron Emission Tomography in Human Cerebral Ischemic Disorders

*J. C. Baron, †M. G. Bousser, †D. Laplane, *D. Comar,
†P. Castaigne, and *C. Kellershorn

*Service Hospitalier Frédéric Joliot, Hôpital d'Orsay 91406, Orsay, France; and
†Hôpital de la Salpêtrière, 47, Bd de l'Hôpital 75013, Paris, France

Despite considerable progress in prevention, no significant therapeutic improvement has been achieved in the management of ischemic completed strokes, which remain a leading cause of morbidity and mortality. Only a better understanding of the pathophysiological phenomena underlying the cerebral ischemic process may lead to differentiation of tissue irreparably condemned to necrosis from tissue that might recover its function following a logically adapted therapeutic action.

In such research, the recent development of positron emission tomography (PET) now allows us to obtain noninvasively, quantitative tomographic images of numerous parameters, such as cerebral blood flow (CBF), cerebral blood volume, oxygen ($CMRO_2$) and glucose metabolism (CMRG).

Among the PET techniques, we chose the ^{15}O continuous inhalation technique because it is particularly well suited to the study of cerebral ischemic disorders and is the only currently available method allowing simultaneous measurement of CBF and $CMRO_2$. Moreover its validity essentially should be preserved in the ischemic brain, which is not the case for other techniques such as combined imaging of CBF and CMRG by intravenous injection of $^{13}NH_3$ and 18 F-fluorodeoxyglucose (16,19,21).

We would like to review briefly the method and present results obtained in three different conditions: cerebral infarction, extra-intracranial arterial bypass surgery, and migrainous infarction.

PRINCIPLE AND METHODS

Principle (18)

Because of the very short half-life (123 sec) of the tracer, a state of "dynamic equilibrium" is reached after 8 to 10 min of continuous inhalation, so that blood and tissue radioactive concentrations are stable. The theoretical model (18,22) states that, because of the total and immediate transfer of the tracer to blood water, the continuous inhalation of $C^{15}O_2$ labels *in vivo* the water of the body, so that the cerebral concentration of $H_2^{15}O$ is proportional to CBF. This relationship is, however, nonlinear so that, for high blood flows, the increase in radioactivity is much smaller than the real increase in CBF (22).

Inhalation of $^{15}O_2$ labels *in vivo* hemoglobin ($Hb^{15}O_2$); tissues take up the tracer in proportion to their oxygen consumption rate and immediately combine it with hydrogen from respiration to locally form labeled water ($H_2^{15}O$). The latter is, however, constantly cleared by effluent flow, leading to the recirculation of the $H_2^{15}O$. The cerebral distribution of equilibrium $H_2^{15}O$ during inhalation of $^{15}O_2$ therefore will be proportional to both $CMRO_2$ and CBF. The theoretical model indicates that the division of the $^{15}O_2$ image by the corresponding $C^{15}O_2$ image eliminates the CBF component and provides a ratio image linearly proportional to the oxygen extraction fraction (OEF):

$$OEF = \frac{Ca - Cv}{Ca}$$

where Ca and Cv are respectively the arterial and venous oxygen contents.

For each brain level studied, a set of three tomographic images is thus obtained: $C^{15}O_2$ (representing CBF), $^{15}O_2$ representing both $CMRO_2$ and CBF and a ratio image $^{15}O_2/C^{15}O_2$ representing OEF.

Method (3)

The patient continuously inhales trace amounts of $C^{15}O_2$ and $^{15}O_2$ consecutively, which are delivered at constant rate and concentration by a medical cyclotron. At equilibrium, axial transverse tomographic images (thickness: 19 mm, lateral resolution: 15 mm) of cerebral radioactive distribution are collected at identical levels using a positron camera. This camera has 6 rows of 11 detectors displayed in a hexagon. All detectors facing each other on opposite rows are paired and equipped with an electronic clock, allowing the exclusive collection of coincident annihilation photons located on a single line. Tomographic reconstruction is then performed by a computer. Three tomographic images (at an angle of 5° with the orbitomeatal line) are obtained during inhalation of each gas. When quantitative studies are done, a femoral puncture is performed to measure blood activities.

Quantitative Studies

To obtain quantitative data, it is necessary to measure accurately the equilibrium radioactive concentrations in both the cerebral regions of interest and the peripheral arterial blood. Simple mathematical formulae are then applied (18–22). The first results obtained in normal subjects (4) showed a 50% underestimation of grey matter CBF and an overestimation of similar magnitude of OEF. These disappointing results led us to design an experimental study to test the validity of the O^{15} continuous inhalation model. This was performed in lightly anesthetized, curarized, and passively ventilated baboons. Numerous physiological parameters were measured at various $PaCO_2$ levels and the relationship between CBF and $PaCO_2$ was studied. Results clearly showed that $C^{15}O_2$ continuous inhalation did allow tomographic measurement of CBF, provided some technological conditions were respected (7) (measurement of true attenuation coefficients, subtraction of random coincidences, ECAT calibration adjusted to the object size....).

In a second set of experiments, it was shown that the calculated OEF was highly correlated with the real OEF measured in cerebral venous blood (12).

New results obtained in seven control patients, taking into account the technological precautions indicated previously, have led to satisfying CBF, $CMRO_2$, and OEF values, when measured in small and homogeneous brain areas (2,12,14). Measurements in larger anatomical areas have led to definition of confidence limits of normal values used as reference in pathological studies (12). The absolute quantification of local CBF and $CMRO_2$ should be still further improved by new PET devices with increased resolution.

HUMAN CEREBRAL ISCHEMIC DISORDERS

Because of the above mentioned difficulties involved in absolute quantitation, only semiquantitative data will be reported in this chapter. On the images obtained, count rates per unit volume were computed for various regions of interest and compared to values obtained from contralateral homologous regions; the side to side difference was considered abnormal if outside the confidence limits defined for roughly similar regions in 17 control studies. Differences in $C^{15}O_2$ and $^{15}O_2/C^{15}O_2$ then represent true differences in CBF and OEF which, however, according to the mathematical model, should be larger.

In the normal brain, $C^{15}O_2$ images represent local CBF, varying according to the amount of grey and white matter in each region so that the main anatomical regions of the brain can be seen (3): Structures with predominantly grey matter appear much more active than those with predominantly white matter. For each brain level considered, there is a close similarity between the $C^{15}O_2$ and $^{15}O_2$ image; the ratio image is homogeneous, indicating that OEF is constant throughout all brain structures. This describes the normal couple between CBF and oxygen metabolism, the former being tightly adjusted to the latter by a constant relationship (Fig. 1).

Cerebral Infarction

Sixty patients suffering from completed hemispheric stroke were studied, 11 of them twice (5,6,10). Fifty five had a single infarct, 4 had two, and 1 had three, making a total of 77 supratentorial infarcts studied. The time of onset varied between 30 hr and 20 yr prior to the investigation; 80% were in the territory of the middle cerebral artery (MCA). Diagnosis was clinically established and confirmed by ancillary diagnostic procedures (including CT scan in 37 patients) or by postmortem study in 5 patients. Patterns observed were as follows:

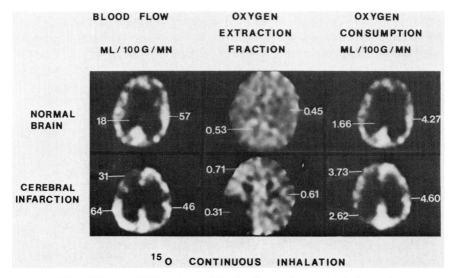

FIG. 1. CBF, OEF, and $CMRO_2$ obtained by the O^{15} continuous inhalation technique in a normal brain **(upper row)** and in an 11-day-old, left middle cerebral artery infarct **(lower row from left to right)**. The brain level studied, identical in the two cases, was situated 6 cm above the orbitomeatal line. It can be seen that in normal brain, CBF and $CMRO_2$ images are similar with an homogeneous OEF, indicating the normal coupling between flow and metabolism. Figures indicate values from white matter (on the left side of the brain) and grey matter (on the right side). By contrast in the stroke patient, there is in the left parietal region (infarcted area) a focal uncoupling with increased CBF, decreased OEF (luxury perfusion) and decreased $CMRO_2$. In the frontal region (noninfarcted), the opposite uncoupling is observed: decreased CBF with increased OEF (misery perfusion).

Infarcted Area

In 51 (94%) of the 54 infarcts occurring less than 31 days previously, there was a focal OEF abnormality, indicating a disruption of the normal flow–metabolism couple. Two opposite patterns of uncoupling were observed.

The most frequently encountered pattern of uncoupling (44 of 54 recent infarcts, i.e., 82%) was a *decrease* of OEF (Fig. 1), implying a focal decrease in arteriovenous difference; this meets the criteria defining Lassen's luxury perfusion syndrome. Areas showing luxury perfusion displayed decreased flow in 54% of cases, normal flow in 33%, and increased flow in 14%.

The second type of disruption of the flow–metabolism coupling was an *increase* in OEF, constantly associated with decreased blood flow. This pattern was observed in 12 of 54 recent infarcts (22%) and, in 6 cases, it coexisted with luxury perfusion in adjacent regions. Such oxygen "hyperextraction" indicates that perfusion is insufficient to meet the metabolic requirements of the tissue. Because it involves a state diametrically contrary to luxury perfusion, we jocularly termed this situation "misery perfusion" (6,9,10). That such focal uncoupling occurred in human infarcts was unknown before the PET era.

Similar results have been obtained by others using the same technique (1,15) or using $^{13}NH_3$ for CBF studies and 18 F-2 DG for glucose metabolism studies (19).

We have shown that the CBF/OEF relationship varied strikingly with the time elapsed after the infarct (6–10) (Figs. 2 and 3). In the first four days, two patterns were encountered: either a very low CBF (no reflow phenomenon ?) with a usually

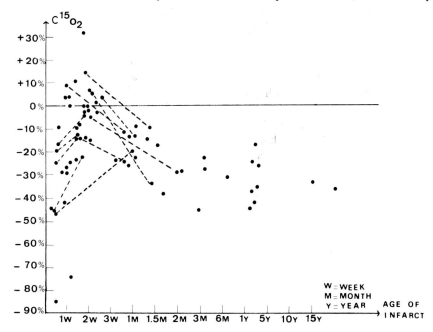

FIG. 2. $C^{15}O_2$ count rate within the infarct relative to the unaffected side (contralateral homologous area) i.e., a percent reflection of the mean change in CBF in 70 infarcts as a function of age of onset. *Broken lines* represent 11 infarcts studied twice. The 0% line indicates a normal CBF *(see text)*.

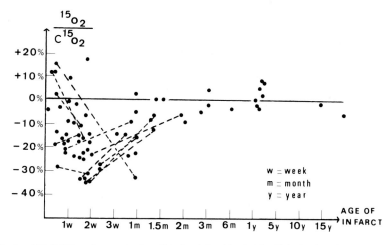

FIG. 3. $^{15}O_2/C^{15}O_2$ ratio count rate within the infarct (as in Fig. 2) indicating the percent change in OEF in 70 infarcts *(see text)*.

increased OEF (misery perfusion), or a variable CBF with a low OEF (luxury perfusion). In a second phase (from day 4 to day 21), a considerable increase in CBF was observed, often up to supranormal values, whereas OEF decreased or remained low, indicating a luxury perfusion. Afterwards, there was a decrease to below normal in CBF and an increase to normal in OEF, indicating progressive removal of necrotic tissue from the infarcted area.

The prognostic correlates of these two types of flow-metabolism uncoupling are still difficult to assess. Correlations between PET scan and CT scan images seem to indicate that regions with a huge early decrease in CBF (with or without misery perfusion) followed by a severe luxury perfusion spontaneously become necrotic. By contrast, the occurrence in the very first days of either a misery perfusion with a slightly decreased CBF or a luxury perfusion with a slightly decreased OEF seems to indicate a favorable tissue prognosis. Although it is far too early to draw therapeutic conclusions, these results suggest that the presence of a moderate misery perfusion might indicate therapeutic intervention aiming at increasing local blood flow in order to accelerate spontaneous recuperation or even to prevent necrosis in some threatened regions.

Adjacent Areas

In regions surrounding the infarcted area in 5 of 51 cases there was a focal hyperemia without luxury perfusion, probably indicating a post- or periischemic

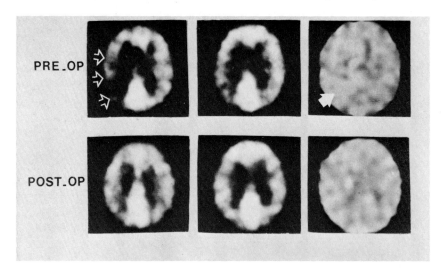

FIG. 4. Preoperative **(upper row)** and postoperative **(lower row)** O^{15} studies in a patient with clinical signs of hemodynamic cerebral ischemia distal to an occluded left internal carotid artery (11) (images taken at a level parallel to, and 6 cm above, the orbitomeatal line). Preoperatively, there is a marked decrease in $C^{15}O_2$ count rate over the left cortical convexity *(arrow frames)* more marked over its posterior part, associated with an increase in $^{15}O_2/C^{15}O_2$ ratio value (OEF) *(filled arrow)*, indicating a misery perfusion. Postoperatively, all images were normal (together with a disappearance of clinical signs).

hypermetabolism. In all cases, CT scan was normal in areas surrounding the infarct. In a few cases, a focal decrease in CBF with normal OEF and CT scan was observed in thalamus or cortical mantle ipsilateral to the infarct, probably indicating a deactivation phenomenon, as already suggested by others (19).

Remote Areas

A statistical study of 42 carotid artery territory infarcts showing neither overt brain herniation nor cerebellar CT scan changes demonstrated in the cerebellar hemisphere contralateral to the infarct a highly significant matched decrease in $C^{15}O_2$ and $^{15}O_2$ activities with a normal OEF (8). This remote metabolic depression is reminiscent of the phenomenon of diaschisis, affecting the cerebral hemisphere contralateral to brain infarction; it is apparently reversible since, in our limited material, it was not observed later than 2 months after the ischemic insult. The most likely hypothesis would attribute the occurrence of this "crossed cerebellar diaschisis" to interruption of neural pathways functionally connecting the sensorimotor cortex to the contralateral cerebellar cortex, i.e., the "cerebrocerebellar loop." This diaschisis could be the early metabolic correlate of the crossed cerebellar atrophy already reported in a few cases of either large or more circumscribed adult-onset cerebral infarction or hemorrhage (8).

Physiological Studies of Superficial Temporal Artery to Middle Cerebral Artery Extra-Intracranial Bypass Surgery

Although superficial temporal artery–middle cerebral artery (STA–MCA) bypass surgery is now widely used, its indications remain controversial and its physiological effects poorly understood. A cooperative study is underway in Paris trying to correlate, before and 1 to 3 months after surgery, in patients selected purely on clinical grounds, CBF and oxygen metabolism data with clinical, angiographic, and CT scan data. The preliminary results of the first 10 patients studied showed two widely different groups of patients and the results can be summarized as follows:

In the first group, patients had clinical signs of hemodynamic cerebral ischemia with postocclusive transient ischemic attacks (TIAs) and/or fluctuating deficits. Before surgery, O_{15} studies showed a functional asymmetry with decreased CBF and an increased or normal OEF predominating in watershed areas (9–11). These two metabolic patterns, i.e., misery perfusion and matched decrease in flow and metabolism, were reversible after surgery, together with a good clinical result. Thus, there is in this group as already shown by others (17,23) a rationale for bypass surgery.

The second group was extremely heterogeneous both clinically and functionally. Patients had no clear signs of cerebral hemodynamic ischemia, and surgery was indicated for "prevention" because of intracranial internal carotid artery or middle cerebral artery stenosis or because of carotid occlusion without postocclusive ischemic events. Before surgery, blood flow and metabolism varied widely from patient to patient but were usually symmetrical. After surgery, there was no clear correlation: The prevention effect was impossible to assess in individual patients; the functional effect was different in each patient; globally there seemed to be a bilateral increase in CBF and oxygen metabolism sometimes predominating on the nonoperated side. These puzzling results are preliminary and need to be confirmed by other studies.

This study has shown that in a small group of highly selected patients (first group), there is a high correlation before surgery between clinical signs of hemo-dynamic cerebral ischemia and decreased blood flow with increased or normal OEF, and after surgery between a good clinical result and a return to symmetry of functional parameters.

Migraine (13)

A patient with a migrainous cerebral infarction was studied 14 days after the onset of symptoms. There was in the infarcted area a decrease in CBF with decreased OEF, indicating a luxury perfusion typical of recent infarction.

More strikingly, functional abnormalities were detected in other areas of the brain distant from the infarcted area. There was an increase in CBF with normal OEF (i.e., "focal hyperemia") in the left temporal lobe and a decrease in CBF with increased OEF (misery perfusion) in the right occipital cortex, suggesting an in-volvement, latent clinically, of the corresponding arterial territories, and thus stress-ing the unusual nature and extent of the underlying process.

SUMMARY

Although only semiquantitative, the preceding results obtained in three different pathologic conditions clearly indicate the usefulness of the ^{15}O continuous inhalation technique as a clinical research tool in the investigation of the pathophysiology of cerebral ischemic disorders. With the advent of both absolute quantitation of CBF and OEF (12) and new PET devices of improved spatial resolution, this technique should gain great importance in neurological research.

REFERENCES

1. Ackerman, R. H., Correia, J. A., Alpert, N. M., Baron, J. C., Gouliamos, A., Grotta, J. C., Brownell, G. L., and Taveras, J. M. (1981): Positron imaging in ischemic stroke disease using ^{15}O labelled compounds. *Arch. Neurol.*, 38:537–543.
2. Alpert, N. M., Correia, J. A., Ackerman, R. H., Finklestein, S., Buananno, F. S., Brownell, G. L., and Taveras, J. M. (1980): Transverse section measurement of cerebral blood flow in man. *J. Nucl. Med.*, 21:22.
3. Baron, J. C., Comar, D., Bousser, M. G., Soussaline, F., Crouzel, C., Plummer, D., Kellershohn, C., and Castaigne, P. (1978): Etude tomographique chez l'homme du débit sanguin et de la consommation d'oxygène due cerveau par inhalation continue d'oxygène 15. *Rev. Neurol.*, 134:545–556.
4. Baron, J. C., Comar, D., Soussaline, F., Todd-Prokopek, A., Bousser, M. G., Castaigne, P., and Kellershohn, C. (1979): Continuous ^{15}O inhalation technique: an attempt to quantify CBF, EO_2 and $CMRO_2$. *Acta Neurol. Scand.*, 60 (*suppl.* 72):194–195.
5. Baron, J. C., Comar, D., Bousser, M. G., Plummer, D., Loc'H, C., Kellershohn, C., and Castaigne, P. (1979): Patterns of CBF and oxygen extraction fraction (EO_2) in hemispheric infarcts:

a tomographic study with the [15]O inhalation technique. *Acta Neurol. Scand.*, 60 (*suppl.* 72):324–325.

6. Baron, J. C., Bousser, M. G., Comar, D., and Kellershohn, N. C. (1980): Human hemispheric infarction studied by positron emission tomography and the [15]O inhalation technique. In *Computerized Tomography*, edited by J. M. Caillé and G. Salamon, p. 231–237. Springer-Verlag, Berlin.

7. Baron, J. C., Naquet, R., Steinling, M., Loc'H, C., and Soussaline, F. (1980): Tomographic measurement of cerebral blood flow with the $C^{15}O_2$ continuous inhalation technique: experimental evidence. *Ann. Neurol.*, 8:99–100.

8. Baron, J. C., Bousser, M. G., Comar, D., and Castaigne, P. (1980): "Crossed cerebellar diaschisis" in human supratentorial brain infarction. *Ann. Neurol.*, 8:128.

9. Baron, J. C., Rey, A., Guillard, A., Bousser, M. G., Comar, D., and Castaigne, P. (1981): Non-invasive tomographic imaging of cerebral blood flow and oxygen extraction fraction in superficial temporal artery to middle cerebral artery anastomosis. In: *Cerebral Vascular Disease*, Vol. 3, edited by J. S. Meyer, H. Lechner, and M. Revich, pp. 58–64. Excerpta Medica, Amsterdam.

10. Baron, J. C., Bousser, M. G., Comar, D., Soussaline, F., and Castaigne, P. (1982): Non invasive tomographic study of cerebral blood flow and oxygen metabolism in vivo: potentials, limitations, and clinical applications in cerebral ischemic disorders. *Eur. Neurol.*, 20:273–284.

11. Baron, J. C., Bousser, M. G., Rey, A., Guillard, A., Comar, D., Castaigne, P. (1982): Reversal of focal "misery-perfusion syndrome" by extra-intracranial arterial by-pass in hemodynamic cerebral ischemia: a case study with 150 positron emission tomography. *Stroke*, 12:454–459.

12. Baron, J. C., Steinling, M., Tanaka, T., Cavalheiro, E., Soussaline, F., and Collard, P. (1981): Quantitative measurement of CBF, OEF, and $CMRO_2$ with the [15]O continuous inhalation technique and positron emission tomography: experimental evidence and normal values in man. In: *Cerebral Blood Flow and Metabolism*, 1 (*suppl.* 1):5–6.

13. Bousser, M. G., Baron, J. C., Iba-Zizen, M. T., Comar, D., Cabanis, E., and Castaigne, P. (1980): Migrainous cerebral infarction: a tomographic study of cerebral blood flow and oxygen extraction fraction with the Oxygen-15 inhalation technique. *Stroke*, 11:145–148.

14. Frackowiak, R. S. J., Lenzi, G. L., Jones, T., and Heather, J. D. (1980): Quantitative measurement of cerebral blood flow and oxygen metabolism in man using [15]O and positron emission tomography: theory, procedure and normal values. *J.C.A.T.*, 4:727–736.

15. Frackowiak, R. S., Jones, T., and Lenzi, G. L. (1981): Cerebrovascular disorders evaluated with positron tomography: preliminary results. In: *Cerebral Vascular Disease*, Vol. 3, edited by J. S. Meyer, H. Lechner, M. Revich, pp. 117–120. Excerpta Medica, Amsterdam.

16. Ginsberg, M. D., and Reivich, M. (1979): Use of the 2-deoxyglucose method of local cerebral glucose utilization in the abnormal brain: evaluation of the lumped constant during ischemia. *Acta Neurol. Scand.*, 60 (*suppl.* 77):226–227.

17. Grubb, R. L., Ratcheson, R. A., Raichle, M. E., Kliefoth, A., and Gado, M. H. (1979): Regional cerebral blood flow and oxygen utilization in superficial temporal-middle cerebral artery anastomosis patients. *J. Neurosurgery*, 50:733–741.

18. Jones, T., Chesler, D. A., and Terpogossian, M. M. (1976): The continuous inhalation of oxygen 15 for assessing regional oxygen extraction in the brain of man. *Br. J. Radiol.*, 49:339–343.

19. Kuhl, D. E., Phelps, M. E., Kowell, A. P., Metter, E. J., Selin, C., and Winter, J. (1980): Effects of stroke on local cerebral metabolism and perfusion: mapping by emission computed tomography ^{18}F-DG and [13]NH$_3$. *Ann. Neurol.*, 8:47–60.

20. Lassen, N. A. (1966): The luxury-perfusion syndrome and its possible relation to acute metabolic acidosis localised within the brain. *Lancet*, ii:1113–1115.

21. Phelps, M. E., Hoffman, E. J., and Coleman, R. E. (1976): Tomographic images of blood pool and perfusion in brain and heart. *J. Nucl. Med.*, 17:603–612.

22. Subramanyam, R., Alpert, N. M., Hoop, B., Brownell, G. L., and Taveras, J. M. (1978): A model of regional cerebral oxygen distribution during continuous inhalation of $^{15}O_2$, $C^{15}O_2$ and $C^{15}O$. *J. Nucl. Med.*, 19:48–53.

23. Thomas, D. J., Jones, T., Lenzi, G. L., Moss, S., Ensell, J. S., and Lumley, J. P. S. (1979): Oxygen utilization and regional cerebral blood flow studies using Oxygen 15 and Xenon 133 in patients before and after superficial temporal to middle cerebral artery anastomosis. In *Cerebral Vascular Diseases*, Vol. 2, edited by J. S. Meyer, H. Lechner, and M. Reivich, pp. 7–11. Excerpta Medica, Amsterdam.

Advances in Stroke Therapy, edited by
F. C. Rose. Raven Press, New York © 1982.

Stroke Trials: The Facts

Rudy Capildeo, S. Haberman, and F. Clifford Rose

Stroke Unit, Department of Neurology, Charing Cross Hospital, London, England

There have been at least 17 acute stroke trials reported in the English literature between the years 1972 and 1981 (1,3,9,11–19,21,22,24,25). Despite recent reviews (2,4), a detailed analysis of each of the trials has not been presented in similar format. The purpose of this chapter is to analyse all 17 trials in the same way, an approach that will highlight the problems of acute stroke trials performed to date. Ten major points have been chosen.

1. *Number of patients assessed*. This figure is essential. If all patients assessed are admitted to the trial, then the selection of patients is automatically open to doubt and the trial probably invalid. If only a small number of patients are excluded, then the selection criteria may not be strict enough. If a large number of patients are assessed and only a small number of patients are included in the trial, then over-selection may have taken place.

2. *Number admitted to trial*. This figure usually corresponds to the authors stated figure but, if patients drop out because of protocol invalidation or for other reasons, their number also has to be given.

3. *Type of study*. This refers to whether the study is double-blind, randomised, placebo, controlled etc.

4. *Patient group*. This indicates the type of stroke being studied. Trials conducted on "stroke" or "acute stroke" are almost certainly doomed to failure since "stroke" is not an acceptable medical diagnosis and the different types e.g., infarct, haemorrhage, etc. (4,5,17) must be properly defined.

5. *Time limit*. This refers to the period allowed in each trial between ictus (onset of the stroke) and initiation of therapy.

6. *Treatment groups*. This is an analysis of the numbers in each treatment group. If the groups are not comparable from the outset, no conclusions can be made.

7. *Duration of treatment*. This is a reflection in part on the type of medication being evaluated.

8. *Method of assessment*. Two types of assessment are easily recognised (a) where individual parameters are measured and evaluated separately (7) and (b)

53

whether individual parameters are added to form a global score. The dangers of global assessment have been demonstrated (6,7).

9. *Duration of follow-up*. This can vary widely in different trials.

10. *Outcome*. Many readers accept the summary of a journal article but its conclusions concerning efficacy of treatment depend upon trial design (7), which means that the preceding major points, 1 through 9, should have been carried out. In this chapter, each of the published trials is tabulated separately.

TABLE 1. *Double-blind study of effects of dexamethasone on acute stroke[a] (Patten, Mendell, Bruun et al., 1972)*

1. Number of patients assessed	38
2. Number admitted to trial	31
3. Type of study	Double-blind
4. Patient group	Acute stroke/LP, EEG, isotype scan
5. Time limit	Less than 24 hr
6. Treatment groups	17 placebo/14 steroid[b]
7. Duration of treatment	17 days
8. Method of assessment	Global
9. Duration of follow-up	17 days
10. Outcome	Dexamethasone better than placebo

[a]From ref. 19.
[b]Dexamethasone.
Comments: This trial is frequently quoted, but it can be criticised on 7 points of our ten points: 1. Number of patients assessed is too few. 2. The number of patients admitted to the trial is too small. 4. The patient group is not adequately defined. 6. Treatment groups were not comparable—three cases of cerebral haemorrhage in the placebo group and two cases of brainstem infarction in the steroid group. 8. Method of assessment was global only. 9. Duration of follow-up was too short. 10. Conclusion is untenable.

TABLE 2. *Double-blind evaluation of glycerol therapy in acute cerebral infarction[a] (Matthew, Meyer, Rivera et al., 1972)*

1. Number of patients assessed	?
2. Number admitted to trial	62
3. Type of study	Double-blind
4. Patient group	54 cerebral infarction, 8 cerebral haemorrhage (CSF, isotope scan)
5. Time limit	Less than 4 days
6. Treatment groups	25 placebo/29 glycerol
7. Duration of treatment	4–6 days
8. Method of assessment	Global
9. Duration of follow-up	9 days—? weeks
10. Outcome	Glycerol better than placebo for cerebral infarction; no difference for cerebral hemorrhage

[a]From ref. 15.
Comments: The following six points can be criticised: 1. All patients assessed were included in the trial. 4. Adding 8 cerebral haemorrhage cases confuses the picture. 5. Time limit is too long. 6. Global assessment only was used. 9. Duration of follow-up is too short. 10. The conclusion cannot be justified.

TABLE 3. *Dexamethasone as treatment in cerebrovascular disease: a controlled study in intracerebral haemorrhage[a] (Tellez and Bauer, 1973)*

1. Number of patients assessed	42
2. Number admitted to trial	40
3. Type of study	Double blind
4. Patient group	Cerebral haemorrhage/LP/angiography
5. Time limit	Within 48 hr
6. Treatment groups	21 control/19 steroid[b]
7. Duration of treatment	10 days
8. Method of assessment	Individual parameters/global
9. Duration of follow-up	14 days
10. Outcome	No significant difference between treatment groups

[a]From ref. 24.
[b]Decadron.
Comments: Despite the negative result, the authors provide a lot of background data. The following four points can be criticised: 1. Number of patients assessed is too few. 2. Number admitted to the trial is too small. 6. Treatment groups were not directly comparable—the control group was "less ill". 9. Duration of follow-up too short.

TABLE 4. *Dexamethasone as treatment in cerebrovascular disease: a controlled study in acute cerebral infarction[a] (Bauer and Tellez, 1973)*

1. Number of patients assessed	54 patients
2. Number admitted to trial	54 patients
3. Type of study	Double-blind
4. Patient group	Cerebral infarction/brainstem infarction/LP
5. Time limit	Within 48 hr
6. Treatment groups	26 placebo (includes 4 brainstem)/28 steroid[b]
7. Duration of treatment	10 days
8. Method of assessment	Individual parameters/global
9. Duration of follow-up	14 days
10. Outcome	No significant difference between patient groups

[a]From ref. 3.
[b]Decadron.
Comments: A lot of background data provided. The following four points can be criticised: 1. Number of patients assessed is too few. 2. Number admitted to the trial is too small in view of patient groups. 4. Patient groups contain different diagnostic groups; the groups were not comparable in terms of severity. 9. Duration of follow-up is too small.

TABLE 5. *Management of completed strokes with dextran 40. A community hospital failure[a] (Spudis, de la Torre, and Pikola, 1973)*

1. Number of patients assessed	167
2. Number admitted to trial	59
3. Type of study	Open study, randomized
4. Patient group	Stroke
5. Time limit	Less than 24 hr
6. Treatment groups	30 dextron/29 control/LP
7. Duration of treatment	3 days
8. Method of assessment	Individual parameters
9. Duration of follow-up	3 weeks
10. Outcome	No significant difference between patient groups

[a]From ref. 22.
Comments: The study took 3 years to complete. The trial can be criticised on the following three points: 3. It is an open study. 4. Patient group is not defined. 9. Duration of follow-up is too short.

TABLE 6. *High-dosage dexamethasone in the treatment of strokes in the elderly[a] (Wright, 1974)*

1. Number of patients assessed	247
2. Number admitted to trial	61
3. Type of study	Uncontrolled
4. Patient group	Stroke in the elderly
5. Time limit	Less than 7 days
6. Treatment groups	247 total/61 steroids[b]
7. Duration of treatment	7 days
8. Method of assessment	Discharges/long stay/deaths
9. Duration of follow-up	3 months
10. Outcome	No significiant effect shown

[a]From ref. 25.
[b]Dexamethasone.
Comments: A large number of patients were initially assessed. The following four points can be criticised: 3. The trial was uncontrolled, comparing one group of steroid treatment patients on one ward with those from others. 4. Patient group was defined clinically. 8. Assessments in terms of disposal or death. 9. Duration of follow-up should probably be longer.

TABLE 7. *Controlled trial of glycerol versus dexamethasone in the treatment of cerebral edema in acute cerebral infarction[a] (Gilsanz, Rebollar, Buencuerpo et al., 1975)*

1. Number of patients assessed	?
2. Number admitted to trial	68
3. Type of study	Controlled, randomized
4. Patient group	61 acute cerebral infarction/LP, isotope scan, 7 intracerebral haemorrhage
5. Time limit	24–48 hr
6. Treatment groups	30 glycerol/30 steroid[b]
7. Duration of treatment	6 days
8. Method of assessment	Global
9. Duration of follow-up	15 days
10. Outcome	Glycerol was significantly better than dexamethasone in cerebral infarction; no difference in intracerebral hemorrhage

[a]From ref. 11.
[b]Dexamethasone.
Comments: The 7 intracerebral hemorrhage cases confuse the study. They were excluded from the results but not the summary. The following five points can be criticised: 1. Number of patients assessed is not indicated. 3. Not a double-blind study. 8. Global assessments only. 9. Duration of follow-up was only 15 days. 10. Conclusions are untenable.

TABLE 8. *Combined dexamethasone and low-molecular weight dextran in acute brain infarction: double-blind study[a] (Kaste, Fogelholm, and Waltimo, 1976)*

1. Number of patients assessed	?
2. Number admitted to trial	40
3. Type of study	Double-blind
4. Patient group	Cerebral infarction/CSF, isotope scan
5. Time limit	24–48 hr
6. Treatment groups	20 placebo/20 active
7. Duration of treatment	14 days
8. Method of assessment	Global
9. Duration of follow-up	29 days
10. Outcome	No significant difference between treatment groups

[a]From ref. 13.
Comments: Patients excluded on purpose before 24 hr. The following four points can be criticised: 1. Number of patients assessed is not indicated. 2. Number of patients admitted to the trial is too small. 8. Global assessment only is performed. 9. Duration of follow-up too short.

TABLE 9. *Controlled trial of intravenous aminophylline in acute cerebral infarction[a] (Geismar, Marquardsen, and Sylvest, 1976)*

1. Number of patients assessed	?
2. Number admitted to trial	79
3. Type of study	Double-blind
4. Patient group	Acute cerebral infarction/LP
5. Time limit	Less than 4 days
6. Treatment groups	39 controls/40 aminophylline
7. Duration of treatment	24 hours
8. Method of assessment	Global
9. Duration of follow-up	3 weeks
10. Outcome	Some improvement in mild/moderate cases but not sustained 3 weeks

[a]From ref. 10.

Comments: This was a 24-hr treatment regime. The following five points can be criticised: 1. Number of patients assessed is not shown. 4. The patient group is not defined as accurately as possible. 5. The time limit is probably too long. 8. Global assessment only. 9. Follow-up is too short.

TABLE 10. *Double-blind trial of glycerol therapy in early stroke[a] (Larsson, Marinovich, and Barker, 1976)*

1. Number of patients assessed	?
2. Number admitted to trial	27
3. Type of study	Double-blind
4. Patient group	"Early stroke"/LP
5. Time limit	Less than 6 hr
6. Treatment groups	12 glycerol/15 dextrose
7. Duration of treatment	10 days
8. Method of assessment	Global
9. Duration of follow-up	10 days
10. Outcome	No significant differences between the treatment groups

[a]From ref. 14.

Comments: This was an attempt to treat stroke as quickly as possible. The following seven points can be criticised: 1. The number of patients assessed is not indicated. 2. Number admitted to the trial is too small. 4. Because of the difficulties of confirming early diagnosis, efforts should have been made to define the patient group as accurately as possible *after treatment had been started*, hence more patients were required for the trial. 6. The treatment groups are too small. 7. Global assessment only. 9. Duration of follow-up too short. 10. Conclusion is not tenable.

TABLE 11. *A blind controlled trial of dextran 40 in the treatment of ischemic stroke[a] (Matthews, Oxbury, Grainer et al., 1976)*

1. Number of patients assessed	?
2. Number admitted to trial	100
3. Type of study	Blind-controlled
4. Patient group	Ischemic stroke/LP
5. Time limit	Less than 48 hr
6. Treatment group	48 control/52 dextran (includes 7 brainstem strokes in each group)
7. Duration of treatment	3 days
8. Method of assessment	Individual parameters
9. Duration of follow-up	6 months
10. Outcome	Severe strokes improved on Dextran 40 (lower mortality) in acute stage, but no difference at 6 months.

[a]From ref. 16.

Comments: This trial was important in that it showed that assessments must be carried out for up to 6 months. It also raised the question whether severe stroke patients, who through treatment may survive, still might be severely handicapped at 6 months. The following two points can be criticised: 1. The number of patients assessed is not indicated. 6. The treatment groups are compounded with brainstem strokes, although the distribution is identical.

TABLE 12. *Steroid therapy in acute cerebral infarction[a] (Morris, 1976)*

1. Number of patients assessed	?
2. Number admitted to trial	53
3. Type of study	Double-blind
4. Patient group	Acute cerebral infarction/LP, isotope scan
5. Time limit	Less than 24 hr
6. Treatment group	27 placebo/26 steroid[b]
7. Duration of treatment	12 days
8. Method of assessment	Global assessment
9. Duration of follow-up	29 days
10. Outcome	Placebo group did slightly better

[a]From ref. 18.
[b]Dexamethasone.
Comments: The following four points can be criticised: 1. Number of patients assessed is not indicated. 2. Number of patients admitted to the trial is small. 8. Global assessment only. 9. Duration of follow-up is too short.

TABLE 13. *New approach to treatment of recent stroke[a] (Admani, 1978)*

1. Number of patients assessed	?
2. Number admitted to trial	91
3. Type of study	Double-blind
4. Patient group	Acute stroke
5. Time limit	1–10 days
6. Treatment groups	44 placebo/47 naftidrofuryl
7. Duration of treatment	12 weeks
8. Method of assessment	Global
9. Duration of follow-up	12 weeks
10. Outcome	Naftidrofuryl significantly better than placebo

[a]From ref. 1.
Comments: The following six points can be criticised: 1. Number of patients assessed is not indicated. 3. Patient group is not defined. 4. The time limit for inclusion was very long. 8. Global assessments only. 9. Duration of follow-up probably too short. 10. Conclusion is untenable (*See* Steiner et al., ref. 21a.)

TABLE 14. *Intravenous glycerol in cerebral infarction: a controlled 4-month trial[a] (Fawer, Justafre, Berger et al., 1978)*

1. Number of patients assessed	64
2. Number admitted to trial	51
3. Type of study	Double-blind
4. Patient group	Cerebral infarction/LP,EEG, isotope scan
5. Time limit	Less than 48 hr
6. Treatment groups	32 placebo/32 glycerol
7. Duration of treatment	6 days
8. Method of assessment	Individual parameters
9. Duration of follow-up	4 months
10. Outcome	Glycerol significantly improved patients with moderate disability, but global performances were transient

[a]From ref. 9.
Comments: There was no real difference between the two treatment groups. The following two points can be criticised: 2. Number admitted to the trial is small. 9. Duration of follow-up is probably too short.

TABLE 15. *Dexamethasone in acute stroke[a] (Mulley, Wilcox, and Mitchell, 1978)*

1. Number of patients assessed	256
2. Number admitted to trial	118
3. Type of study	Double-blind
4. Patient group	Acute stroke
5. Time limit	Less than 48 hr
6. Treatment groups	57 placebo/61 dexamethasone
7. Duration of treatment	14 days
8. Method of assessment	Various parameters
9. Duration of follow up	1 year
10. Outcome	No significant difference between the treatment groups

[a]From ref. 17.

Comments: The main criticism of this trial was that the patient group was not defined. The authors' conclusion that dexamethasone is not indicated for a heterogeneous group of patients with stroke is true. The trial should have been directed towards identifying patient groups that might benefit from dexamethasone, hence it is a necessary prerequisite to define the patient group as accurately as possible from the outset.

TABLE 16. *Clinical and statistical comparison of different treatments in 300 patients[a] (Santambrogio, Martinotti, Sardella et al., 1978)*

1. Number of patients assessed	300
2. Number admitted to trial	166
3. Type of study	Randomised
4. Patient group	Cerebral infarction/LP
5. Time limit	Less than 24 hr
6. Treatment groups	Hydergine 33 /dexamethasone 34/mannitol 28/placebo 32
7. Duration of treatment	10 days
8. Method of assessment	Global
9. Duration of follow-up	10 days
10. Outcome	No significant difference

[a]From ref. 21.

Comments: The following five points can be criticised: 3. The study was not double-blind. 6. Despite the large number of patients assessed, 166 patients included in the trial, the effect of having four treatment groups, with numbers in each ranging between 28 and 34, is that small numbers of patients are being compared and (not surprisingly) the outcome is no significant difference between the treatment groups. 8. Global assessment only. 9. The duration of follow-up is too short. 10. The conclusion is untenable.

TABLE 17. *The effect of ornithine alpha-ketoglutarate in stroke[a] (Griffith, Dorf, James et al., 1979)*

1. Number of patients assessed	50
2. Number admitted to trial	45
3. Type of study	Double-blind
4. Patient group	Acute stroke
5. Time limit	96 hours
6. Treatment groups	Placebo/23/22 ornithine alpha ketoglutarate
7. Duration of treatment	5 days
8. Method of assessment	Global/Individual parameters
9. Duration of follow-up	10 days
10. Outcome	Treatment group better day 5; no difference day 10

[a]From ref. 12.

Comments: The following points can be criticised: 1. Too few patients were assessed. 2. The number of patients admitted to the trial was too small. 4. The patient group was not adequately defined. 7. Duration of treatment was probably too short. 9. Duration of follow-up was too short.

DISCUSSION

1. *Number of patients assessed*. Only five studies indicated the number of patients included in the trial and the actual number of patients assessed before selection to the trial: Fawer et al.: 51/64 (9), Mulley et al.: 118/256 (16), Santambrogio: 166/300 (21), Spudis: 59/167 (22), and Wright: 61/247 (25). Two further studies indicated dropouts after selection for the trial (19,22). Ten studies gave no information concerning this point.

2. *Number admitted to trials*. Fourteen trials had less than 100 patients. The numbers in the other three trials are: Matthews: 100 (16), Mulley: 118 (17), and Santambrogio: 166 (21). It is hardly surprising that there is little positive information on acute stroke treatment when the trials are so small.

3. *Type of study*. Twelve trials were double-blind.

4. *Patient group*. No acute stroke trial has yet been reported when CT scanning has been used to either confirm the diagnosis or for the purposes of matching. In seven trials, stroke was defined only on clinical criteria (1,10,11,17,21,24,25). This means that cerebral infarction could not have been distinguished from cerebral haemorrhage or even cerebral tumor with any certainty. The other trials used either cerebrospinal fluid examination and/or isotope scanning to establish the diagnosis as far as possible.

5. *Time limit*. This depends upon the action of the drug being used. Some treatments may need to be started as soon as possible whereas others may be started after 24, 48, or even 72 hr. Of the 17 trials reviewed, only the trial by Larsson (14) attempted to initiate treatment within 6 hr. In contrast, Admani (1) included patients up to 10 days after the ictus. Three studies specifically waited until they knew that the neurological deficit was still present after 24 hr, i.e. admission to the trial was between 24 and 48 hr (3,13,22), which would exclude transient ischaemic attacks. In our opinion, treatment should be given as soon as possible providing it is safe and efficacious; patients recovering within 24 hr then can be excluded from the trial.

6. *Treatment groups*. It is imperative that the two groups to be compared be identical, as far as possible, so that the factor to be studied (drug treatment) is the only variable. The trials by Bauer and Tellez (3) indicate the problems of not having properly matched groups from the outset. Randomisation will not match patient groups adequately when numbers are small, so that randomisation plans are necessary to ensure matched groups (7).

7. *Duration of treatment*. Seven trials gave medication for only 7 days and then the regimes differed widely. Duration of treatment should be directly related to the actions of the drug.

8. *Method of assessment*. Eleven of the trials used a global assessment, basically a total score made up of a series of subsets. This method is statistically unsound. It assumes that change in the subsets is always in the same direction, which may not be the case. One trial measured outcome in terms of disposal, i.e., discharges, referral to a long-stay institution, or death (25).

9. *Duration of follow-up.* It has already been pointed out in the trial of Matthews et al. (16) that follow-up must be continued for at least 6 months. Only one other study followed up patients for a longer period, i.e., Mulley et al. (17), who followed patients for 1 year. Twelve trials assessed patients for only 4 weeks.

10. *Outcome.* The methodology of all the trials analysed in this chapter are open to major criticism. Only three trials (3,16,18) attempted to:

a) Define the patient group

b) Perform a double-blind controlled study comparing active agent against placebo

c) Initiate treatment within 48 hr

d) Include over 50 patients.

These three trials, by Bauer and Tellez, Matthews et al., and Norris have different methodological problems.

CONCLUSIONS

A satisfactory stroke trial has yet to be done. It is necessary to design new stroke trials using CT scanning for defining the patient groups. The possibility of multi-centre trials must be considered.

A working party should be set up to standardise methods for assessing the acute stroke patient and a new classification of stroke may help towards this aim (5,6).

There needs to be a basic understanding of the problems of stroke management.

Finally, it follows that *no definite statement can be made as to the efficacy, or lack of it, of any therapeutic regime that has been tried to date.*

REFERENCES

1. Admani, A. K. (1978): New approach to treatment of recent stroke. *Br. Med. J.*, 2:1678–1679.
2. Anderson, D. C., and Cranford, R. G. (1979): Current concepts of cerebrovascular disease. Stroke: corticosteroids in ischaemic stroke. *Stroke*, 10:68–71.
3. Bauer, R. B., and Tellez, H. (1973): Dexamethasone as treatment in cerebrovascular disease. 2. A controlled study in acute cerebral infarction. *Stroke*, 4:541–546.
4. Buonanno, F., and Toole, J. F. (1981): Management of patients with established cerebral infarction. *Stroke*, 12:7–16.
5. Capildeo, R., Haberman, S., and Rose, F. C. (1977): New classification of stroke: Preliminary communication. *Br. Med. J.*, 2:1578–1580.
6. Capildeo, R., Haberman, S., and Rose, F. C. (1978): New classification of stroke. *Q. J. Med.*, 47:177–196.
7. Capildeo, R., and Rose, F. C. (1978): The design of an acute stroke trial. In: *Baclofen: Spasticity and Cerebral Pathology.* Edited by A. M. Jukes. Cambridge Medical Publications Ltd., Northampton, England.
8. Capildeo, R., and Rose, F. C. (1979): The assessment of neurological disability. In: *Progress in Stroke Research I,* edited by R. M. Greenhalgh and F. Clifford Rose. Pitman Medical, Tunbridge Wells, United Kingdom.
9. Fawer, R., Justafre, J. C., Berger, J. P., and Schelling, J. L. (1978): Intravenous glycerol in cerebral infarction: a controlled 4-month trial. *Stroke*, 9:484–486.
10. Geismar, P., Marquardsen, J., and Sylvest, J. (1976): Controlled trial of intravenous aminophylline in acute cerebral infarction. *Acta Neurol. Scand.*, 54:173–180.
11. Gilsanz, V., Rebollar, J. L., Buencuerpo, J., and Chantres, M. T. (1975): Controlled trial of glycerol versus dexamethasone in the treatment of cerebral oedema in acute cerebral infarction. *Lancet*, 1:1049–1051.
12. Griffith, D. N. W., Dorf, G., James, I. M., and Woollard, M. L. (1979): The effect of ornithine alpha-ketoglutarate in stroke. In: *Progress in Stroke Research I.*, edited by R. M. Greenhalgh and F. Clifford Rose. Pitman Medical, Tunbridge Wells, United Kingdom.

13. Kaste, M., Fogelholm, R., and Waltimo, O. (1976): Combined dexamethasone and low-molecular weight dextran in acute brain infarction: double-blind study. *Br. Med. J.*, 2:1409–1410.

14. Larsson, O., Marinovich, W., and Barker, K. (1976): Double-blind trial of glycerol therapy in early stroke. *Lancet*, I:832–834.

15. Mathew, N. T., Meyer, J. S., Rivera, V. M., Charney, J. Z., and Hartmann, A. (1972): Double-blind evaluation of glycerol therapy in acute cerebral infarction.

16. Matthews, W. B., Oxbury, J. M., Grainger, K. M. R., and Greenhall, R. C. D. (1976): A blind controlled trial of dextran 40 in the treatment of ischaemic stroke. *Brain*, 99:196–206.

17. Mulley, G., Wilcox, R. G., and Mitchell, J. R. A. (1978): Dexamethasone in acute stroke. *Br. Med. J.*, 2:994–996.

18. Norris, J. W. (1976): Steroid therapy in acute cerebral infarction. *Arch. Neurol.*, 33:69–71.

19. Patten, B. M., Mendell, J., Bruun, B., Curtin, W. and Carter, S. (1972): Double-blind study of the effects of dexamethasone on acute stroke. *Neurology (Minneap.)*, 22:377–383.

20. Rose, F. C., and Capildeo, R. (1981): *Stroke: The Facts*. Oxford University Press, Oxford, England.

21. Santambrogio, S., Martinotti, R., Sardella, F., Porro, F., and Randazzo, A. (1978): Is there a real treatment for stroke? Clinical and statistical comparison of different treatments in 300 patients. *Stroke*, 9:130–132.

22. Spudis, E. V., de la Torre, E., and Pikola, L. (1973): Management of completed strokes with dextran 40. A community hospital failure. *Stroke*, 4:895–897.

23. Steiner, T. J., Capildeo, R., and Rose, F. C. (1979): New approach to treatment of recent stroke. *Br. Med. J.*, 2, 412.

24. Tellez, H., and Bauer, R. B. (1973): Dexamethasone as treatment in cerebrovascular disease. 1. A controlled study in intracerebral haemorrhage. *Stroke*, 4:547–555.

25. Wright, W. B. (1974): High-dosage dexamethasone in the treatment of strokes in the elderly. *Gerontol. Clin.*, 16:88–91.

Advances in Stroke Therapy, edited by
F. C. Rose. Raven Press, New York © 1982.

Acute Medical Therapy of Ischemic Strokes and the Role of Prostaglandins

F. M. Yatsu and B. M. Coull

*Department of Neurology, Comprehensive Stroke Center of Oregon,
Oregon Health Sciences University, Portland, Oregon 97201*

Four pathological mechanisms contributing to the various stroke syndromes provide therapeutic considerations for both acute and preventive therapies as well as
a basis for future therapeutic strategies. These four pathophysiological mechanisms
include: a) arterial wall pathology, b) blood constituent abnormalities, c) cardiogenic
emboli, and d) the brain parenchyma's exquisite vulnerability to ischemic insults.
Current therapeutic modalities either under study or available for each of these four
areas will be discussed, but particular emphasis will be placed on the value and
theoretical potentials for the role of prostaglandins.

ARTERIAL WALL PATHOLOGY

Recognition of the importance of arterial wall pathology in the genesis of most
stroke syndromes represents a major advance in our understanding of cerebrovascular disease. In particular, knowledge of the crucial role of atherosclerosis and
attendant risk factors has led to the development of important medical and surgical
therapies for patients at risk for stroke. Current research into the basic mechanism
of atherogenesis will extend our knowledge to the molecular links to atherosclerotic
cerebrovascular disease and no doubt result in more specific and effective therapies.
As efforts of the last several decades have defined the role of extracranial cerebrovascular disease, exciting new developments such as that of computed positron
emission tomography (PET) promise to elucidate the important role of the intracranial microcirculation in strokes.

The generally recognized reduced incidence of strokes in the western world over
the past three decades is attributed largely to more effective control of hypertension,
the major risk factor for strokes (15). In addition to the control of hypertension
which requires large scale educational acceptance by both the general public and
the medical profession, efforts to reduce the impact of atherosclerosis are the next
item on the agenda for stroke prevention.

Evidence now indicates that atherosclerosis is multifactorial, and the causes
include not only hypertension but hyperlipidemia, smoking, cardiac diseases, and

diabetes mellitus. Reduction or modification of these risk factors should further impact the occurrence of strokes.

Several sources confirm a 25% decline in the incidence of stroke during the past 35 years. The Framingham study, with a follow-up of 5,209 men and women over a 24-year follow-up period and disclosing an occurrence of 345 strokes (38), and a 29 year retrospective study to 1974 from the Mayo Clinic (9), clearly demonstrate the declining incidence. Soltero et al. (30) found similar statistical data as did Haberman et al. (12) with results obtained from England and Wales.

The important role of hypertension control in reducing stroke mortality and cardiac disease is clearly demonstrated by Svardsudd and Tibblin (33) in their analysis and 13.5-year follow-up of 855 randomly selected 50-year-old men from the general population of Gotenborg, Sweden. They found a direct correlation between stroke morbidity and degree of hypertension. Similar data linking hypertension and stroke are given by the study of Rabkin et al. (25) from Canada from a cohort of 3,983 healthy men followed for a 26-year period ending 1974. Finally, Furlan et al. (8) discovered an inverse relationship between the incidence of intracerebral hemorrhage and the treatment of hypertension in a 32 year retrospective analysis of the population surrounding Rochester, Minnesota between 1945 and 1976. During that analysis period, the yearly incidence rate per 100,000 fell from 15.7 to 6.7.

Whether long-term effects in reducing the impact of atherosclerosis can be made by decreasing risk factors is yet problematical, but interest in its application is gaining increasing acceptance. In fact, strategies to reduce blood cholesterol and smoking as preventive measures appear to be making a statistical impact (24). That atheroma-regression can be achieved in patients already exhibiting the effects of atherosclerosis is bolstered by experimental studies using subhuman primates (37), but application of these studies to humans appears premature.

We are testing the hypothesis that reduced lysosomal cholesterol-ester hydrolase is a risk factor for atherosclerosis, presumably because its deficiency leads to an increased accumulation of intraarterial cholesterol esters. In our study of 24 stroke and transient ischemic attack (TIA) patients compared to age-matched controls, the lysosomal cholesterol-ester hydrolase in mononuclear cells is significantly reduced in stroke and TIA patients ($1,048 \pm 117$ pmol/mg protein/hr versus $2,205 \pm 164$, $p < 0.005$). Our data suggest that a genetic basis may play a role in atherogenesis in the customary stroke patient, a factor not previously appreciated and furthermore, that individuals with depressed levels of lysosomal cholesterol-ester hydrolase may be particularly vulnerable to atherogenesis because of their "cholesterol intolerance," perhaps remediable by strict reduction of dietary cholesterol (42).

Since improvement in the microcirculation adjacent to a thrombotic stroke might avert irreversible ischemic damage or reduce the extent of infarction, efforts to enhance the microcirculation warrant further study. Several studies suggest that aminophylline may have such a role. Geismar et al. (10) observed an unsustained beneficial effect of aminophylline when administered to acute stroke patients. Estrin (6) reported that a 63-year-old man with a right hemiparesis and nonfluent aphasia recovered dramatically 10 hr later following 250 mg of intravenous aminophylline for an acute asthmatic attack. Britton et al. (4) in a double-blind controlled study of aminophylline administered at a mean of 40 hr after stroke, found no statistical benefit when compared to placebo patients. They gave a 230 mg loading dose followed by a steady infusion at 0.5 mg/kg/hr for up to 4 hr. In accordance with other observations in the literature, we have encountered the occasional acute stroke patient who improves following an intravenous aminophylline dose of 5.6 mg/kg weight given over 15 to 20 min within the first day of ischemic stroke. The optimal intravenous dose of aminophylline in ischemic stroke is unknown, but we believe that if an effect is to be obtained, improvement should be prompt. Aminophylline in high dosages may produce convulsions, and should be administered with caution to patients with cardiac disease, especially myocardial ischemia. For this reason, we have found the drug to have limited usefulness in acute cerebral infarction.

According to the Poiseuille-Hagen formula, fluid flow through a cylindrical tube is directly related to pressure and inversely proportional to viscosity (11). Because of autoregulatory mechanisms for cerebral blood flow, this relation does not strictly pertain to normal physiologic conditions but is of crucial importance when cerebral vascular autoregulation is impaired. Acute stroke is one such instance in which regional vascular autoregulation is impaired and perfusion to an ischemic brain region can be increased by raising mean arterial pressure or reducing blood viscosity. In particular, vasopressor therapy in normotensive stroke patients may provide a useful mechanism for improving the microcirculation around a thrombotic infarction (29). These considerations have not as yet received extensive clinical application. Wise et al. (36) found in a nonrandomized study that 5 of 13 nonhypertensive patients improved neurologically when their diastolic pressures were elevated from between 85 and 100 mm mercury. The authors recommend using intravenous lev-ophed, but we have found intravenous dopamine as effective and with fewer complications. Although no prospective, randomized study has been made for the benefits of vasopressor therapy, it also should be considered under certain circumstances, particularly with normotensive patients and in patients developing complications during cerebral angiography.

Reduction of blood viscosity provides another mechanism for improving the microcirculation around a thrombotic stroke. Whole blood viscosity is influenced by multiple factors which include plasma proteins, blood platelets, hematocrit, red blood cell deformation and flow velocity. Hematocrit is perhaps the simplest of these factors to manipulate and can be lowered by use of hemodilution, thereby reducing blood viscosity (11). Low molecular weight dextrans have received much attention for this purpose, since they are retained in plasma for appreciable periods and reduce blood viscosity (28). The beneficial effect of hemodilution by low molecular weight dextran has been demonstrated in experimental animal stroke models (5,32). Unfortunately, these encouraging experimental results have not been followed by similar clinical success. Mathews et al. (17) in a randomized controlled trial using dextran 40 to treat acute ischemic stroke within 48 hr of onset found no long-term benefit compared to placebo. Acute stroke mortality was reduced by the treatment but neurological function was not improved. The authors point out that diagnostic limitations were likely to produce considerable variation within the study population. Based on experimental studies in dogs, recently, Wood et al. (39) have advocated combination volume expansion and hemodilution for treatment of focal cerebral ischemia. Proper clinical trials in stroke patients to support this approach are lacking.

In summary, a number of strategies to manipulate the rheology of a damaged microcirculation in ischemic infarction has shown theoretical or experimental promise but benefit to stroke patients from any one or combination of treatments remains to be proved.

BLOOD CONSTITUENT ABNORMALITIES

Although abnormalities in platelet function and coagulation, reflected as platelet hyperaggregability and hypercoagulable states, may exist in stroke syndromes, objective abnormalities in the majority of stroke patients do not exist and may be considered as paraphenomena according to Miettinger (20). However, normal platelet function as well as the coagulation cascade are most likely triggered by pathological changes in the arterial wall such as an ulcerated atheroma. Efforts to minimize platelet reactivity and the coagulation cascade with antiplatelet aggregation drugs and anticoagulation, respectively, have become widely accepted treatment strategies to avert thrombotic strokes, particularly in patients with warning symptoms of TIAs of brain. Furthermore, the heightened promise of preventing strokes by manipulation of platelet adhesion and aggregation as well as coagulation has galvanized sophisticated research investigation to the promising threshold of more specific and effective therapies for stroke prevention.

For the medical management of TIAs of brain, presumed to be due primarily to platelet emboli, evidence has accumulated on the efficacy of aspirin as an antiplatelet aggregation drug which will reduce the incidence of retinal and cerebral infarctions. Fields et al. (7) found that 1,200 mg aspirin daily reduced TIAs of brain and a trend toward a reduction of thrombotic strokes and retinal infarctions. The cooperative Canadian study under Barnett (3) evaluated 585 patients for the effectiveness of aspirin, sulfinpyrazone, or neither of these drugs in both carotid and vertebral basilar TIAs and reversible ischemic deficits or "threatened strokes" in a follow-up average of 26 months. In their analysis, only men were accorded a 48% reduction in the risk of strokes and stroke death. On the basis of an analysis of inapparent end-point differences of stroke occurrence for patients on aspirin and no therapy, arguments have ensued on the actual benefits of aspirin. Despite these statistical arguments, it is the conventional view that aspirin is indicated for medical therapy of TIAs.

Because of the potential of maximizing the antiplatelet aggregation effects by combining aspirin with dipyridamole affecting the prostaglandin and cyclic AMP systems in platelets, respectively, Fields has orchestrated a North American study to assess the value of 320 mg aspirin given four times a day along with placebo or dipyridamole, the latter in the dose of 75 mg four times a day. The result of this study, which will eventually include approximately 1,000 patients, will become available within three or four years.

Recent studies of Moncada and Vane (21) and Masotti et al. (16) suggest that low-dose aspirin (3.5 mg/kg given daily or up to every three days) may be more effective than 8 to 10 mg/kg/day since the protective antiaggregant prostaglandin, prostacyclin (PGI_2), synthesized in the arterial wall, is relatively unaffected with low-dose aspirin. Meanwhile, low-dose aspirin will inhibit platelet synthesis of thromboxane A_2 (TXA_2) the most potent aggregant known. Although not yet investigated in a randomized, prospective study, it would be reasonable to commence initial medical therapy in patients with TIAs of brain with low-dose aspirin and dipyridamole (50–75 mg three times daily) until more definitive data are forthcoming.

Because prostacyclin has been suggested by Moncada and Vane (21) as the protective prostaglandin that prevents platelet aggregation and is also a known disaggregant and a potent vasodilator, we have developed a protocol approved by Upjohn to infuse prostacyclin (4–8 ng/kg/min/24 hr) in acute thrombotic strokes, multiple TIAs in nonsurgical candidates and in embolic strokes of cardiogenic origin. In order to monitor the degree of platelet aggregation and the balance between PGI_2 and TXA_2, serial assays for the stable metabolites of PGI_2 and TXA_2 will be carried out along with assays of platelet aggregation. These include platelet factor 4, beta thromboglobulin, and circulating platelet aggregates (CPA). A similar study infusing PGI_2 is being conducted by John Hallenbeck of the Bethesda Naval Hospital.

We anticipate that these studies should provide insights into the molecular mechanisms accounting for stroke aggregation and improvement. In addition to these studies, more specific pharmacologic manipulation of platelet function augurs well in providing specific therapies that may be more effective in reducing the effects of thrombotic strokes. For example, specific inhibition of TXA synthetase by an imidazole compound offers the hope of greater specificity while compounds inhibiting catabolism of PGI_2 may also prove useful (23,24). Efforts to develop prostacyclin agonists are also promising. Short-term anticoagulation is recommended for TIAs by some authorities and includes the use of intravenous heparin at the onset followed by coumadin for perhaps six months (19,27). Our own preference is to avoid heparin unless antiplatelet aggregation therapy is ineffective and the patient is experiencing frequent TIAs. When heparin is used, constant infusion is preferable, starting with a bolus of 5,000 units and using 1,000 units/hr to maintain the partial thromboplastin time at 2 to 2.5 times control value.

Long-term anticoagulation, particularly over 1 year, is associated with an alarming increased incidence of intracerebral hemorrhage and should be avoided (13,25).

CARDIOGENIC CAUSES FOR CEREBRAL EMBOLI

Atrial fibrillation and myocardial infarction are associated with an increased incidence of cerebral embolization, and anticoagulation is generally recognized to reduce reembolization (14,18). Prophylactic anticoagulation in these conditions is similarly expected to reduce the risk of embolization but no prospective study has been undertaken. Theoretically, thrombus formation within the heart with atrial fibrillation and following myocardial infarction should be detectable, but bidirectional echocardiography or laboratory tests for hypercoagulable states are frequently insensitive. Nevertheless, strong consideration should be given to prophylactic therapy in these two at-risk population groups. Recently, evidence has been obtained that sulfinpyrazone reduces the incidence of cerebral embolization in patients with mitral stenosis (31).

BRAIN PARENCHYMAL VULNERABILITY TO ISCHEMIC ATTACKS

"Pharmacological protection" to avert ischemic brain infarction has been demonstrated in experimental animal studies, but whether similar strategies can be applied to stroke patients is uncertain. Barbiturates such as pentobarbital are used widely with head trauma associated with increased intracranial pressure (26), but similar investigations have not been made systematically in strokes. A recent abstract (40) suggests that in patients with raised intracranial pressure from stroke, high-dose pentobarbital does not benefit outcome. Agnoli et al. (2), however, show an apparent benefit for patients treated with pentobarbital. In a prospective, double-blind study in 26 patients given low-dose phenobarbital (60–100 mg t.i.d. for 2 days within the first 12–24 hr of stroke), we found no significant benefit (41). Whether larger doses of shorter acting barbiturates would be more beneficial remains unclear and will require further study.

Results of agents such as naftidrofuryl purporting to improve cerebral metabolism have not been impressive (1). Similarly, the use of steroids or Mannitol in acute strokes, other than averting herniation, has shown no beneficial effects (22).

SUMMARY

With a better understanding of the various pathophysiological mechanisms of stroke syndromes, more rational and highly specific forms of therapy are and will become available in minimizing ischemic effects of stroke. Particularly exciting are insights into platelet physiology, the regulation of the hemostatic mechanism, and the role of prostaglandin in minimizing the primary and secondary effects of platelet aggregation. In the final analysis, the best form of stroke therapy is stroke prevention; current inroads in hypertension control and the potentials for atherosclerosis reduction are making significant impacts.

ACKNOWLEDGMENT

This work was supported by grants from NIH, NINCDS Contract No. N01-NS-8-2387.

REFERENCES

1. Admani, A. K. (1978): New approach to treatment of recent stroke. *Br. Med. J.*, 2:1678–1678.
2. Agnoli, A., Palesse, N., Ruggieri, S., Leonardis, G., and Benzi, G. (1979): Barbiturate treatment of acute stroke. In: *Advances in Neurology, Vol. 25*, edited by M. Goldstein, L. Bolis, C. Fieschi, S. Gorini, and C. H. Millikan, pp. 269–274. Raven Press, New York.
3. Barnett, H. J. M., Gent, M., Sackett, D. L., and the Canadian Cooperative Study Group (1978): A randomized trial of aspirin and sulfinpyrazone in threatened stroke. *N. Engl. J. Med.*, 299:53–59.
4. Britton, M., DeFaire, V., Holmes, C., Miah, K., and Rane, A. (1980): Lack of effect of theophylline on the outcome of acute cerebral infarction. *Acta Neurol. Scand.*, 62:116–123.
5. Cyrus, A. E., Close, A. S., Foster, L. L., Brown, D. H., and Ellison, E. H. (1962): Effect of low molecular weight dextran on infarction after experimental occlusion of the middle cerebral artery. *Surgery*, 52:25–31.
6. Estrin, W. J. (1978): Treatment of acute cerebral ischemia with intravenous aminophylline. *Ann. Neurol.*, 3:372.
7. Fields, W. S., Lemak, N. A., Frankowski, R. F., and Hardy, R. J. (1977): Controlled trial of aspirin in cerebral ischemia. *Stroke*, 8:301–310.
8. Furlan, A. J., Whisnant, J. P., and Elveback, L. R. (1979): The decreasing incidence of primary intracerebral hemorrhage: A population study. *Ann. Neurol.*, 5:367–373.
9. Garraway, W. M., Whisnant, J. P., Furlan, A. J., Phillips, II, L. H., Kurland, L. T., and O'Fallon, W. M. (1979): The declining incidence of stroke. *N. Engl. J. Med.*, 300:449–452.
10. Geismar, P., Marquardsen, J., and Sylvest, J. (1976): Controlled trial of intravenous aminophylline in acute cerebral infarctions. *Acta Neurol. Scand.*, 54:173–180.
11. Gottstein, V., Held, K., and Sedlemeyer, I. (1972): Cerebral and peripheral blood flow as affected by induced hemodilution. In: *Hemodilution Theoretical Basis and Clinical Application*, edited by K. Messmer and H. Schmid-Schonbein. pp. 247–263. Karger, Basel.
12. Haberman, S., Capildeo, R., and Rose, F. C. (1978): The changing mortality of cerebrovascular disease. *Q. J. Med.*, 47:71–88.
13. Haerer, A. F., Gotschall, R. A., Conneally, P. M., Dyken, M. L., Poskanzer, D. C., Price, T. R., Swanson, P. D., and Calanchini, P. R. (1977): Cooperative study of hospital frequency and character of transient ischemic attacks. III. Variations in treatment. *J.A.M.A.*, 238:142–146.
14. Hinton, R. C., Kistler, J. P., Fallon, J. T., Fredidlich, A. L., and Fisher, C. M. (1977): Influence of etiology of atrial fibrillation on incidence of systemic embolism. *Am. J. Cardiol.*, 40:509–513.
15. Levy, R. I. (1979): Stroke decline: implications and prospects. *N. Engl. J. Med.*, 300:490–491.
16. Masotti, G., Galanti, G., Poggesi, L., Abbate, R., and Neri Serneri, G. G. (1979): Differential inhibition of prostacyclin production and platelet aggregation by aspirin. *Lancet*, ii:1213–1216.
17. Mathews, W. B., Oxbury, J. M., Grainger, K. M. R., and Greenhall, R. C. D. (1976): A blind controlled trial of dextran 40 in the treatment of ischemic stroke. *Brain*, 99:193–206.
18. McDevitt, E. (1972): Anticoagulant therapy in cerebral vascular disease. In: *Handbook of Clinical Neurology Vol. 12*, edited by P. J. Vinken and C. W. Bruyn, pp. 456–467. Elsevier, New York.
19. McDowell, F. H., Millikan, C. H., and Goldstein, M. (1980): Treatment of impending stroke. *Stroke*, 11:1–3.
20. Miettinger, K. L., Nyman, D., Kjellin, K. G., Siden, A., and Soderstrom, C. E. (1979): Factor VIII related to antigen, antithrombin III, spontaneous platelet aggregation and plasminogen activator in ischemic cerebrovascular disease. *J. Neurol. Sci.*, 41:31–38.
21. Moncada, S., and Vane, J. R. (1979): Arachidonic acid metabolites and the interactions between platelets and blood vessel walls. *N. Engl. J. Med.*, 300:1142–1147.
22. Mulley, G., Wilcox, R. G., and Mitchell, J. R. A. (1978): Dexamethasone in acute stroke. *Br. Med. J.*, 2:994–996.
23. Prostacyclin in therapeutics (1981): *Lancet*, ii:643–644 (editorial).
24. Puska, P., Virtamo, J., Tuomilehto, J., Maki, J., and Neittaanmaki, L. (1978): Cardiovascular risk factor changes in a three year follow-up of a cohort in connection with a community programme (the North Karelin project). *Acta Med. Scand.*, 204:381–388.
25. Rabkin, S. W., Mathewson, F. A. L., and Tate, R. B. (1978): The relation of blood pressure to stroke prognosis. *Ann. Int. Med.*, 89:15–20.
26. Rockoff, M. A., Marshall, L. F., and Shapiro, H. M. (1979): High-dose barbiturate therapy in humans: A clinical review of 60 patients. *Ann. Neurol.*, 6:194–199.

27. Sandok, B. A., Furlan, A. J., Whisnant, J. P., and Sundt, T. M. (1978): Guidelines for the management of transient ischemic attacks. *Mayo Clin. Proceed.*, 53:665–674.
28. Seaman, G. V. F., Hissen, W., Lino, L., and Swank, R. L. (1965): Physicochemical changes in blood arising from dextran infusions. *Clin. Sci.*, 29:293–304.
29. Slater, R., Reivich, M., Goldberg, H., Banks, R., and Greenberg, J. (1977): Diaschisis with cerebral infarction. *Stroke*, 8:684–690.
30. Soltero, I., Leu, K., Cooper, R., Stamler, J., and Garside, D. (1978): Trends in mortality from cerebrovascular diseases in the United States. 1960 to 1975. *Stroke*, 9:549–558.
31. Steele, P., and Rainwater, J. (1980): Favorable effect of sulfinpyrazone on thromboembolism in patients with rheumatic heart disease. *Circulation*, 62:462–465.
32. Sundt, T. M., and Waltz, A. G. (1967): Hemodilution and anticoagulation. *Neurology*, 17:230–238.
33. Svardsudd, K., and Tibblin, G. (1979): Mortality and morbidity during 13.5 years follow-up in relation to blood pressure. The study of men born in 1913. *Acta Med. Scand.*, 205:483–492.
34. Tyler, H. M., Saxton, C. A. P. D., and Parry, M. J. (1981): Administration to man of UK-37, 248-01, a selective inhibitor of thromboxane synthetase. *Lancet*, i:629–632.
35. Whisnant, J. P., Cartilidge, N. E. F., and Elveback, L. R. (1978): Carotid and vertebral-basilar transient ischemic attacks: Effect of anticoagulants, hypertension and cardiac disorders on survival and stroke occurrence—a population study. *Ann. Neurol.*, 3:107–115.
36. Wise, G., Sutter, R., and Burkholder, J. (1972): The treatment of brain ischemia with vasopressor drugs. *Stroke*, 3:135–140.
37. Wissler, R. W. (1979): Evidence for regression of advanced atherosclerotic plaques. *Artery*, 5:398–408.
38. Wolf, P. A., Kannel, W. B., and Dawber, T. R. (1978): Prospective investigations: The Framingham study and the epidemiology of stroke. In: *Advances in Neurology, Vol. 19*, edited by B. S. Schoenberg, pp. 107–120. Raven Press, New York.
39. Wood, J. H., Snyder, L. L., Simeone, F. A., Golden, M. A., and Fink, E. A. (1981): Cerebrovascular and cardiac responses to intravascular volume expansion following focal cerebral ischemia. *Stroke*, 12:130.
40. Woodcock, J., and Ropper, A. H. (1981): High-dose barbiturates in patients with nontraumatic brain swelling. *Neurology*, 31:56.
41. Yatsu, F. M., and Coull, B. M. (1980): *(unpublished observations).*
42. Yatsu, F. M., Hagemenas, F. C., and Manaugh, L. C. (1980): Cholesterol ester hydrolase activity in human symptomatic atherosclerosis. *Lipids*, 12:1019–1022.

Advances in Stroke Therapy, edited by
F. C. Rose. Raven Press, New York © 1982.

Naftidrofuryl

T. J. Steiner and F. Clifford Rose

Department of Neurology, Charing Cross Hospital, London, England

INTRODUCTION AND PHARMACOLOGY

Developed originally in the *Laboratoires Oberval*, naftidrofuryl was a product of the search for a substance with antihypercholesterolaemic activity. Its synthesis, along with a number of related molecules, was reported in 1966 (28). Though weakly cholesterolytic, when its pharmacology was later described (10) it became clear that the molecule had other activity of greater significance. This substance is now marketed as Praxilene throughout most of Europe, but in Germany as Dusodril.

The actions listed in Table 1 are ordered for convenience rather than importance. Naftidrofuryl is highly spasmolytic, inhibiting, for instance, the contractile effects on isolated smooth muscle preparations of acetylcholine, histamine, 5-hydroxy-tryptamine, and oxytocin (30). At the same time, it is a potent direct vasodilator, papaverine-like but several times more powerful in some preparations, and acts with greater effect on vessels of skeletal muscle than on those of myocardium and with lesser effect on skin and cerebral cortex (12). *In vivo*, blood pressure is altered very little (10,30).

Other actions of naftidrofuryl include a) local anaesthetic, with a potency of the same order as procaine, b) analgesic, through a strong antibradykinin effect, c) autonomic ganglion-blocking, less potent than hexamethonium, d) weakly anti-atherogenic, by inhibiting synthesis of lipids, especially serum β-lipoproteins, so lowering serum lipid as well as cholesterol levels, and e) platelet disaggregating,

TABLE 1. *Main pharmacological actions*
of naftidrofuryl

Spasmolytic
Vasodilator
Local anaesthetic
Analgesic
Autonomic ganglion blocking
Antiatherogenic
Inhibits platelet aggregation
Alters cellular energy metabolism

with a potency *in vitro* comparable to that of dipyridamole. It has no observed effect on coagulation. Its actions on the heart lead to mild, negative chronotropia and dromotropia (10), but the ECG is unaltered with usual dosages.

METABOLIC ACTIVATION

The pharmacological profile of naftidrofuryl obviously suggests use in the treatment of arterial insufficiency syndromes and other ischaemic conditions. A number of theoretically desirable activities, though unrelated, occur together in a way that indicates naftidrofuryl is particularly useful for these illnesses. Soon after its original synthesis, naftidrofuryl was being used in open trials in acute and chronic cerebrovascular disease (8,17,25), and it has been widely promoted for peripheral arterial disease.

However, if the basis of its therapeutic application was initially its vasodilator activity, this soon gave way to the concept of a metabolic activator molecule as measurements of markers of cellular energy metabolism indicated enhancement of cellular oxidative activity. In man (Table 2), experiments measuring pyruvate, glucose, lactate, glycerol, and ketone bodies in exercising normal muscle (26) indicate that there is activation of succinic dehydrogenase, an enzyme within the tricarboxylic acid cycle. In resting ischaemic muscle (9), naftidrofuryl increases ADP and ATP formation with reduction in lactate levels. Similar experiments with biopsy cannot be carried out on human cerebral tissue, but some animal experiments have been done. In normal brain (Table 2), naftidrofuryl appears to promote glucose consumption, increase the supply of ATP, and reduce levels of lactate (21).

CEREBRAL ISCHAEMIA AND THERAPEUTIC USE

In view of the evidence, can the activity of naftidrofuryl be used to protect ischaemic brain against the metabolic effects of anoxia? Naftidrofuryl injected directly into the carotid artery has little effect on local cerebral blood flow as measured by ^{133}Xe clearance (24), but Okao and others (23) reported a transient increase in dogs, following intravenous injection of 2 mg/kg, both in cerebral blood flow estimated by heat clearance and in available oxygen measured by platinum

TABLE 2. *Metabolic activation by naftidrofuryl*

Exercising normal muscle in man
Enhancement of cellular oxidative activity by
activation of succinic dehydrogenase
Resting ischaemic muscle in man
Increased ADP and ATP formation
Reduced lactate levels
Cerebral energy metabolism in animals
Increase in supply of ATP
Promotion of glucose consumption
Fall in lactic acid levels

electrode. The effect on blood flow was comparable to that of 10% CO_2 inhaled for 4 or 5 min, and acute cerebral edema and intracranial hypertension interfered with this action. Animal models of cerebral ischaemia have unfortunately been little used with naftidrofuryl, but such evidence as they have produced does suggest that protection of ischaemic cerebral tissue is possible (22). Larsen et al. (18) embolised rats with microspheres via the carotid artery to produce cerebral ischaemia (16). Some had been pretreated for 3 weeks with naftidrofuryl, 20 mg/kg/day intraperitoneally, and a moderate but significant reduction in mortality was demonstrated in these. Though the authors were pleased since some protective effect was indicated, this was clearly not a good model for any clinically encountered situation.

Therapeutic possibilities are dependent on pharmacokinetics, but knowledge for naftidrofuryl is incomplete. It may be taken orally, intramuscularly, where absorption is significantly delayed (11), or intravenously, by bolus or infusion. After oral administration in man, peak plasma levels are achieved after about 1 hr, high concentrations being found in the lungs, liver, kidneys, heart, and brain. Biliary transit occurs, with significant enterohepatic recirculation (11). The half-life in plasma is about 1 hr, with hydrolysis by pseudocholinesterase, but very little is known of the activity of its metabolites (15).

On the other hand, its use in a variety of clinically encountered conditions over fifteen years has demonstrated that naftidrofuryl is safe both in acute and chronic use, with few side-effects, none of which are of major concern: skin rashes have been few and minor; mild gastrointestinal upset may occur uncommonly (7). Evidence that intravenous naftidrofuryl gives rise to severe infusion thrombophlebitis (29) has been disputed (13,20).

CLINICAL TRIALS

The therapeutic employment of any drug is ultimately determined by how the substance fares under clinical trial. Table 3 shows the trials so far published on naftidrofuryl with placebo controls in patients with cerebrovascular disease; all were double-blind and used only oral naftidrofuryl, in doses between 50 and 200 mg t.d.s., 100 mg t.d.s. being the most common. In the first five listed, variously defined groups of elderly patients with chronic cerebrovascular syndromes were treated and assessed with emphasis on psychological testing and functional scores.

TABLE 3. *Published controlled studies of naftidrofuryl in vascular impairment of cerebral function (variously defined)*

Study	Date	N	Result	Significance
Judge and Urquhart (14)	1972	24	Some improvement	Yes
Bouvier et al. (4)	1974	51	Improved	?
Cox (6)	1975	32	Improved	Yes
Bargheon (2)	1975	108	Improved	?
Brodie (5)	1977	60	Some improvement	Yes
Admani (1)	1978	91	Improved	Yes

In the first three (4,6,14), only hospital in-patients participated, but of the other two, one used residents in a nursing home (2), and one was GP-managed (5).

The last trial (1), from Sheffield, England, was limited to conscious patients with "recent ischaemic cerebral infarction" and provides the only information of any objective value regarding use of naftidrofuryl in stroke.

Looking at all the trials together (Table 3), one has to be impressed by the unanimity of the results, briefly summarised as the effect of treatment with nafti-drofuryl compared to placebo. On the other hand, while many clinical trials that are less than first-rate are published without comment, each one of these has been criticised in print (3,27). While this does not necessarily negate the positive findings, it is a pity that the total effort expended has been dissipated among many studies with nonuniform aims, so that it remains difficult to assess the agent's worth satisfactorily. It seems likely that naftidrofuryl is useful in improving cerebral function in the elderly, confused, chronically cerebrovascular diseased patient.

As the Sheffield trial (1) (for lack of another) currently has to form the basis for judging the use of naftidrofuryl in acute stroke, it has a greater significance than it might otherwise warrant. Its major conclusions are summarised in Table 4: reduced death rate attributable to stroke, reduced length of stay in hospital, better neuro-logical and functional recovery. It is informative to reconsider these claims without reiterating the methodological objections to the trial (27). "Death attributable to stroke" was not defined. Seven of the 22 deaths occurring during the follow-up period of only 12 weeks were adjudged not due to stroke; that is, the occurrence of death at that particular time was to be considered coincidental. This seems far-fetched, and it is unlikely that this is what Admani actually meant, but it is improper otherwise to exclude these cases from the analysis of outcome, and the difference between treated and placebo groups for all deaths was not statistically significant. In terms of bed occupancy, 24 of 44 control patients were discharged during the trial follow-up, and only 23 of 47 treated patients. To make the extraordinary claim of reduced bed occupancy by the treated group (the "salient finding" of the trial), Admani counted only the days in hospital of these patients discharged within the 12 weeks. At the end of that time, it can be calculated that there were still 22 patients in hospital upon whose eventual fate no comment was passed, and 15 (two-thirds) of these long-stay patients were on naftidrofuryl. The conclusion regarding recovery was based upon a summation of sub-scores for numerous assessed neu-rological and neurophysical variables according to a defined scale. This technique has gained apparent respectability through widespread use in the last decade, but offends the most fundamental laws of statistics. This particular scale exacted the

TABLE 4. *Naftidrofuryl in acute stroke*

"Reduces death rate attributable to stroke..."
"Increases extent of recovery..."
"Reduces acute bed occupancy..."

Compiled from ref. 1.

same penalty for nystagmus as for inability to cook or for having hallucinations, and awarded 5 times as many points for sensory function as for power in either affected limb (i.e., 20 points gained if no sensory loss; 8 points forfeited if totally hemiplegic).

Although the conclusions of the Sheffield trial would have been no more valid in any case than the trial design, the rationale for the use of naftidrofuryl in acute ischaemic stroke is good. Dead brain is irreparable, as all know, but the concept of an intermediary critical ischaemia, which many have found attractive for some time, now can be demonstrated by PET scanning (19). Figure 1 illustrates a left cerebral ischaemic episode some 8 hr old that proceeded to infarction; there is high relative oxygen extraction in a hypoperfused area. In other words, this is living brain tissue, scavenging for oxygen that is in short supply. Protection of such tissue by some means may be the only feasible approach to the treatment of acute cerebral infarction, and to the Hippocratic challenge: "It is impossible to remove a strong attack of apoplexy and not easy to remove a weak attack." In considering whether naftidrofuryl can do this, it has to be remembered that it is a potent vasodilator; the whole question of vasodilators in acute ischaemic stroke is an uneasy one still unresolved by clinical trials.

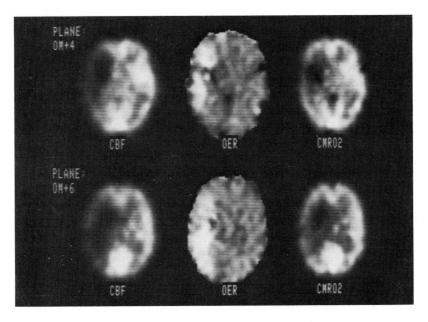

FIG. 1. PET scan of a 67-year-old man with onset 8 hr earlier of right hemiparesis and dysphasia, clinically diagnosed as left middle cerebral artery territory infarction. A CT scan performed 6 hr after onset was normal. The high oxygen extraction ratio (OER) in the left middle cerebral artery distribution indicates a relative excess of metabolic demand for oxygen over supply, identifying a condition that has been termed "critical perfusion" (19). (We are grateful to the Physics Isotopes Section, MRC Cyclotron Unit, Hammersmith Hospital, London, for this scan of one of our patients.)

What is certain is that further and better clinical trials of naftidrofuryl are required. Our own double-blind trial is in its fourth and probably final year of recruiting. We are using it against placebo in matched cases of CT scan-proven acute cerebral hemisphere infarction. Patients on active treatment receive 10 days' continuous intravenous infusion at 600 mg daily, then oral medication at 300 mg daily for 9 months. Assessment is over a minimum of 1 year, and will be reported after the end of 1982.

CONCLUSIONS

Meanwhile, no recommendation about the use of naftidrofuryl in acute ischaemic stroke can be made. This may be less the fault of the drug than of the poor quality of the experimental work that has endeavoured to support it. Much of this work is now being repeated in hospitals and laboratories in the United Kingdom. There is no doubt that the substance deserves an adequate clinical trial, and the results are being awaited with considerable interest.

ACKNOWLEDGMENTS

The trial of naftidrofuryl in acute cerebral hemisphere infarction referred to in this chapter is supported by Lipha Pharmaceuticals, Limited, United Kingdom.

REFERENCES

1. Admani, A. K. (1978): New approach to treatment of recent stroke. *Br. Med. J.*, 2:1678–1679.
2. Bargheon, J. (1975): Essai en double aveugle du Praxilène en gériatrie. *Gaz. Med. Fr.*, 82:4755–4758.
3. Beghi, E. (1979): Naftidrofuryl. In: *Drug Treatment and Prevention in Cerebrovascular Disorders*, edited by G. Tognoni and S. Garattini, pp. 211–222. Elsevier-North Holland Biomedical Press, Amsterdam.
4. Bouvier, J. B., Passeron, O., and Chupin, M. P. (1974): Psychometric study of Praxilene. *J. Int. Med. Res.*, 2:59–65.
5. Brodie, N. H. (1977): A double-blind trial of naftidrofuryl in treating confused elderly patients in general practice. *Practitioner*, 218:274–278.
6. Cox, J. R. (1975): Double-blind evaluation of naftidrofuryl in treating elderly confused hospitalised patients. *Gerontol. Clin.*, 17:160–167.
7. Editorial (1979): Naftidrofuryl (Praxilene) in peripheral vascular disease. *Drug. Ther. Bull.*, 17:83–84.
8. Eichhorn, O. (1969): Zur Behandlung der ischämischen Hirnschädigung. *Med. Welt.*, 42:2314–2318.
9. Elert, O., Niebel, W., Krause, E., and Satter, P. (1976): Beeinflussung des Energiestoffwechsels der minderdurchbluteten Extremitätenmuskulatur durch Naftidrofuryl. *Therapiewoche*, 26:3947–3950.
10. Fontaine, L., Grand, M., Chabert, J., Szarvasi, E., and Bayssat, M. (1968): Pharmacologie générale d'une substance nouvelle vasodilatatrice, le naftidrofuryl. *Chim. Thér.*, 6:463–469.
11. Fontaine, L., Belleville, M., Lechevin, J. C., Silie, M., Delahaye, J., and Boucherat, M. (1969): Étude du métabolisme du naftidrofuryl chez l'animal et chez l'homme. *Chim. Thér.*, 1:44–49.
12. Hagihara, Y., Satoh, M., Takane, H., and Ohta, Y. (1973): Action of naftidrofuryl oxalate on the peripheral circulation. *Folia Pharmacol. (Jpn.)*, 69:721–728.
13. Heidrich, H. (1978): Incidence of thrombophlebitis with naftidrofuryl. *Br. Med. J.*, 1:618–619.
14. Judge, T. G., and Urquhart, A. (1972): Naftidrofuryl—a double blind cross-over study in the elderly. *Curr. Med. Res. Opinion*, 1:166–172.

15. Kitagawa, H., Nakata, R., and Yano, H. (1973): Metabolic studies on naftidrofuryl oxalate (LS 121) in rats. *Oyo Yakuri*, 7:1231–1240.
16. Kogure, K., Busto, R., Scheinberg, P., and Reinmuth, O. M. (1974): Energy metabolites and water content in rat brain during the early stage of development of cerebral infarction. *Brain*, 97:103–114.
17. Labet, R. (1970): Action du Praxilène sur les accidents vasculaires cérébraux. *Vie Méd.*, 3645–3650.
18. Larsen, R. G., Dupeyron, J. P., and Boulu, R. G. (1978): Modèle d'ischémie cérébrale expérimentale par microsphères chez le rat. Étude de l'effet de deux extraits de Ginkgo biloba et du naftidrofuryl. *Therapie*, 33:651–660.
19. Legg, N. J., Wise, R. J. S., and Frackowiak, R. S. J. *(this volume)*.
20. MacLellan, D. G. (1977): Intravenous naftidrofuryl. *Br. Med. J.*, 2:267 (Letter).
21. Meynaud, A., Grand, M., and Fontaine, L. (1973): Effect of Naftidrofuryl upon energy metabolism of the brain. *Arzneim.-Forsch.*, 23:1431–1436.
22. Meynaud, A., Grand, M., Belleville, M., and Fontaine, L. (1975): Effet du naftidrofuryl sur le métabolisme énergétique cérébral chez la souris. *Therapie*, 30:777–788.
23. Okao, S., Nagao, S., Manabe, T., Akioka, T., Mizukawa, N., Matsumoto, K., Iwatsuki, K., and Nishimoto, A. (1973): The effects of the vasodilator (Praxilene) on the cerebral haemodynamics in acute intracranial hypertension and cerebral oedema. *Jpn. Circ. J.*, 37:999–1007.
24. Péchadre, J. C., and Simard, D. (1974): A la lumière des effets du naftidrofuryl sur le débit sanguin cérébral. *Rev. Neurol.*, 130:301–307.
25. Porot, M., and Lajoinie, J. (1971): Action du Naftidrofuryl sur les troubles neuro-psychiatriques des accidents vasculaires cérébraux. *Vie Méd.*, 2:(27), 3205–3207.
26. Shaw, S. W. J., and Johnson, R. H. (1975): The effect of Naftidrofuryl on the metabolic response to exercise in man. *Acta Neurol. Scand.*, 52:231–237.
27. Steiner, T., Capildeo, R., and Clifford Rose, F. (1979): New approach to treatment of recent stroke. *Br. Med. J.*, 1:412 (letter).
28. Szarvasi, E., Bayssat, M., Fontaine, L., and Grand, M. (1966): Quelques nouvelles structures naphtaléniques à activité antispasmodique. *Bull. Soc. Chim. France*, 6:1838–1846.
29. Woodhouse, C. R. J., and Eadie, D. G. A. (1977): Severe thrombophlebitis with Praxilene. *Br. Med. J.*, 1:1320.
30. Yanagita, T., Iizuka, H., and Takeda, K. (1972): General pharmacological effects of naftidrofuryl oxalate. *Oyo Yakuri*, 6:509–521.

Advances in Stroke Therapy, edited by
F. C. Rose. Raven Press, New York © 1982.

Effects of I.V. Hydergine on rCBF in Man Following Infarction in the Middle Cerebral Artery Territory

J. M. Orgogozo, A. M. Bidabe, P. Floras, and J. M. Caillé

Unité de Pathologie Vasculaire Cérébrale, Department of Neuroradiology, Hôpital Pellegrin, Université de Bordeaux II, Bordeaux, France

Drugs that markedly increase cerebral blood flow, either by directly affecting the muscular layer of the arterioles, like papaverine (12,17), or by changing pH around arterioles, like acetazolamide (5), have proven to be of little or no benefit in animal stroke models or in clinical trials. As with increasing $PaCO_2$, these drugs have been shown to steal blood away from the ischaemic lesion, with possible deterioration in the clinical condition. On the other hand, induced reduction of $PaCO_2$ has been found to have no useful effects in stroke patients (3) despite the fact that an "inverse steal" effect—i.e. a steal of blood from nonaffected to affected areas—can be obtained with this procedure (16). Hydergine (co-hydergocrine mesylate, BAN), a natural mixture of four dihydrogenated ergot peptides, has little demonstrable effect on brain circulation, and no steal effect has been observed with it (13). In animal models, this drug protects against the consequences of experimental cerebral ischemia, a protection attributed (7) to blockade of α-adrenergic synapses in the brain, with resulting metabolic effects similar to those of barbiturates (19). As a pilot study before a formal clinical trial, we examined the acute effects of I.V. Hydergine on regional cerebral blood flow (rCBF) and systemic arterial blood pressure (BP) in patients with a recent infarction in the middle cerebral artery (MCA) distribution.

PATIENTS AND METHODS

Ten patients were selected according to the following criteria: a) infarction in middle cerebral artery distribution documented by CT scan, b) onset of stroke less than 8 days before the study, c) absence of stupor or coma at time of the study, d) age below 75 years, e) indication present for carotid arteriography, f) no occlusion of the appropriate internal carotid artery (as evidenced from Doppler examination).

Regional cerebral blood flow was measured with the intracarotid xenon injection method using a 16 individual detector system that allows calculation of the initial slope index of the 10-min height-over-area ratio and of the grey and white matter flows by compartmental analysis. The 10-min height-over-area was chosen for this study because other, deterministic methods are less valid in cases of brain lesions, particularly infarction.

Two dosages of Hydergine were used: 0.9 mg/70 kg in five patients and 1.2 mg/70 kg in the other five. The first measurement of rCBF was made more than 5 min after angiography. At the end of this procedure which takes about 20 min, the drug dissolved in 100 ml glucose 5% was administered within 5 min by drip; 10 min after the end of the infusion, a second rCBF determination was made. Just before, during, and after each measurement, systolic blood pressure was recorded; $PaCO_2$ was determined in an arterial blood sample (Radiometer, Copenhagen) at the beginning of each rCBF run.

Clinical, CT scan, and angiography data for each patient were reported on a data sheet along with BP, $PaCO_2$, and rCBF measurements. Only data from nine patients could be used, because of technical problems in the calculation of rCBF in one. Some of these data are presented in Table 1. Patients 1 to 5 received 0.9 mg Hydergine/70 kg; patients 6 to 9 received 1.2 mg/70 kg.

RESULTS

The changes in BP, $PaCO_2$, mean, and regional CBF from the resting studies to the test studies were similar with both dosages used.

$PaCO_2$

Having no effect on respiration or on general oxidative metabolism, Hydergine would not be expected to affect $PaCO_2$. In fact this variable was controlled in order

TABLE 1. *Patients*

Patient no.	Sex	Age	CT scan	Angiography
1	F	54	Left parietal cortical hypodensity	Complete proximal MCA occlusion
2	F	70	Cortical atrophy, without clear focal lesion	Intracerebral atheroma Delayed filling of an MCA branch
3	F	60	Large left frontotemporal hypodensity	Occlusion of prerolandic and rolandic arteries
4	F	68	Left temporal hypodensity	Delayed filling of the superficial MCA branches
5	M	68	Large right temporoparietal hypodensity	Complete proximal MCA occlusion
6	M	49	Large hypodensity in the left MCA territory	No obstruction or atheroma of the MCA (embolism?)
7	M	51	Large hypodensity in the right MCA territory	Complete proximal MCA ccclusion
8	M	52	Right occipital hypodensity	Delayed filling of the parietooccipital MCA branches
9	F	57	Hypodensity in the left subcortical MCA territory	No occlusion or atheroma of the cervicocranial arteries

MCA—Middle cerebral artery

to make sure that changes in CBF would not have been due to changes in $PaCO_2$. As shown in Table 2, there were no systematic changes in $PaCO_2$, the mean values for the whole group being 4.9 kPa before, and 5.0 kPa after drug administration.

Blood Pressure

Although Hydergine has been used as a mild hypotensive agent in the past, we found no marked effect on arterial blood pressure in this series, except in one case (from 180 to 150 mm Hg systolic pressure), the only one to have been hypertensive at the time of the measurement (Table 2). These results were a little surprising, considering the relatively high doses administered by direct I.V. injection. All the patients were supine at the time of the investigation, and were not allowed to sit up in bed until 3 hr after drug administration.

Mean Cerebral Blood Flow

Changes in mean CBF were quite different from patient to patient, but only in three cases (patients 2, 8, and 9) did they reach the threshold of 15%, which corresponds to a significant difference at the $p < 0.05$ level in our laboratory (*unpublished data* on 30 test-retest studies). These changes were not systematic, as seen in Table 3, and the mean change for the whole group is almost nil. The reduction of mean CBF observed in patient 8 can be explained by the fall in systolic BP because of loss of autoregulation at the acute stage of brain infarction. Contrariwise, the increase in mean CBF in patient 9 occurred despite reduction of $PaCO_2$ with no change in BP, and could therefore be ascribed to the drug. In patient 2, mean CBF decreased by 16% despite a small increase in both BP and $PaCO_2$. In the two patients with a 10% (not significant) variation of CBF, the effect of the

TABLE 2. *Effects of I.V. Hydergine on systolic BP and on $PaCO_2$ in acute brain infarction*

Patient no.	Systolic BP (mm Hg)		$PaCO_2$ (kPa)	
	Before	After	Before	After
1	160	160	5.3	5.3
2	130	140	4.8	5.1
3	130	120	4.1	4.6[a]
4	160	160	4.5	5.0[a]
5	160	160	4.3	4.5
6	120	120	4.5	4.2
7	100	100	5.9	5.6
8	180	150[b]	5.3	5.6
9	140	140	5.5	5.0[a]

Dosage: 0.9 mg/70 kg (1 to 5) and 1.2 mg/70 kg (6 to 9).
[a]Change of more than 10%.
[b]Change of more than 10 mm Hg.

TABLE 3. *Effect of I.V. Hydergine on mean CBF in acute brain infarction*

Patient no.	CBF (height over area in ml/min/100 g)		% Variation
	Before	After	
1	34.5	35	0
2	35.2	29.6	− 16
3	40.7	42	+ 3.2
4	38.8	35	− 9.8
5	25.4	26.8	+ 5.5
6	31.6	34.6	+ 9.5
7	27.1	27.1	0
8	65.4	55.1	− 15.7
9	31.6	36.3	+ 14.8
		Mean:	− 1%

Dosage: 0.9 mg/70 kg (cases 1–5) and 1.2 mg/70 kg (cases 6–9).

TABLE 4. *Effect of I.V. Hydergine on rCBF in acute M.C.A. brain infarction*

Patient no.	Control rCBF (ml/min/100 g)		Change with drug (%)	
	Focal	Extrafocal	Focal	Extrafocal
1	28.5	36.7	− 3.5	+ 2.7
2	30.9	36.3	− 14.5	− 17
3	52.9	38.8	+ 2.4	+ 3.8
4	43.2	36.5	− 13.5	− 9.4
5	18.2	27.5	+ 17.6	+ 5.4
6	50/23.5	30.3	− 4/+ 12	+ 8.6
7	24	29	0	0
8	99.5	48	− 15.5	− 15.8
9	30	36	+ 23	+ 12.5
		Mean:	+ 0.4%	− 1%

drug may have been obscured by the observed changes in $PaCO_2$ which increased in case 4 (with reduction of CBF) and decreased in case 6 (with increase of CBF). However, it is clear that the changes in mean CBF with these dosages of Hydergine are neither important nor consistent.

Regional Cerebral Blood Flow

To study changes in rCBF we considered separately the "focal areas," as defined by CT scan, angiography, and the result of the first rCBF measurement, and the "nonfocal areas," i.e., the rest of the hemisphere studied. It can be seen in Table 4 that, when compared to nonfocal areas, focal areas can have reduced flow (cases 1, 2, 5, 7, 9), increased flow (luxury perfusion; cases 3, 4, 8), or a mixture of increased and decreased flow (case 6). All but one (case 8) of the extrafocal flows were below the normal values for our laboratory (20). After administration of 0.9 to 1.2 mg/70 kg Hydergine, significant changes occurred in six cases: a marked focal rCBF increase in two cases with low focal flow (cases 5 and 9), a marked focal rCBF decrease in two cases with high focal flow (cases 4 and 8), and a combination of rCBF increase and decrease was observed in the areas of, respectively, low and high focal flow in case 6. No change was seen in cases 1, 3, and 7, and in only one instance was there further rCBF decrease in an already ischemic focal area (case 2). Looking simultaneously at the focal and extrafocal areas, it can be seen that no case qualifies for a steal syndrome (i.e. a significant focal rCBF decrease accompanying a significant extrafocal increase). No inverse steal occurred either, although in some cases, the rCBF increase is more marked in focal than in nonfocal areas (cases 5 and 9). On the whole, the effects of Hydergine resulted in a more homogeneous pattern of rCBF by reduction of flow in the hyperemic areas, and an increase in ischemic foci.

Side Effects

No acute or delayed side effects of the drug were reported. The only patient with a moderate fall in systolic BP showed no deterioration of his condition during this time.

DISCUSSION

Despite some contradictory reports (9,14), most investigators have found little or no effect of Hydergine on mean CBF in man, neither in patients without structural brain lesions, nor in cases of cerebrovascular disease (1,6,8,13,18). Kohlmeyer and Blessing (11) found an increase in CBF with a dose of 0.6 mg Hydergine I.V., but not with 0.9 mg. Our study confirms this last point, and shows that no effect on rCBF is obtained by increasing the dose to 1.2 mg/70 kg. This peculiar type of dose–effect relationship (more effect with smaller dose) should be clarified by studies with smaller and larger doses. In the study of Olesen and Skinhøj (18), doses of 0.3 to 0.9 mg I.V. are mentioned but without comments on the possible dose-dependent effect on CBF.

Our results on rCBF confirm what had been observed by Kohlmeyer and Blessing (11) in less precisely defined focal brain lesions: With the drug, rCBF decreases in hyperemic foci and increases in ischemic foci, while the nonfocal areas remain virtually unchanged. This "smoothing" effect also has been observed by Depresseux (4) with Vincamine, and attributed by him to a decrease and an equalization of cerebral hemodynamic resistance. In older studies, McHenry et al. (14) found no steal effect with Hydergine, while in the study of Olesen and Skinhøj (18), a decrease in rCBF in ischemic foci occurred only during a fall in systemic blood pressure with rapid I.V. injection of the drug. We believe that the lack of drug-induced hypotension in our group of patients as compared to previous investigations is due to the choice of the 5-min injection instead of a bolus injection and to our maintaining the patients supine during the whole procedure.

The lack of effect of I.V. Hydergine on arterial BP and on mean CBF in our patients with an acute middle cerebral artery territory infarction is an interesting observation in view of its use in the treatment of acute stroke: the adverse effects of a fall in BP (2) and of marked increases of CBF leading to a steal phenomenon (10) are better documented than other possible benefits from a drug with metabolic effects. Indeed, drugs with a papaverine-like action are looked at with suspicion since the report of Olesen and Paulson (17), and the need to avoid hypotensive episodes has followed the discovery of loss of autoregulation in acute cerebral ischemia (15).

CONCLUSION

This clinical, pharmacological study shows that at doses of 0.9 to 1.2 mg/70 kg, Hydergine is a safe drug in patients suffering from acute cerebral infarction. The effect of smoothing out the heterogeneity of the rCBF pattern, previously described by Kohlmeyer and Blessing (11), reflects a possible beneficial effect on the microcirculation of ischemic brain, but the verification of this speculation still needs a properly designed clinical trial.

REFERENCES

1. Agnoli, A., Battistini, N., Bozzao, L., and Fieschi, C. (1965): Drug action on regional cerebral blood flow in cases of acute cerebrovascular involvement. *Acta Neurol. Scand.*, 41:*(Suppl.)* 14:142–144.
2. Cantu, R. C., Ames, A., Digiacinto, G., and Dixon, J. (1969): Hypotension: a major factor limiting recovery from cerebral ischemia. *J. Surg. Res.*, 9:525–529.
3. Christensen, M. S., Paulson, O. B., Olesen, J., Alexander, S. C., Skinhøj, E., Dam, W. H., and Lassen, N. A. (1973): Cerebral apoplexy (stroke) treated with or without prolonged artificial hyperventilation. 1. Central circulation, clinical course and cause of death. *Stroke*, 4:568–619.
4. Depresseux, J. (1978): The effect of Vincamine on the regional cerebral blood flow in man. *Eur. J. Neurol.*, 17:100–107.
5. Ehrenreich, D. L., Burns, R. A., Alman, R. W., and Fazekas, J. F. (1961): Influence of acetazolamide on cerebral blood flow. *Arch. Neurol.*, 5:125–129.
6. Gottstein, U. (1965): Pharmacological studies of total cerebral blood flow in man with comments on the possibility of improving regional cerebral blood flow by drugs. *Acta Neurol. Scand.*, 41:*(Suppl.)* 14:136–141.
7. Gygax, F., Ruf, G., Wiernsperger, N., and Baumann, T. (1979): Effect of adrenergic blockade on cerebral ischemia. In: *Brain and Heart Infarct, Vol. II*, edited by K. J. Zülch, et al. Springer-Verlag, Berlin.
8. Herrschaft, H. (1975): The efficacy and course of action of vaso- and metabolic-active substances on regional cerebral blood flow in patients with cerebro-vascular insufficiency. In: *Blood Flow and Metabolism of the Brain*, edited by M. Harper et al. Churchill-Livingstone, Edinburgh.
9. Heyck, H. (1961): Der Einfluss der ausganglage auf sympathikolytische Effekte am Hirnkreislauf bei cerebrovascular Erkrankungen. *Arztl. Forsch.*, 15:243–251.
10. Hossmann, K. A., Lechtape-Grüter, H., and Hossmann, V. (1973): The role of cerebral blood flow for the recovery of the brain after prolonged ischemia. *J. Neurol.*, 204:281–299.
11. Kohlmeyer, K., and Blessing, J. (1978): Zur Wirkung von Dihydroergocristin-methansulfonat auf den Hirnkreislauf des Menschen im Akutversuch. *Arzneim. Forsch./Drug Res.*, 28:1788–1797.
12. McHenry, L. C., Jaffe, M. E., Kawamura, J., and Goldberg, M. I. (1970): Effect of papaverine on regional blood flow in focal vascular diseases of the brain. *N. Engl. J. Med.*, 282:1167–1171.

13. McHenry, L. C., Jaffe, M. E., Kawamura, J., et al. (1971): Hydergine effect on cerebral circulation in cerebrovascular disease. *J. Neurol. Sci.*, 13:475–480.
14. Marc-Vergnes, J. P., Bes, A., Charlet, J. P., et al. (1974): Pharmacodynamie de la circulation cérébrale. *Pathologie-Biologie*, 22:815–825.
15. Olesen, J. (1973): Quantitative evaluation of normal and pathological cerebral blood flow regulation to perfusion pressure: changes in man. *Arch. Neurol.*, 28:143–149.
16. Olesen, J. (1974): Cerebral blood flow. Methods for measurement, regulation, effects of drugs and changes in disease. *Acta Neurol. Scand.*, 50:*(Suppl.)* 57:1–80.
17. Olesen, J., and Paulson, O. B. (1971): The effect of intra arterial papaverine on the regional cerebral blood flow in patients with stroke or intracranial tumor. *Stroke*, 2:148–159.
18. Olesen, J., and Skinhøj, E. (1972): Effects of ergot alcaloids (Hydergine) on cerebral haemodynamics in man. *Acta Pharmacol. (Kbn.)*, 31:75–85.
19. Smith, A. L. (1977): Barbiturate protection in cerebral hypoxia. *Anesthesiology*, 47:285–293.
20. Vernhiet, J., Renou-Bidabe, A. M. Orgogozo, J. M., Constant, P., and Caillé, J. M. (1978): Effects of a Diazepam-Fentanyl mixture on cerebral blood flow and oxygen consumption in man. *Br. J. Anaesth.*, 50:165–169.

Advances in Stroke Therapy, edited by
F. C. Rose. Raven Press, New York © 1982.

Early Medical Management of Aneurysmal Subarachnoid Haemorrhage

R. D. Illingworth and D. A. Lane

Departments of Neurosurgery and Haematology, Charing Cross Hospital, London

Although rupture of an intracranial aneurysm causes early death in 40% of patients (11,41), in the remainder, the bleeding ceases spontaneously, the site of bleeding is sealed by a plug of platelets and fibrin, and clot surrounds the aneurysm (12). Blood in the subarachnoid space stimulates fibrinolytic activity, which is not normally present in the cerebrospinal fluid (CSF) (57), and this may be a factor in the recurrent bleeding from which one-third of survivors of the first haemorrhage will die within the following 6 weeks (38,41). Intracranial surgery can prevent recurrent haemorrhage by obliterating the aneurysm but does not otherwise assist in recovery unless a large intracerebral haematoma can be removed (23).

In the last 20 years, much neurosurgical effort has been directed towards improving the results of aneurysm surgery, and improved techniques in both surgery and anesthesia, in particular, the use of the operating microscope, and more experience in patient selection, have resulted in published operative mortalities of under 5% (18,20,24,27,66). These figures have been obtained for patients who have recovered from the effect of the initial subarachnoid haemorrhage (SAH) and who have been operated on at least one week after the bleeding has occurred. Few surgical series have looked at the overall or management mortality of patients admitted to neurosurgical departments and, where they have done so, much higher overall mortalities have been reported despite improving surgical results (1,63). The problem is that some patients, already damaged irretrievably by the haemorrhage before admission, will die whatever is done, and others will die either of recurrent haemorrhage or of progressive neurological deterioration due to ischaemia, before surgery can be undertaken. Early operation results in higher mortality (13,29,63,67), and the timing of operation in relation to the SAH remains crucial to the outcome (13,22). Similarly, a poor neurological state is also associated with a higher postoperative mortality (7,55).

No way as yet exists to improve patients who have been gravely damaged by the effect of their first haemorrhage other than by removing intracerebral clots, and there appears to be no certain way of preventing or treating the progressive neurological deterioration due to cerebral ischaemia that may affect patients before or after operation, and can be the commonest cause of death (24). Early operation as yet has not been shown to reduce overall mortality in patients admitted to neurosurgical departments, and most surgeons have, until recently, elected to delay operation until patients are felt to be in optimum condition and to give antifibrinolytic drugs in the hope of preventing recurrent SAH.

The antifibrinolytic drugs epsilon aminocaproic acid and amino-methylcyclohexane carboxylic acid (tranexamic acid) are widely used in the preoperative management of patients with aneurysmal SAH, but there is no agreement about their effectiveness. Although some publications have maintained that such management has reduced the incidence of recurrent bleeding (1,8,9,16,33,35–37,39,43,46–48,52,58,61), other series have denied this (4,14,15,17,44,49,51,62). In this chapter, we review what is known of the hematological basis of fibrinolysis inhibition in the management of SAH, and also review and discuss the previous published clinical series.

REGULATION OF FIBRINOLYSIS

A concept that recurs in the study of human blood coagulation is that a balance exists between the formation of blood clots and the dissolution of these clots by the fibrinolytic enzyme system (5). Thrombin is the enzyme responsible for clot formation while the major fibrinolytic enzyme is plasmin. Because sensitive and specific radioimmunoassay methods can detect activation products of thrombin and plasmin in normal individuals (28), it seems reasonable to suppose that such a balance may be normally operative at a basal level. Support for this has been obtained from the demonstration that a small percentage of normal fibrinogen is catabolised by limited thrombin (40) and plasmin (34) action in the circulation. During vessel injury, the coagulation and fibrinolytic systems are stimulated and the putative balance is disturbed, initially so that coagulation predominates over fibrinolysis and the wound is surrounded by a platelet and fibrin plug. Following this, fibrinolysis predominates, contributing to the processes of tissue repair. Many of the relationships existing between the two systems are yet to be elucidated, but much information has been obtained in the last 10 years about their interdependency, and it is instructive to review briefly what is known of the main components and molecular mechanisms of physiological and pathological fibrinolysis.

The terminal reactions that take place when the coagulation system is activated involve the conversion of the inactive plasma protein prothrombin to a serine protease, thrombin, which has a relatively narrow proteolytic specificity. The primary target of thrombin is circulating fibrinogen which is transformed to fibrin monomer. Associated with this reaction is the release of two peptides, fibrinopeptides, A and B, which signal the onset of fibrin formation (6). Fibrin monomer in low concentrations circulates as "soluble fibrin" but may form a clot readily should its concentration become high enough. Thrombin also activates factor XIII to an active form that can catalyze the covalent crosslinking of fibrin. This further reduces its solubility and increases its resistance to haemodynamic shear forces (50).

An activator of the fibrinolytic enzyme system is known to be present in endothelial cells and is released into the circulation in normal and pathological situations. Release of activator does not necessarily cause plasmin action. This is partly because of the presence of a fast-acting plasma inhibitor of plasmin called alpha$_2$-antiplasmin (10) which rapidly neutralizes any free plasmin that is generated. Also, fibrin formation seems to be essential before plasmin can act proteolytically. Recent work has suggested that the reason for the requirement of fibrin in the initiation of fibrinolysis is that both the activator and plasminogen bind to fibrin (65). This serves to localise the fibrinolytic response onto fibrin clots. Detailed biochemical information on the structure of the fibrinolytic activator is lacking because of the difficulties in purifying adequate amounts of protein, and the mechanisms involved in its binding to fibrin are not well understood, although more is known about the plasminogen and fibrin reactions.

Plasminogen is comprised of a single polypeptide chain that is cleaved in two chains—a "light" and "heavy" chain—during its conversion to plasmin by activator (Fig. 1). These two polypeptide chains remain covalently associated because of the presence of interchain disulphide bonds (53). The light chain contains the active site responsible for dissolving the clot. The heavy chain region contains five "kringle" or "lysine binding" structures that are involved in the binding of plasminogen to fibrin (Fig. 2). It has been shown that as fibrin is formed, plasminogen becomes specifically incorporated into the clots by means of the interaction of the lysine binding sites and the fibrin molecule (45). Both the fibrinolytic activator and plasminogen are therefore brought into close proximity on their natural substrate and a localised activation takes place, producing plasmin which then breaks down fibrin into lower molecular weight, soluble fragments.

Why then does the fast-acting plasmin inhibitor, alpha$_2$-antiplasmin, not prevent fibrin-bound plasmin from degrading the clot? It seems that the reaction between alpha$_2$-antiplasmin and plasmin in part is mediated through the same lysine binding sites on plasmin that bind to fibrin. Once plasminogen or plasmin is located on the fibrin network the lysine binding sites on the heavy chain are inaccessible to alpha$_2$-antiplasmin (6).

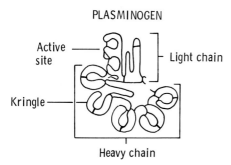

PLASMINOGEN

Active site — Light chain

Kringle —

Heavy chain

FIG. 1. Model of the plasminogen molecule constructed from knowledge of its primary structure. Plasminogen is comprised of a single polypeptide chain that is split into light and heavy polypeptide chains when it is converted into plasmin. The kringles or lysine binding sites are located on the heavy chain, and these structures mediate binding of plasminogen to fibrin. The active site of plasmin responsible for digestion and dissolution of fibrin is contained in the light chain. Adapted from Sottrup-Jensen et al. (53).

PLASMINOGEN

Activator

PLASMINOGEN ACTIVATION

Fibrin array

FIBRINOLYSIS

Fibrin breakdown

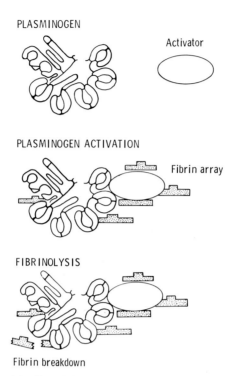

FIG. 2. Localization of the fibrinolytic process on fibrin. Circulating plasminogen and activator specifically bind onto a fibrin clot as it forms from circulating fibrinogen. Activator then converts plasminogen to plasmin. The major inhibitor of plasmin, alpha$_2$-antiplasmin, is unable to neutralise the plasmin because the plasmin and alpha$_2$-antiplasmin reaction is initially mediated through the kringle structures which are bound onto the fibrin. Plasmin then digests the fibrin clot, and any plasmin that is released into the circulation is rapidly inhibited by alpha$_2$-antiplasmin and therefore cannot digest circulating fibrinogen.

MECHANISM OF ACTION OF ANTIFIBRINOLYTIC AGENTS

The fibrinolytic inhibitors, epsilon aminocaproic acid and tranexamic acid, interact with the components of the fibrinolytic system in a number of ways. It was believed initially that they exerted their antifibrinolytic activity by inducing a conformational change in plasminogen, thereby inhibiting its activation (2), but it is now thought that this is incorrect (21).

Two situations may be considered: First, the naturally occurring physiological activator (that has high affinity for fibrin) binds onto a fibrin clot together with plasminogen (which binds with its lysine binding sites, as mentioned above) and promotes a localised fibrinolysis. This fibrinolysis may be totally inhibited by epsilon aminocaproic acid or tranexamic acid at relatively low concentrations (approximately 1 μM or 0.013 mg/100 ml). This is because these agents bind with high affinity to the lysine binding sites on plasminogen, displacing it from fibrin and the fibrin bound activator.

In the second situation, fibrinolysis is induced by the exogenous fibrinolytic activators streptokinase or urokinase. A complex, concentration-dependent retardation of fibrinolysis then occurs when the antifibrinolytic agents are added. When the high-affinity lysine binding sites are saturated with the antifibrinolytic agents by the specific interaction mentioned above, no alteration in fibrinolysis occurs. This strongly suggests that exogenous activation of fibrinolysis occurs independently of plasminogen binding to fibrin. At higher concentrations of inhibitors (10 μM or 0.13 mg/100 ml), they induce a conformational change in plasminogen, but rather than inhibiting fibrinolysis, this actually facilitates plasmin generation and clot lysis. As the concentration of inhibitors are further raised (100 μM or 1.3 mg/100 ml), marked inhibition occurs which is probably due to a direct interference with formed plasmin. This comparison of the inhibition of fibrinolytic activators has therefore suggested that the antifibrinolytic agents have a much weaker and less specific effect on fibrinolysis when exogenous activators are employed to induce fibrinolysis (21).

The above description of the mechanism of action of antifibrinolytic agents is a simplified account. Once fibrinolysis is initiated and plasmin generated, a modified form of plasminogen may be produced by plasmin cleavage. Normal "native" plasminogen has glutamic acid as an NH_2 terminal amino acid, and plasmin cleaves a low molecular weight fragment from this region of the molecule to form a lower molecular weight derivative with lysine as NH_2 terminus (64). Lys-plasminogen has increased affinity for fibrin and is more readily activated to plasmin (56). Greater concentrations of antifibrinolytic agents are therefore necessary to dissociate the Lys-plasminogen complex with fibrin. Also, as detailed earlier, the alpha$_2$-antiplasmin inhibition of free plasmin is dependent upon the lysine binding sites of plasmin. If these sites are blocked by antifibrinolytic agents binding with high affinity, any reaction that alpha$_2$-antiplasmin may have with plasmin may be impeded.

FIBRINOLYSIS AND TISSUE REPAIR

Little is known of the role of fibrinolysis in the later stages of wound repair. Presumably, when blood vessels are damaged and fibrin and blood platelets plug the wound, a series of regenerative processes are initiated to repair the damaged vessel. There is much current interest in the finding that blood platelets secrete a growth factor that stimulates the proliferation of endothelial cells (19). At the same time as endothelial regeneration occurs, proteases within and outside the vessels break down the clot, but usually at a rate compatible with vessel integrity. The nature of these proteases is ill defined. That plasminogen activator is stored in endothelial cells suggests a role for plasminogen activation to plasmin, but other proteases of broader specificity have been shown to be able to degrade fibrinogen and fibrin. Chymotrypsin-like and elastase-like proteases isolated from human granulocytes produce terminal degradation products of fibrinogen with similar antigenic and structural properties to those produced by plasmin (42). These proteases are not inhibited by epsilon aminocaproic acid and tranexamic acid. Because these processes are so poorly defined, the possible role of fibrinolytic inhibitors in therapeutic control of wound healing must remain the subject of speculation and sound clinical research. When SAH patients are studied, a further consideration must be that the defect responsible for rebleeding may be related to the vessel wall abnormality that caused the original haemorrhage, rather than the fibrinolytic mechanisms.

Despite the above objections, it should be noted that antifibrinolytic agents have been used to prevent bleeding in certain groups of patients (32). Beneficial effects of inhibiting fibrinolysis have been reported in urinary tract disorders and in the control of menorrhagia. The antifibrinolytic agent is thought to act in these two latter situations by inhibiting the high local concentrations of activator found in the kidney and endometrium, respectively. Theoretical considerations relating to the balance of coagulation and fibrinolysis have been advanced as a rationale for the use of antifibrinolytic agents in haemophilia, but the published evidence concerning its value is conflicting.

REVIEW OF PUBLISHED CLINICAL SERIES

The problem in evaluating the effect of antifibrinolytic drugs in preventing recurrent haemorrhage after SAH is the variability of the natural outcome. Although the risk of fatal rebleeding depends on the time since the last haemorrhage (41) and the clinical grade of the patient (1,3), the recurrence of such bleeding in any patient appears to be fortuitous. It follows that in every clinical study of the effects of any treatment of aneurysmal SAH, the treated patients must be compared with a carefully matched series of control patients, and the numbers involved must be large enough to eliminate results due to chance. Matching of treated patients and controls is more important than random selection or double blind studies, and the validity of such matching can be assessed by using the prediction tables of Alvord (3).

Although in the last 15 years twenty-four papers have been published on the use of antifibrinolytic drugs in preventing recurrent SAH, there is no broad agreement. Sixteen publications have stated that such treatment is effective (1,8,9,16,33,35–37,39,43,46–48,52,58,61), but eight have denied this (4,14,15,17,44,49,51,62). Recent papers have tended to be less favourable, suggesting that with time, doubt has increased rather than lessened. The sixteen previously published series describing the effectiveness of antifibrinolytic drugs are summarized in Table 1. It will be seen that only five have control groups of untreated patients (8,9,16,33,48), and in three of these series, the number of patients in each group is twenty-five or less (8,16,33). The two largest series with control groups (9,48) show large differences in the rebleeding rates between the treated and control patients, but in one (9), 29% of the patients included did not have aneurysms, and in neither study is information given about the period during which patients were at risk of rebleeding.

The eight publications reporting no benefit from the use of antifibrinolytic agents are summarised in Table 2. Seven have control groups (4,14,15,17,44,51,62), but in three, the numbers are small (15,17,62). The two largest series from the two

TABLE 1. Previous publications describing the effectiveness of antifibriolytic treatment in aneurysmal subarachnoid haemorrhage

Study	Drug[a], daily dose	Treated patients				Control patients				Matched series	Double blind
		N	Rebleeds (Deaths)	Cerebral ischaemia (Deaths)	DVT[a] (PE)	N	Rebleeds (Deaths)	Cerebral ischaemia (Deaths)	DVT (PE)		
Mullan and Dawley (35)	EACA, 24 g	35[b]	2 (1)	0	0						No
Norlen and Thulin (39)	EACA, 16–20 g / AMCA, 30–40 mg/kg	14	0	1 (1)	[c]						
Gibbs and Corkill (16)	AMCA, 3 g	25	[c] (1)	0	[c]	22	[c]	(4)	0	No[d]	No
Ransohoff et al. (46)	EACA, 24 g	50	6 (5)	[c]	[c]						
Tovi (58)	AMCA, 4–6 g	34	6 (2)	(2)	0						
Smith and Upchurch (52)	EACA, 24 g	21	1	[c]	1						
Nibbelink (36)	EACA, 24–36 g / AMCA	242[e]	[c] (5.8%)	[c]	[c]	[e]	[c]	[c]	[c]	No	No
Nibbelink et al. (37)	EACA, 24–36 g / AMCA 8–16 g	471	11.6% (27)	16.8%	1.1% (0.4%)						
Utley and Richardson (61)	EACA, 24 g / AMCA, 12 g	42 / 182	8 (7) / 22 (14)	[c] / [c]	(1) / 0						
Sengupta et al. (48)	EACA, 24 g	66	0	1	1 (1)	76	17 (4)	0	0	No[d]	No
Post et al. (43)	EACA, 24–36 g	85	10 (4)	(1)	3 (0)						
Schisano (47)	EACA, 24 g / AMCA, 2–4 g	58	1 (1)	(9)	[c]						
Chandra (8)	AMCA, 6 g	20	1 (1)	10	0	19	4 (5)	0	0	No[d]	Yes
Maurice-Williams (33)	AMCA, 6 g	25	6 (3)	0	2	25	14 (10)	2	2	No	No
Chowdhary et al. (9)	EACA, 36 g	83[f]	3 (1)	8	5% (1)	82[f]	22 (10)	0	5% (1)	No[d]	No
Adams et al. (1)	EACA, 36 g / AMCA, 12 g	249	33[g] (14)[g]	0 (17)							

[a]EACA = Epsilon amino caproic acid; AMCA = Amino methylcyclohexane carboxylic acid (Tranexamic acid); DVT = deep vein thrombosis; PE = pulmonary embolism.

[b]Thirty patients had aneurysms.

[c]Not stated.

[d]Insufficient data.

[e]This study compared deaths in patients treated with antifibrinolytic drugs (5.8%) with those in patients with induced hypotension (28.9%), and in those with antifibrinolytics plus hypotension (23.8%). Total patients in all grades 242.

[f]The treated group includes 20 patients without aneurysms, and the control group 28 without aneurysms.

[g]Results at 14 days after SAH.

TABLE 2. Previous publications describing the noneffectiveness of antifibrinolytic treatment in aneurysmal subarachnoid haemorrhage

Study	Drug[a], daily dose	Treated patients				Control patients				Matched series	Double blind
		N	Rebleeds (deaths)	Cerebral ischaemia (deaths)	DVT (PE)	N	Rebleeds (deaths)	Cerebral ischaemia (deaths)	DVT (PE)		
Gibbs and O'Gorman (15)	EACA, 36 g	32	8 (8)	[b]	[b]	22	8 (8)	[b]	[b]	No	No
Girvin (17)	EACA[b]	39	14 (6)	3 (1)	[b]	27	4 (3)	1 (1)	[b]	No	No
Shaw and Miller (49)	EACA, 36 g	9	5	[b]	[b]					No	No
Profeta et al. (44)	EACA, 10–15 g	135	[c]	[b]	[b]	166	[c]	[b]	[b]	No	No
Van Rossum et al. (62)	AMCA, 6 g	25[d]	5 (4)	[b]	0	26[d]	4 (3)	[b]	0	No	Yes
Fodstad (14)	AMCA, 4–6 g	23	1 (1)	(2)	2	23	9 (3)	0	1	No	Yes
Shucart et al. (51)	EACA, 36 g	30	6 (5)	(5)	2 (4)	29	7 (5)	(2)	3 (1)	No	No
Ameen and Illingworth (4)	EACA, 36 g	45	11 [b]	[b]	[b]	55	4 [b]	[b]	[b]	No	No
	EACA, 24 g	100	7 (4)	18 (8)	12 (4)	100	15 (6)	15 (4)	7 (5)	Yes	No

[a]EACA = Epsilon amino caproic acid; AMCA = Amino methycyclohexane carboxylic acid (tranexamic acid); DVT = deep vein thrombosis; PE = pulmonary embolism.

[b]Not stated.

[c]No difference between control and treated groups, but no details given.

[d]Only 11 patients in treated group and 13 in control group had aneurysms on angiography.

groups, both of at least one hundred patients in the treatment and control groups, report no benefit from the use of antifibrinolytic agents (4,44). In the series of Ameen and Illingworth (4), 100 patients treated with epsilon aminocaproic acid 24 g daily were compared with 100 control patients treated otherwise similarly. The study was retrospective, and the two groups were consecutive rather than concurrent. The study was not blind, but the patients were very carefully matched and the Alvord prediction tables (3) were used to verify that the anticipated outcome in the two groups was similar. Table 3 shows that although the incidence of rebleeding was reduced in the treated group, this benefit was more than compensated for by an increase in deaths from cerebral ischaemia. It is not always easy to determine clinically whether a patient's deterioration has been due to rebleeding or to cerebral ischaemia but, in this study, the mortality in the treated patients was higher than in the control groups, indicating clearly no overall benefit. The differences in rebleeding and cerebral ischaemia rates between the two groups were not statistically significant.

There is some evidence to suggest that antifibrinolytic drugs actually may influence the outcome adversely by contributing to a higher incidence of cerebral ischaemia such as has been described above. In the previous publications, cerebral ischaemia has been mentioned as a problem in four series. Schisano (47) describes cerebral ischaemia in 10 patients, with 9 of 57 deaths (17.2%) treated with antifibrinolytic drugs, and Maurice-Williams (33) had 8 patients with cerebral ischaemia of 25 in the treated group (32%), as against 2 of 25 in the controls (8%). The high incidence of cerebral ischaemia in the treated group of Maurice-Williams (33) may be due to the drugs being used for 6 weeks as a substitute for operation. Fodstad (14) describes 12% of deaths from cerebral ischaemia in treated patients as against 4% in controls. In the series of Ameen and Illingworth (4) the incidence of cerebral ischaemia was 18%, similar to that described by Schisano (47). Girvan (17) reports deaths from cerebral ischaemia in 3 of 37 treated patients (7.7%); Tovi (58) reports 2 cases, and Norlen and Thulin (39) and Sengupta et al. (48) 1 each. No incidence is recorded in the series of Chowdhary et al. (9). Venous thromboembolic complications also have been described (4,9,33,37,43,48), but the numbers are small. It also has been suggested that an increased incidence of hydrocephalus can be due to the use of antifibrinolytic drugs (26).

DISCUSSION

Although antifibrinolytic drugs are readily absorbed from the gastrointestinal tract (14,31), rapidly achieve a therapeutic level in the blood if given by intravenous

TABLE 3. *Results of pre-operative management of aneurysmal SAH: EACA 24 g daily*

Patients	N	Rebleeds	(Deaths)	Cerebral ischaemia	(Deaths)	DVT	PE	(Deaths)	Total deaths
Treated	100	7	(4)	18	(8)	12	4	(1)	13
Control	100	15	(6)	15	(4)	7	5	(1)	11

From ref. 4, with permission of the publisher.

injection (14), and pass the blood–brain barrier (60), their effectiveness in the prevention of recurrent aneurysmal SAH does not appear to be well established by clinical studies (4). Fibrinolytic activity in CSF is immediately activated by intra-cranial haemorrhage (59) and although antifibrinolytic drugs can interfere with this process, their ability to do so may be impaired when given some time after the haemorrhage. The drugs break the binding of the proteolytic enzyme plasmin to fibrin and inactivate free plasmin, but in aneurysmal SAH, may not gain sufficient access to the clot around the aneurysm to prevent progressive dissolution. Although reduction of fibrinogen degradation products in CSF can be demonstrated in patients taking antifibrinolytic agents, the levels may remain raised (33,57) indicating that some breakdown of clot is still occurring. With more detailed studies of management mortality, it is becoming clear that control of recurrent SAH is not in itself sufficient to greatly influence the total mortality, since cerebral ischaemia is at least as significant a cause of death and disability in patients after SAH. Of course, it would be possible to prevent most deaths due to recurrent haemorrhage by operating on all patients within the first 48 hr after SAH, but the recently reported results of such early surgery (29,63,67) did not support its effectiveness in the reduction of such mortalities. It appears that the reduced mortality from rebleeding may be more than offset by an increased postoperative mortality. In a previously published, personal series of 170 patients with aneurysmal subarachnoid haemorrhage (24), the operative mortality in 143 patients was 2.8% against a mortality of 20 of 27 in the remaining nonoperated patients. This gives a total management mortality of 14.1% (24 of 170). Nine of these deaths occurred from rebleeding and 11 from cerebral ischaemia (Table 4A). Assuming that one-half of deaths from rebleeding could be prevented by early operation and that the deaths from cerebral ischaemia remained the same, to produce the same case mortality, an operative mortality of 5.1% would be required (Table 4B). If all deaths from rebleeding could be prevented by early operation and the other figures remained the same, an operative mortality

TABLE 4. Actual (A) and notional (B and C) management and operative mortality in 170 patients with aneurysmal SAH

Series	Deaths from rebleeding	Deaths from cerebral ischaemia	Management mortality	(%)	Operative mortality	(%)
(A) 72–1978 Series (24)	9/170	11/170	24/170	(14.1)	4/143	(2.7)
(B) 1/2 rebleed deaths	4.5/170	11/170	24/170	(14.1)	8.5/165.5	(5.1)
(C) No rebleed deaths	0/170	11/170	24/170	(14.1)	13/170	(7.6)

(A) Deaths from rebleeding and cerebral ischaemia, and the management and operative mortality in the series of 170 patients with aneurysmal SAH (24).

(B) Operative mortality that would have been needed to produce the same management mortality in the series if one-half the deaths from rebleeding had been prevented by earlier operation.

(C) Operative mortality that would have been needed to produce the same management mortality if operation had been performed sufficiently early to eliminate all deaths from rebleeding. Deaths from cerebral ischaemia have been assumed to remain the same in B and C.

of 7.6% would be required (Table 4C). Recent published series have described operative mortalities of 13% (63), 16% (29), and 16.7% (67), for good grade patients operated on in the first 2 or 3 days after SAH, which does not suggest that earlier operation would have produced better results in the series mentioned previously. There is evidence that the risk of rebleeding is actually greater in poor grade patients (1,54). It may be more logical to aim for early operation in those patients (63), although it equally could be argued that the operative mortality in these patients will be prohibitively high and that instead, one should aim for late operation when the risk of cerebral ischaemia has largely passed (4). The risk of rebleeding in good grade patients is relatively small. In the cooperative study (30), rebleeding occurred in 17% of patients in the first 2 weeks after SAH, and Jane et al. (25) describe rebleeding in 10 to 15% of patients within the first 10 days. Sundt and Whisnant (54) report 12% rebleeds in the first 10 days in conscious patients, and Adams et al. (1), 9.2% in grades 1 and 2.

In each of these studies, one-third of those that rebled died, giving a mortality of 3 or 4% from rebleeding in good grade patients in the first 10 days. If these good grade patients are operated on at 10 days, very low operative mortalities can be achieved. It is by no means clear that earlier operation, eliminating the risk of rebleeding, can produce better results.

As a result of our reviews of the normal process of fibrinolysis and the action of antifibrinolytic agents and of the published clinical series, we can come to three conclusions:

a) Knowledge of the mechanism of fibrinolysis inhibition is incomplete and its role in the prevention of recurrent aneurysmal SAH is therefore not well defined.

b) There is no unanimity in the published clinical series as to the effectiveness of fibrinolysis inhibition in the prevention of recurrent haemorrhage, and the weight of evidence in the larger, more recent series tends not to favour its effectiveness.

c) Prevention of early, recurrent haemorrhage, while an important part of the management of SAH, is not the only challenge to be met, since progressive, neurological deterioration due to cerebral ischaemia remains at least as large a problem in clinical practice.

It is not yet clear that operation for ruptured intracranial aneurysm in the first 2 days after SAH can be expected to produce a reduction in overall mortality, compared to operation in the second week. Much still needs to be learned about preoperative management if results are to be improved.

ACKNOWLEDGMENT

Acknowledgments to Mrs. V. Roberts for much secretarial assistance.

REFERENCES

1. Adams, P., Kassell, N. F., Torner, J. C., Nibbelink, D. W., and Sahs, A. L. (1981): Early management of aneurysmal subarachnoid hemorrhage: a report of the cooperative aneurysm study. *J. Neurosurg.*, 54:141–146.

2. Alkjaersig, N., Fletcher, A. P., and Sherry, S. (1959): E-aminocaproic acid: an inhibitor of plasminogen activation. *J. Biol. Chem.*, 234:832–837.

3. Alvord, E. C., Loeser, J. D., Bailey, W. L., and Copass, M. K. (1972): Subarachnoid haemorrhage due to ruptured aneurysms. A simple method of estimating prognosis. *Arch. Neurol.*, 27:273–284.

4. Ameen, A. A., and Illingworth, R. (1981): Antifibrinolytic treatment in the preoperative management of subarachnoid haemorrhage caused by ruptured intracranial aneurysm. *J. Neurol. Neurosurg. Psychiat.*, 44:220–226.

5. Astrup, T. (1956): Fibrinolysis in the organism. *Blood*, 11:780–781.

6. Blomback, B., Hessel, B., Hogg, D., and Therkildsen, L. (1978): A two step fibrinogen-fibrin transition in blood coagulation. *Nature*, 275:501–505.

7. Botterell, E. H., Lougheed, W. M., Scott, J. W., and Vandewater, S. L. (1956): Hypothermia, and interruption of carotid, or carotid and vertebral circulation, in surgical management of intracranial aneurysms. *J. Neurosurg.*, 13:1–42.

8. Chandra, B. (1978): Treatment of subarachnoid haemorrhage from ruptured intracranial aneurysms with tranexamic acid. A double blind clinical trial. *Ann. Neurol.*, 3:502–504.

9. Chowdhary, U. M., Carey, P. C., and Hussein, M. M. (1979): Prevention of early recurrence of spontaneous subarachnoid haemorrhage by epsilon aminocaproic acid. *Lancet*, i:741–743.

10. Collen, D., and Wiman, B. (1978): Fast acting plasmin inhibitor in human plasma. *Blood*, 51:563–569.

11. Crawford, M. D., and Sarner, M. (1965): Ruptured intracranial aneurysm: community study. *Lancet*, ii:1254–1257.

12. Crompton, M. R. (1966): Recurrent haemorrhage from cerebral aneurysms and its prevention by surgery. *J. Neurol. Neurosurg. Psychiatry*, 29:164–170.

13. Drake, C. G. (1971): Ruptured intracranial aneurysms. *Proc. R. Soc. Med.*, 64:477–481.

14. Fodstad, H. (1979): Tranexamic acid (AMCA) in Aneurysmal Subarachnoid Haemorrhage. *J. Clin. Pathol.*, 33:(Suppl.) 14:68–73.

15. Gibbs, J. R., and O'Gorman, P. (1967): Fibrinolysis in subarachnoid haemorrhage. *Postgrad. Med. J.*, 43:779–784.

16. Gibbs, J. R., and Corkill, A. G. L. (1971): Use of an antifibrinolytic agent (tranexamic acid) in management of ruptured intracranial aneurysms. *Postgrad. Med. J.*, 47:199–200.

17. Girvin, J. P. (1973): The use of antifibrinolytic agents in the preoperative management of ruptured intracranial aneurysms. *Trans. Am. Neurol. Assoc.*, 98:150–152.

18. Guidetti, B. (1973): Results of 98 Intracranial aneurysms operations performed with the aid of an operating microscope. *Acta. Neurochir. (Wein)*, 29:65–71.

19. Heldin, C-H., Westermark, B., and Wasteson, A. (1981): Platelet-derived growth factor. Isolation by a large scale procedure and analysis of subunit composition. *Biochem. J.*, 193:907–913.

20. Hollin, S. A., and Decker, R. E. (1977): Microsurgical treatment of internal carotid artery aneurysms. *J. Neurosurg.*, 47:142–149.

21. Hoylaerts, M., Lijnen, H. R., and Collen, D. (1981): Studies on the mechanism of the antifibrinolytic action of tranexamic acid. *Biochem. Biophys. Acta*, 673:75–85.

22. Hunt, W. E., and Hess, R. M. (1968): Surgical risk as related to time of intervention in the repair of intracranial aneurysms. *J. Neurosurg.*, 28:14–19.

23. Illingworth, R. (1979): Surgical treatment of ruptured intracranial aneurysms. *Am. Heart J.*, 98:269–271.

24. Illingworth, R. D. (1979): Surgical management of subarachnoid haemorrhage due to ruptured intracranial aneurysm. In: *Progress in Stroke Research 1.* Edited by R. M. Greenhalgh and F. C. Rose, pp. 377–386. Pitman Medical, Tunbridge Wells, United Kingdom.

25. Jane, J. A., Winn, H. R., and Richardson, A. E. (1977): The natural history of intracranial aneurysms: rebleeding rates during the acute and long term period and implications for surgical management. *Clin. Neurosurg.*, 24:176–184.

26. Knibeslöl, M., Karaday, A., and Tovi, D. (1976): Echoencephalographic study of ventricular dilatation after subarachnoid haemorrhage, with special reference to the effect of antifibrinolytic treatment. *Acta Neurol. Scand.*, 54:57–70.

27. Krayenbühl, H. A., Yasargil, M. G., Flamm, E. S., and Tew, J. M. (1972): Microsurgical treatment of intracranial saccular aneurysms. *J. Neurosurg.*, 37:678–686.

28. Lane, D. A. (1981): Fibrogen derivatives in plasma. *Br. J. Haematol.*, 47:329–335.

29. Ljunggren, B., Brandt, L., Kågström, E., and Sundbarg, G. (1981): Results of early operations for ruptured aneurysms. *J. Neurosurg.*, 54:473–479.

30. Locksley, H. B. (1966): Report on the co-operative study of intracranial aneurysms and suba-rachnoid haemorrhage. Section V, part II. Natural history of subarchnoid haemorrhage, intra-cranial aneurysms and arteriovenous malformations. *J. Neurosurg.*, 25:321–368.

31. McNicol, G. P., Fletcher, A. P., Alkjaersig, N., and Sherry, S. (1962): The absorption, distribution and excretion of epsilon aminocaproic acid following oral or intravenous administration to man. *J. Lab. Clin. Med.*, 59:15–25.

32. McNicol, G. P., and Douglas, A. S. (1972): Thrombolytic therapy and fibrinolytic inhibitors. In: *Human Blood Coagulation, Haemostasis and Thrombosis*, edited by R. Biggs. Blackwell Scientific Publications, Oxford.

33. Maurice-Williams, R. S. (1978): Prolonged antifibrinolysis: An effective non-surgical treatment for ruptured intracranial aneurysms? *Br. Med. J.*, 1:945–947.

34. Mosesson, M. W. (1974): Fibrinogen catabolic pathways. *Sem. Thromb. Hemostas.*, 1:63–84.

35. Mullan, S., and Dawley, J. (1968): Antifibrinolytic therapy for intracranial aneurysms. *J. Neu-rosurg.*, 28:21–23.

36. Nibbelink, D. W. (1974): Antihypertensive and antifibrinolytic therapy following subarachnoid haemorrhage from ruptured intracranial aneurysm. *Stroke*, 5:432–433.

37. Nibbelink, D. W., Torner, J. C., and Henderson, W. G. (1975): Intracranial aneurysms and sub-arachnoid haemorrhage. A co-operative study. Antifibrinolytic therapy in recent onset subarachnoid haemorrhage. *Stroke*, 6:622–629.

38. Nishioka, U. (1966): Report on the co-operative study of intracranial aneurysms and subarachnoid haemorrhage. Section VII, part I. Evaluation of the conservative management of ruptured intra-cranial aneurysms. *J. Neurosurg.*, 25:574–592.

39. Norlen, G., and Thulin, C-A. (1969): The use of antifibrinolytic substances in ruptured intracranial aneurysms. *Neurochirurgia (Stuttg.)*, 12:100–102.

40. Nossel, H. L., Yudelman, I., Canfield, R. E., Butler, V. P., Spandonis, K., Wilner, G. D., and Qureshi, G. D. (1974): Measurement of fibrinopeptide A in human blood. *J. Clin. Invest.*, 54:43–53.

41. Pakarinen, S. (1967): Incidence, aetiology and prognosis of primary subarachnoid haemorrhage. *Acta Neurol. Scand.*, 43:(Suppl.) 29.

42. Plow, E. F., and Edgington, J. S. (1978): Comparative characterisation of products of plasmin and leukocyte protease cleavage of human fibrinogen. *Thromb. Res.*, 12:653–665.

43. Post, K. D., Flamm, E. S., Goodgold, A., and Ransohoff, J. (1977): Ruptured intracranial aneu-rysms, case morbidity and mortality. *J. Neurosurg.*, 46:290–295.

44. Profeta, G., Castellano, F., Guarnieri, L., Ogliano, A., and Ambrosio, A. (1975): Antifibrinolytic therapy in the treatment of subarachnoid haemorrhage caused by arterial aneurysm. *J. Neurosurg. Sci.*, 19:77–78.

45. Rakoczi, I., Wiman, B., and Collen, D. (1978): On the biological significance of the specific interaction between fibrin, plasminogen and antiplasmin. *Biochim. Biophys. Acta*, 540:295–300.

46. Ransohoff, J., Goodgold, A., and Benjamin, M. V. (1972): Pre-operative management of patients with ruptured intracranial aneurysms. *J. Neurosurg.*, 36:525–530.

47. Schisano, G. (1978): The use of antifibrinolytics in aneurysmal subarachnoid haemorrhage. *Surg. Neurol.*, 10:217–222.

48. Sengupta, R. P., So, S. C., and Villarego-Ortega, F. J. (1976): Use of epsilon aminocaproic acid (EACA) in the pre-operative management of ruptured intracranial aneurysms. *J. Neurosurg.*, 44:479–484.

49. Shaw, D. M., and Miller, J. D. (1974): Epsilon aminocaproic acid and subarachnoid haemorrhage. *Lancet*, ii:847.

50. Shen, L. L., McDonagh, R. P., McDonagh, J., and Hermans, J. (1977): Early events in the plasmin digestion of fibrinogen and fibrin. *J. Biol. Chem.*, 252:6184–6189.

51. Shucart, W. A., Hussain, S. K., and Cooper, P. R. (1980): Epsilon-aminocaproic acid and re-current subarachnoid haemorrhage. *J. Neurosurg.*, 53:28–31.

52. Smith, R. R., and Upchurch, J. J. (1973): Monitoring antifibrinolytic therapy in subarachnoid haemorrhage. *J. Neurosurg.*, 38:337–344.

53. Sottrup-Jensen, L., Claeys, H., Zajdel, M., Petersen, T. E., and Magnusson, S. (1978): The primary structure of human plasminogen isolation of two lysine-binding fragments and one mini-plasminogen by elastase-catalysed-specific limited proteolysis. In: *Progress in Chemical Fibri-nolysis and Thrombolysis, Vol. 3*, edited by J. F. Davidson, R. M. Rowan, M. M. Samama, P. C. Desnoyers. Raven Press, New York.

54. Sundt, T. M., and Whisnant, J. P. (1978): Subarachnoid haemorrhage from intracranial aneurysms: surgical management and natural history of disease. *N. Engl. J. Med.*, 299:116–122.
55. Symon, L. (1976): Subarachnoid haemorrhage from intracranial aneurysm and angioma. In: *Cerebral Arterial Disease*, edited by R. W. R. Russell, pp. 231–261. Churchill Livingstone, Edinburgh, London, and New York.
56. Thorsen, S. (1975): Differences in the binding of fibrin and native plasminogen and plasminogen modified by proteolytic degradation. Influence of 6-aminocarboxylic acids. *Biochim. Biophys. Acta*, 393:55–65.
57. Tovi, D. (1972): Studies on Fibrinolysis in the Central Nervous System with special reference to Intracranial Haemorrhage and to the effect of Antifibrinolytic Drugs. *Umeå University Medical Dissertations, No. 8.*
58. Tovi, D. (1973): The use of antifibrinolytic drugs to prevent early recurrent aneurysmal subarachnoid haemorrhage. *Acta Neurol. Scand.*, 49:163–175.
59. Tovi, D., and Nilsson, I. M. (1972): Increased fibrinolytic activity and fibrinogen degradation products after experimental intracerebral haemorrhage. *Acta Neurol. Scand.*, 48:403–415.
60. Tovi, D., and Thulin, C-A. (1972): Ability of tranexamic acid to cross blood-brain barrier and its use in patients with ruptured intracranial aneurysms. *Acta. Neurol. Scand.*, 48:257.
61. Utley, D., and Richardson, A. E. (1974): Epsilon-amino-caproic acid and subarachnoid haemorrhage. *Lancet*, ii:1080.
62. Van Rossum, J., Wintzen, A. R., Endtz, L. J., Schoen, J. H. R., and De Jonge, H. (1977): Effect of tranexamic acid on rebleeding after subarachnoid haemorrhage. A double-blind controlled clinical trial. *Ann. Neurol.*, 2:242–245.
63. Weir, B., and Aronyk, K. (1981): Management mortality and the timing of surgery for supratentorial aneurysms. *J. Neurosurg.*, 54:146–150.
64. Wiman, B., and Wallen, P. (1975): Structural relationship between "Glutamic Acid" and "Lysine" forms of human plasminogen and their interaction with the NH_2 terminal peptide as studied by affinity chromatography. *Eur. J. Biochem.*, 50:489–495.
65. Wiman, B., and Collen, D. (1978): Physiological mechanism of fibrinolysis. *Nature*, 272:549–550.
66. Yasargil, M. G., and Fox, J. L. (1975): The microsurgical approach to intracranial aneurysms. *Surg. Neurol.*, 3:7–14.
67. Yoshimoto, T., Uchida, K., Kaneko, U., Kayama, T., and Suzuki, J. (1979): An analysis of follow-up of results of 1000 intracranial saccular aneurysms with definitive surgical treatment. *J. Neurosurg.*, 50:152–157.

Advances in Stroke Therapy, edited by
F. C. Rose. Raven Press, New York © 1982.

Risk Factors for Cerebrovascular Disease

S. Haberman*, R. Capildeo, and F. Clifford Rose

*Neuroepidemiology Unit, Department of Neurology, Charing Cross Hospital, London,
and *Actuarial Science Unit, The City University, London, England*

Risk factors are defined as those factors associated with a high incidence risk of disease. Their study can provide valuable information concerning the aetiology and management of disease and constitutes one of the principal activities of analytical epidemiology.

The study of the occurrence of natural experiments is necessarily the domain of this branch of epidemiology since, during the course of their lives, different individuals are exposed to a variety of disparate factors or conditions, some of which may play an important role in the occurrence of disease.

The classification of a risk factor does not necessarily indicate a direct, causal relationship. Although the relationship may be indirect, it still may be possible to make a significant impact on the occurrence of, or mortality from, the disease by dealing with this association, e.g., the association between cigarette smoking and the incidence of heart disease.

DESCRIPTIVE EPIDEMIOLOGY

Descriptive epidemiology of stroke concerns the observation of the disease as it arises in human populations, and the major findings concern those demographic and environmental factors that appear to be associated with increased incidence of, or mortality from, cerebrovascular disease (Table 1).

The almost exponential increase in incidence rates and in national mortality rates with age is well documented (31).

TABLE 1. *Demographic and environmental factors associated with cerebrovascular disease*

Age
Sex
Geographic location
Racial and ethnic factors
Meteorological variables
Water softness

A thorough investigation of the sex differences in stroke incidence rates, national stroke mortality rates and survival rates after stroke has been carried out and reported in detail elsewhere (17). Differences in national mortality rates can be attributed to sex differences in the underlying incidence figures, the major excess in incidence being about 30% overall but varying with the pathological type of stroke: for cerebral infarction there is a male excess of about 45%; for intracerebral haemorrhage, the sex differences are negligible; for subarachnoid haemorrhage, there is a female excess of about 100% (14) (Table 2). The level of the male excess is substantially less than the striking sex ratio for heart disease (45), as shown in the Framingham Study (Table 3).

The marked geographical variation in mortality and incidence of stroke is well documented within the United States as well as between different countries; e.g., in a comparison of stroke mortality rates between countries in the years 1966 to 1967 at ages 55 to 64 for men, Kuller (30) reported a seven-fold variation between Switzerland (71 per 100,000) and Japan (519 per 100,000). Within the United States for the years 1969 to 1971, the variation at ages 55 to 64 for men can be illustrated by the stroke death rate from a low mortality region (Denver, Colorado: 93 per 100,000) and a high mortality region (Savannah, Georgia: 142 per 100,000).

Geographical variations between countries in stroke death rates generally have been substantiated either by pathological studies revealing a greater extent of atherosclerosis of the cerebral arteries, or by community-based surveys of incidence and prevalence, or both. These investigations showed that cerebral infarction was the predominant pathological type of stroke, and that differences between countries

TABLE 2. *Sex differences in stroke incidence rates*

Type of stroke	Male/female ratio of weighted average of age-adjusted incidence rates
All strokes	1.30
Cerebral infarction	1.45
Intracerebral haemorrhage	1.00
Subarcachnoid haemorrhage	0.50

TABLE 3. *Sex ratio of incidence rates for cardiovascular disease (whites only): (Framingham study: 18-year follow-up)*

Condition	Male/female incidence rate at ages		
	45–54	55–64	65–74
Sudden death due to coronary artery disease	6.0	6.8	1.8
Myocardial infarction	5.9	4.9	2.1
Angina pectoris	1.8	1.3	0.8

do not appear to be due to an excess of cerebral haemorrhage in certain populations, as has been suggested by analyses of death certificates.

The marked variations in stroke death rates within countries have been noted and extensively studied for the United States and Japan. Many investigators have attributed such differences to artefacts related to variations in certification practices and in selection of the underlying cause of death on a certificate or to differences in diagnostic accuracy among certifying physicians. Two major studies (1,29) have attempted to evaluate these differences in the United States by re-evaluating the causes of death in selected areas, but found that the differentials persisted.

Many studies have reported on racial and ethnic variations in stroke mortality and incidence rates, e.g., the differences in stroke death rates among Japanese compared to other populations. Japanese migrants to Hawaii and California have much lower rates than Japanese in Japan (55). Allowing for the tendency for migrants to come from southern Japan where the death rates are low, the study suggests that the differences in death rates between countries have a major environmental, rather than genetic, component.

Within the United States, stroke death rates are much higher for blacks than for whites, especially in the southern part of the country. These differences are present for both sexes, decrease with advancing age, and seem to be narrowing over time (35). As an example, there is a 15-fold difference in 1969 to 1971 stroke death rates at ages 45 to 54 for white men in Denver (21 per 100,000) and black men in Savannah (379 per 100,000). Those studies comparing stroke incidence rates for blacks and whites report a higher incidence for the former, especially in the younger age groups (6,19).

The seasonal variation in stroke mortality and incidence has been reviewed in detail (16), and there is conclusive evidence that the pattern is related inversely to ambient temperature. Low temperature may be related to raised blood pressure which could explain the high risk of stroke in northern Japan. Other meteorological variables that have been considered are humidity and atmospheric pressure (or altitude, which may be inversely related to blood pressure levels).

Although numerous studies have been published on the relationship between water hardness and cardiovascular (in particular stroke) mortality, the relationship remains controversial (43), but a recent United Kingdom study reported a 10 to 15% higher mortality rate (after adjustment for other factors) in areas with very soft water relative to areas with medium-hard water (40).

GENERAL CONSIDERATIONS IN STUDIES OF RISK FACTORS

There are two principal experimental designs of analytical epidemiological studies. The case control study (Fig. 1) begins with a group of individuals with stroke (cases) and a comparable group without stroke (controls), and their current status or past history for factors differentially distributed in the two groups is explored. For any given risk factors, the relative risk (the ratio of the risk of stroke in those with the factor present to the risk of stroke in those without the factor) can be

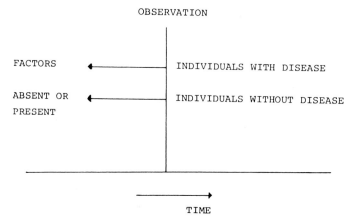

FIG. 1. Format for a retrospective study.

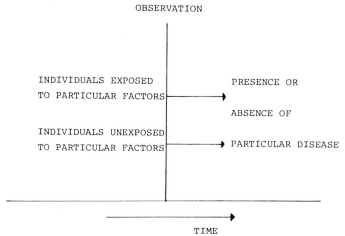

FIG. 2. Format for a prospective study.

calculated. Such studies usually can be carried out quickly and fairly cheaply. The advantages and disadvantages of this type of research strategy are described in detail elsewhere (32). One problem is the inability of these studies to provide an estimate of absolute risk (i.e. the risk of stroke in those with a given risk factor).

To measure absolute risk, a prospective study design is required (Fig. 2). This begins with a group (or cohort) with a particular factor (believed to be related to stroke, the disease of interest) and a group without the factor. The two groups are observed over a period of time to see how many persons develop a stroke, and the frequency of stroke in the two groups are compared. These studies typically are lengthy and expensive e.g., the Framingham (Massachusetts) investigation where observations were begun in 1950 on an original cohort of approximately 5,000 men and women, ages 30 to 62 at entry, who were then followed with standardised biennial examinations.

The usual cohort study begins in the present and continues into the future but, under certain circumstances, it may be possible to begin observation at some point in the past and investigate disease outcome in the present and future. This is possible if cohorts of those with and without a given risk factor were examined and interviewed in a standardised manner in the past to determine health and exposure status, and the two groups then must be studied longitudinally in a uniform, standardised manner—a 'retrolective' study (8) e.g., the study of college students from Harvard University and the University of Pennsylvania (38). This approach has the advantage of reducing the time and expense associated with prospective studies, but it is most unusual to find cohorts of individuals who have been examined, questioned, and observed in a standardised manner over many years, so that a retrolective study may have to rely on cohorts examined and followed in a fairly uniform manner. This probably will not achieve the level of standardisation available with prolective prospective studies that begin in the present and continue into the future.

For stroke, the case-control approach is restricted by the real or apparent changes in a risk factor following a stroke, and the necessity of restricting measurement to survivors only. The short-term case fatality may be as high as 30 to 40% (34), and the bias associated with observing survivors only is related to the pathological type of stroke, degree of residual disability, and age at onset.

The main drawback of a prospective approach is the relatively low stroke incidence rate at younger ages, but there is evidence that risk factors measured in the remote past may be better predictors of stroke than levels determined closer to the time of onset, so that long-term follow up may be a necessity. Clearly the progression of cerebral atherosclerosis takes many years and the elevated risk factors necessarily must be present over an extended period. On the other hand, some factors (e.g. increased platelet aggregation) may be present for a brief period only before onset and may be missed by a prospective study unless measurements are performed regularly.

The majority of the results discussed in this chapter have been derived from two major prospective investigations, namely Framingham and Rochester (Minnesota).

With both case-control and cohort investigations, it is important to specify the pathological type of cerebrovascular disease and the location and extent of vascular lesions in as much detail as possible, e.g., a given risk factor may be an important predictor of cerebral infarction but have no predictive value for subarachnoid haemorrhage secondary to ruptured aneurysm. Further the topographic distribution of cerebral atherosclerosis in relation to cerebral infarction may differ between populations (41) and lead to problems if risk factors are different.

In evaluating the results of studies, five considerations are important:

1. Is the risk factor related to a particular type of stroke?
2. Is the risk factor important only for certain demographic sections of the population?

3. Do increased levels of the factor correspond to increased risk of the disease (i.e. a dose-response relationship)?

4. Is there a threshold level of the risk factor below which there is no increased risk?

5. Does the removal or reduction of the risk factor correspond to a reduction in the incidence of the disease?

The fifth consideration has clear, important implications, not only for primary prevention but also for providing aetiological clues.

RISK FACTORS

The accumulated data suggest that one can build up a picture of the stroke-prone individual: Recent reports from the Framingham study indicate that we may identify 10% of the asymptomatic population in whom 50% of all strokes will occur (52). The evidence that has emerged from epidemiological studies has suggested that there are five significant risk factors for stroke in adults, and an additional four where the evidence is equivocal (Table 4). We shall discuss these risk factors in turn.

Hypertension

Of the currently identified risk factors, hypertension is the most significant; this holds true for cerebral infarction, intracerebral haemorrhage, and subarachnoid haemorrhage (53). Some investigators report a linear relationship between the level of blood pressure (systolic or diastolic) and risk of stroke, which applies to both sexes and all age groups included in the Framingham study (23). Others, however, believe that the relationship is more complex. The Framingham experience indicated that the first casual blood pressure at the initial examination was an adequate predictor of subsequent stroke risk, but subsequent blood pressure measurements, pulse pressures, or mean arterial pressure yielded little additional information (23).

Table 5 indicates the risk of cerebral infarction relative to persons of the same sex and age group who were normotensive, e.g., among men aged 50 to 59 who had high blood pressure levels at examination, the incidence rate of cerebral infarction was 6.4 times that for normotensive men of the same age. The definitions are: those with blood pressure of 160/95 or more on two examinations are classified

TABLE 4. *Recognised risk factors for stroke in adults*

Definite evidence	Equivocal evidence
Hypertension	Blood lipids
Diabetes mellitus	Obesity
Heart disease	Cigarette smoking
Transient ischaemic attacks	Exogenous oestrogens
Blood haemoglobin	

TABLE 5. *Relative risk of cerebral infarction by hypertensive status (Framingham study: 24-year follow-up)*

	Age at examination		
	50–59	60–69	70–79
Men			
Normal	1.0	1.0	1.0
Borderline	2.2	2.8	3.8
High	6.4	7.1	3.5
Women			
Normal	1.0	1.0	1.0
Borderline	2.1	1.9	1.9
High	5.9	10.0	4.6

as hypertensive, and those with blood pressure 140/90 or less are normotensive, with the remainder classified as borderline. Table 5 illustrates a clear dose-response relationship with a particularly increased risk at ages 60 to 69.

The relationship between hypertension and stroke also has been studied in Japan (27) with results consistent with those from the Framingham study. The higher levels of blood pressure among the United States black population and its high risk of stroke is also consistent with these results. The geographical variations in stroke mortality and incidence are highly correlated with regional variations in blood pressure (30) in Japan but not in the United States (44), nor does the correlation between increased blood pressure and increased stroke morbidity and mortality rates hold for Japanese–United States comparisons. Japanese residing in California have higher blood pressure than Japanese living in either Hawaii or Japan, yet they have lower stroke prevalence and mortality rates than their counterparts in Hawaii or Japan (33).

The application of blood pressure control programmes would be expected to reduce the risk of stroke. This has been confirmed by many studies [e.g., (49)]. Therapy was most successful in those with markedly elevated blood pressure, but clinical trials of treating patients with mild (48) and moderate (47) hypertension also resulted in reduced incidence of strokes of all types.

Diabetes Mellitus

The association between diabetes mellitus and cerebral infarction is well documented. A high percentage of death certificates on which stroke is listed as the underlying cause of death also consider diabetes mellitus a contributing cause (28). Kessler (25) followed up diabetic patients over a number of years and found an increasing stroke mortality rate relative to age-matched controls, findings which are supported by studies of stroke mortality. Many case-control investigations report a high prevalence of diabetes mellitus among stroke patients when compared to controls (10).

The Framingham study (24) reports a higher risk of cerebral infarction among persons with diabetes mellitus present than among nondiabetics. From Table 6, for example, we see that the incidence of cerebral infarction among diabetic women aged 60 to 69 is five times that for nondiabetic women of the same age. Adjusting for the presence of other major risk factors, the relative risk of cerebral infarction among diabetics is reduced to 2 (24). The Rochester investigation found an incidence rate of all stroke among diabetics that was 1.7 times that of the general population (39). Since the general population includes both diabetics and nondiabetics, we would expect the risk relative to nondiabetics to be higher than 1.7. There is no evidence that treatment of the diabetes (through diet, oral hypoglycaemic agents, or insulin) reduced the risk of stroke (11).

Variations in the prevalence of diabetes or in blood glucose levels cannot explain geographic differences in stroke mortality or morbidity but, in a regional study in the United States, a consistent trend was found between blood glucose levels and the local stroke risk (44) 1 hr after ingestion of 50 g of oral glucose. The same study reported that blacks had higher blood glucose values than whites, which is also consistent with the higher stroke risk.

Heart Disease

Over the first 24 years of observation of the Framingham cohort (54), there occurred 204 ischaemic strokes. A number of electrocardiographic abnormalities are associated with increased risk of cerebral infarction (Table 7). Evidence of left ventricular hypertrophy results in a risk 10.0 times that for persons of the same age and sex with no such evidence. Relative risk is similarly 4.2 in those with ST-T wave abnormalities and 2.5 for intraventricular block. The presence of coronary heart disease (coronary insufficiency, angina pectoris, and myocardial infarction) carries a risk of 3.0, the corresponding figures for congestive heart failure being 9.0, for rheumatic heart disease and atrial fibrillation 25.0, and for atrial fibrillation alone 8.5.

All of these relative risks are significantly higher than 1 ($p < .001$). For those persons with rheumatic heart disease alone, the relative risk is 2.4: This is not significant ($p > .05$), but the index is based on only seven observed ischaemic

TABLE 6. *Relative risk of cerebral infarction by diabetic status (Framingham study: 24-year follow-up)*

	Age at examination		
	50–59	60–69	70–79
Men			
Diabetes absent	1.0	1.0	1.0
Diabetes present	4.0	4.0	0.7
Women			
Diabetes absent	1.0	1.0	1.0
Diabetes present	1.3	5.0	3.0

TABLE 7. *Relative risk of cerebral infarction by cardiac status (Framingham study: 22-year follow-up)*

ECG abnormalities	
LVH	10.0
ST-T	4.2
IVB	2.5
Coronary heart disease	3.0
Congestive heart failure	9.0
Rheumatic heart disease and atrial fibrillation	25.0
Atrial fibrillation alone	8.5
Rheumatic heart disease alone	2.4

strokes. The figures quoted include no adjustment for hypertensive status, but a significantly high risk is present for all these factors in normotensives, hypertensives and those with borderline hypertension. The presence of coronary heart disease or of congestive heart failure also was noted to decrease markedly the probability of survival following a stroke, and this finding has been supported by other studies (7,9,18).

Transient Ischaemic Attacks

The Rochester study (50) has shown that about 10% of patients experiencing a completed stroke recall a previous history of transient ischaemic attacks (TIAs). Some case control studies [e.g., (5)] have reported corresponding figures as high as 50% among hospitalised patients, but this may be attributed to selection bias. Many longitudinal studies have reported on the prognosis of TIA patients, with particular emphasis on the risk of subsequent stroke, but comparison is impeded by the varying definitions of TIA (based on duration of symptoms), varying ages of patients analysed, and varying periods of follow-up. Of 27 studies reporting the natural history of TIAs, Brust (3) found that 13 used a definition of TIA based on symptoms of less than 24 hr duration, 6 used a shorter cut-off, 3 allowed neurologic residua beyond 24 hr, and 5 did not report the criterion used. The Rochester study showed that the risk of completed stroke was a function of the time interval following the initial TIA (51). If we compare the actual probability of a stroke occurring from the TIA experience with the expected probability derived from the stroke incidence rates obtained from the experience of the total population of Rochester and adjusted for the age and sex distribution of those with TIAs, we obtain the figures shown in Table 8. The ratio of actual to expected probability falls from 17.3 in the first year after TIA to about 5.0 in later years. In fact over one-half of all strokes occurring in the TIA cohort occurred within 1 year of the first TIA.

Blood Haemoglobin

Increased levels of blood haemoglobin have been related to coronary heart disease, the relationship being particularly notable in frank polycythemia. Levels of blood

TABLE 8. *Relative risk of stroke by TIA history (Rochester study: 25-year analysis)*

Interval of time since TIA (years)	Actual/expected[a] stroke incidence rate
0–1	17.3
1–2	8.9
2–10	5.1

[a]Based on Rochester stroke incidence rates.

TABLE 9. *Relative risk of cerebral infarction by blood haemoglobin concentration (Framingham study: 24-year follow-up)*

	Age at examination		
	40–49	50–59	60–69
Men			
Under 15 g %	1.0	1.0	1.0
At or over 15 g %	1.5	2.1	1.9
Women			
Under 14 g %	1.0	1.0	1.0
At or over 14 g %	4.4	1.6	3.3

haemoglobin within the normal range are also significantly related to the incidence of cerebral infarction. The Framingham study (21) has shown that at or above 15 g % blood haemoglobin concentration in men and at or above 14 g % in women, the incidence of cerebral infarction is significantly higher ($p < .01$). Relative to persons with lower concentrations and of the same age, the risk is between 1.5 and 4.4 times higher (Table 9). However this significant extra risk is diminished when allowance is made for other risk factors, namely hypertension, diabetes, electrocardiographic abnormalities, cholesterol, and cigarette smoking.

Blood Lipids

The relationships between dietary intake of fat and cholesterol and between serum cholesterol levels and cerebral infarction are much less clear cut than for heart disease.

The distributions of dietary intake of fat and cholesterol are not related to the stroke death rate when comparing countries, for example Japan and United States. Also there is no relationship between serum cholesterol levels and stroke death rates among population samples in different areas of Japan (26), or between different areas of the United States (44). Cholesterol levels are similar between blacks and whites despite the apparent differences in stroke death rates and extent of cerebral atherosclerosis. Japanese in Hiroshima had much lower cholesterol levels than those in either Hawaii or California, but they had higher stroke mortality rates (36).

Among the Framingham cohort, the risk of cerebral infarction was related to serum cholesterol levels only for men in the youngest age group studied, 50 to 59 (53): Men in this age group with cholesterol levels between 220 and 260 (i.e. moderate) had a significant risk of cerebral infarction ($p < .05$) 1.8 times that of men of the same age with a cholesterol level below 220 (Table 10). No such relationship was found in women. In other community investigations, e.g., the Evans County study (19), no clear or consistent relationships were found between serum cholesterol and the incidence rate of subsequent stroke. If the relationship holds true for only younger individuals as suggested by the Framingham data, this could explain the lack of consistent findings in those studies that have dealt with older populations. The correlation is no better with other lipid components, including triglyceride-rich pre-β lipoproteins and cholesterol-rich β-lipoprotein (22).

Obesity

The relationship between obesity and stroke is equivocal. Obesity is a major risk factor for elevated blood pressure and diabetes. Weight change is associated with an increase in both cholesterol and triglyceride levels, but obesity is only weakly related to serum cholesterol levels (2). Therefore, the fundamental question is whether obesity is an independent risk factor for stroke, but there is no consistent international pattern between obesity and stroke mortality (2). In Japan, there was no relationship between the prevalence of obesity and stroke mortality rates. The three-area geographic study in the United States (44) found no consistent correlation between obesity indices and stroke mortality or incidence rates, although black women had greater incidence of obesity than white women. Data from the Evans County community study (19) and the follow-up of college students from Harvard and Pennsylvania (38) do not help, as neither sets are adjusted for the subsequent development of diabetes or hypertension prior to the stroke. Obesity (as measured by relative weight) was found to be related to the risk of cerebral infarction in the Framingham cohort for both sexes, with the excess risk reaching statistical significance for women only (53). In the Framingham cohort, obese hypertensives had

TABLE 10. *Relative risk of cerebral infarction by serum cholesterol level (Framingham study: 24-year follow-up)*

Serum cholesterol level (mg/dl)		Age at examination		
		50–59	60–69	70–79
Men				
Low	< 220	1.0	1.0	1.0
Moderate	220–259	1.8	0.4	0.3
High	≥ 260	3.5	1.3	1.0
Women				
Low	< 220	1.0	1.0	1.0
Moderate	220–259	0.7	0.4	0.3
High	≥ 260	1.1	0.5	0.4

higher stroke incidence rates than nonobese hypertensives (12). In Japan, a much higher percentage of hypertensives are not obese compared to the United States (30). In the high stroke mortality rate areas of Japan, the hypertensives are mainly thin, and it is possible that in these populations, a marked increase in salt intake and perhaps protein and vitamin deficiences are major risk factors for hypertension. The interrelationship between obesity, hypertension, diabetes, and subsequent risk of stroke still needs clarification.

Cigarette Smoking

Like blood lipids and obesity, there is no consistent evidence linking cigarette smoking and stroke, a risk clearly different from that for coronary heart disease and peripheral vascular disease.

An extensive review of the literature on the relationship between stroke and cigarette smoking has been published elsewhere (15). There is no evidence of a relationship between cigarette smoking and international differences in stroke mortality nor between cigarette smoking and geographic variations in stroke morbidity and mortality within the United States (44). No relationship was reported in the Hiroshima community based study (20) nor in the Washington County cohort and case control studies (37), although a positive relationship between cigarette smoking and subsequent mortality was found in the study of former college students (38).

For the Framingham cohort, Table 11 shows the risk of cerebral infarction relative to persons of the same age and sex who were nonsmokers at examination: Men aged 50 to 59 who smoked 20 or more cigarettes per day had a risk of cerebral infarction 2.2 times greater than men of the same age who were nonsmokers. These figures show neither a consistent relationship nor any significant differences. The analysis takes into account changes in smoking habits over the 24 years of follow-up.

TABLE 11. *Relative risk of cerebral infarction by cigarettes smoked (Framingham study: 24-year follow-up)*

No. smoked per day	Age at examination		
	50–59	60–69	70–79
Men			
Nonsmokers	1.0	1.0	1.0
Under 20	2.7	1.1	2.7
20 and over	2.2	0.9	0.9
Women			
Nonsmokers	1.0	1.0	1.0
Under 20	0.4	0.4	1.6
20 and over	0.6	1.2	5.2[a]

[a]Small numbers.

Exogenous Oestrogens

Regarding exogeneous oestrogens, case control studies have shown that oral contraceptives increase the incidence of stroke (4,46), which has been postulated as being due to increased thrombogenesis, increased blood pressure, and increased blood glucose associated with the use of exogeneous oestrogens. Since a study of stroke incidence among all female residents of Rochester from ages 15 to 49 in the years just prior to and following the introduction of oral contraceptives failed to demonstrate any change in the stroke rate (42), further studies are needed for clarification.

CONCLUSIONS

The major risk factors for the incidence of stroke are hypertension, diabetes, heart disease, TIAs, and blood haemoglobin. When we compare simply the position for stroke and heart disease we find that only some of the risk factors are shared (Table 12).

Further analysis is needed to investigate these differences and the possibility that the aetiologies of the two conditions are different (13). One hypothesis suggested for the absence of definite relationships between stroke and blood lipids, obesity, and cigarette smoking is that since high cholesterol levels, obesity, and heavy smoking are highly correlated with coronary heart disease, those with hypercholesterolaemia, severe obesity, and/or heavy smoking habits may die of a myocardial infarction before developing clinically apparent cerebrovascular disease (13).

Alternatively, stroke and heart disease may have different precipitating factors: While a stroke can be due only to the loss of functioning tissue, the symptoms of coronary vasoocclusive disease can be due to either the loss of functioning tissue or to disorders of rhythm, as well as be precipitated by "overstress" associated with obesity, lack of exercise, cigarette smoking, or nutritional factors (e.g., a diet high in saturated fat), factors that cannot be conclusively implicated in the pathogenesis of cerebrovascular disease (13).

TABLE 12. *Comparison of risk factors for stroke and heart disease*

Definite evidence for both
Hypertension
Diabetes mellitus
Blood haemoglobin
Definite evidence for stroke alone
Heart disease
Transient ischaemic attacks
Definite evidence for heart disease alone
Blood lipids
Obesity
Cigarette smoking

REFERENCES

1. Acheson, R. M., Nefzger, M. D., and Heyman, A. (1973): Mortality from stroke among US veterans in Georgia and 5 western states. *J. Chron. Dis.*, 26:405–414.
2. Blackburn, H., Taylor, H. L. and Keys, A. (1970): The electrocardiogram in predicting a five-year coronary heart disease incidence among men aged 40 through 59. In: *Coronary Heart Disease in Seven Continents*, edited by A. Keys, pp. 154–211. American Heart Association, New York.
3. Brust, J. C. M. (1977): Transient ischaemic attacks: natural history and anticoagulation. *Neurology*, 27:701–707.
4. Collaborative Group for the Study of Stroke in Young Women (1974): Oral contraception and increased risk of cerebral ischemia or thrombosis. *N. Engl. J. Med.*, 288:871–878.
5. David, N. J., and Heyman, A. (1960): Factors influencing the prognosis of cerebral thrombosis and infarction due to atherosclerosis. *J. Chron. Dis.*, 11:394–404.
6. Eckstrom, P. T., Brand, F. R., Edlavitch, S. A., and Parrish, H. M. (1969): Epidemiology of stroke in a rural area. *Public Health Rep.*, 84:878–882.
7. Fairfax, A. J., Lambert, C. D., and Leatham, A. (1976): Systemic embolism in chronic sinoatrial disorder. *N. Engl. J. Med.*, 295:190–192.
8. Feinstein, A. (1973): Clinical Biostatistics XX. The epidemiologic trohoc, the ablative risk ratio and 'retrospective research.' *Clin. Pharmacol. Ther.*, 14:291–307.
9. Friedman, G. D., Loveland, D. B., and Ehrlich, S. P. (1968): Relationship of stroke to other cardiovascular disease. *Circulation*, 38:533–541.
10. Gertler, M. M., Leetma, H. E., Rusk, H. A., Covalt, D. A., Saluste, E., and Rosenberger, J. (1969): Profile of covert ischemic heart and ischemic thrombotic cerebrovascular diseases. *NY State J. Med.*, 69:2664–2666.
11. Golden, M. G., Knatterud, G. L., and Prout, T. E. (1971): Effects of hypoglycemic agents on vascular complications in patients with adult-onset diabetes. III. Clinical implications of UGDP results. *JAMA*, 218:1400–1410.
12. Gordon, T., and Kannel, W. B. (1976): Obesity and cardiovascular disease: the Framingham study. *Clin. Endocrinol. Metab.*, 5:367–375.
13. Haberman, S., Capildeo, R., and Clifford Rose, F. (1978): The changing mortality of cerebrovascular disease. *Q. J. Med.*, 47:71–88.
14. Haberman, S., Capildeo, R., and Clifford Rose, F. (1981): Sex differences in the incidence of cerebrovascular disease. *J. Epidemiol. Comm. Health*, 35:45–50.
15. Haberman, S., Capildeo, R., and Clifford Rose, F. (1981): Smoking: a risk factor for stroke. In: *Smoking and Arterial Disease*, edited by R. M. Greenhalgh, pp. 17–28. Pitman Medical, Tunbridge Wells, United Kingdom.
16. Haberman, S., Capildeo, R., and Clifford Rose, F. (1981): Seasonal variation in cerebrovascular disease mortality. *J. Neurol. Sci.*, 52:25–36.
17. Haberman, S., Capildeo, R. and Clifford Rose, F. (1981): Sex differences in stroke. In: *Hormones and Vascular Disease*, edited by R. M. Greenhalgh, chapter 36. Pitman Medical, Tunbridge Wells.
18. Harrison, D. C., Fitzgerald, J. W., and Winkle, R. A. (1976): Ambulatory electrocardiography for diagnosis and treatment of cardiac arrythmias. *N. Engl. J. Med.*, 294:373–380.
19. Heyman, A., Karp, H. R., Heyden, S., Bartel, A., Cassel, J. C., and Tyroler, H. A. (1971): Cerebrovascular disease in the biracial population of Evans County, Georgia. *Arch. Intern. Med.*, 128:949–955.
20. Johnson, K. G., Yano, K., and Kato, H. (1967): Cerebral vascular disease in Hiroshima, Japan. *J. Chronic. Dis.*, 20:545–559.
21. Kannel, W. B., Gordon, T., Wolf, P. A., and McNamara, P. M. (1972): Haemoglobin and the risk of cerebral infarction: the Framingham study. *Stroke*, 3:409–420.
22. Kannel, W. B., Gordon, T., and Dawber, T. R. (1974): Role of lipids in the development of brain infarction: the Framingham study. *Stroke*, 5:679–685.
23. Kannel, W. B., Dawber, T. R., Sorlie, P., and Wolf, P. A. (1976): Components of blood pressure and risk of atherothrombotic brain infarction: the Framingham study. *Stroke*, 7:327–331.
24. Kannel, W. B., and McGee, D. L. (1979): Diabetes and cardiovascular disease: the Framingham study. *JAMA*, 241:2035–2038.
25. Kessler, I. I. (1971): Mortality experience of diabetic patients: a 26 year follow-up study. *Am. J. Med.*, 51:715–724.
26. Komachi, Y., Iida, M., Takahashi, H., Tominaga, S., Shimamoto, T., Chikayama, Y., and Ozawa, H. (1967): Studies on serum lipids of Japanese cerebrovascular diseases, with special

reference to serum total cholesterol and triglyceride levels. *Ann. Rep. Centre Adult Disease*, 7:35–47.

27. Komachi, T., Iida, M., Shimamoto, T., Chikayama, Y., Takahashi, H., Konishi, M., and Tominaga, S. (1971): Geographic and occupational comparisons of risk factors in cardiovascular diseases in Japan. *Jpn. Circ. J.*, 35:189–207.

28. Kuller, L. H., and Seltser, R. (1967): Cerebrovascular disease mortality in Maryland. *Am. J. Epidemiol.*, 86:442–450.

29. Kuller, L. H., Bolker, A., Saslaw, M. S., Paegel, B. L., Sisk, C., Borhani, N., Wray, J. A., Anderson, H., Peterson, D., Winkelstein, W. Jr., Cassel, J., Spiers, P., Robinson, A. G., Curry, H., Lilienfeld, A. M., and Seltser, R. (1969): Nationwide cerebrovascular disease mortality study. *Am. J. Epidemiol.*, 90:536–578.

30. Kuller, L. H. (1978): Epidemiology of stroke. In: *Advances in Neurology, Vol. 19, Neurological Epidemiology: Principles and Clinical Applications*, edited by B. S. Schoenberg, pp. 281–311. Raven Press, New York.

31. Kurtzke, J. F. (1969): *Epidemiology of Cerebrovascular Disease*, chapter 5. Springer Verlag, New York.

32. Lilienfeld, A. M. (1976): *Foundations of Epidemiology*. Chapters 8 and 9. Oxford University Press, New York.

33. Marmot, M. G., Syme, S. L., Kagan, A., Kato, H., Cohen, J. B., and Belsky, J. (1975): Epidemiologic studies of coronary heart disease and stroke in Japanese men living in Japan, Hawaii and California: prevalence of coronary and hypertensive heart disease and associated risk factors. *Am. J. Epidemiol.*, 102:514–525.

34. Matsumoto, N., Whisnant, J. P., Kurland, L. T., and Okazaki, H. (1973): Natural history of stroke in Rochester, Minnesota, 1955 through 1969: an extension of a previous study, 1945 through 1954. *Stroke*, 4:20–29.

35. Miller, G. D., and Kuller, L. H. (1973): Trends in mortality from stroke in Baltimore, Maryland: 1940–1941 through 1968–1969. *Am. J. Epidemiol.*, 98:233–242.

36. Nichaman, M. Z., Hamilton, H. B., Kagan, A., Grier, T., Sacks, S. T., and Syme, S. L. (1975): Epidemiologic studies of coronary heart disease and stroke in Japanese men living in Japan, Hawaii and California: distribution of biochemical risk factors. *Am. J. Epidemiol.*, 102:491–501.

37. Nomura, A., Comstock, G. W., Kuller, L., and Tonascia, J. A. (1974): Cigarette smoking and strokes. *Stroke*, 5:483–486.

38. Paffenbarger, R. S., and Williams, J. L. (1967): Chronic disease in former college students V. Early precursors of fatal stroke. *Am. J. Public Health*, 57:1290–1300.

39. Palumbo, P. J., Elveback, L. R., and Whisnant, J. P. (1978): Neurologic complications of diabetes mellitus: transient ischaemic attack, stroke and peripheral neuropathy. In: *Advances in Neurology Vol. 19: Neurological Epidemiology: Principles and Clinical Applications*, edited by B. S. Schoenberg, pp. 593–601. Raven Press, New York.

40. Pocock, S. J., Shaper, A. G., Cook, D. G., Packham, R. F., Lacey, R. F., Powell, P., and Russell, P. F. (1980): British regional heart study: geographic variations in cardiovascular mortality, and the role of water quality. *Br. Med. J.*, 2:1243–1249.

41. Resch, J. A., and Okabe, N. (1969): Cerebral atherosclerosis. *Geriatrics*, 24:111–123.

42. Schoenberg, B. S., Whisnant, J. P., Taylor, W. F., and Kempers, R. D. (1970): Strokes in women of childbearing age: a population study. *Neurology*, 20:181–189.

43. Sharrett, A. R., and Feinleib, M. (1975): Water constituents and trace elements in relation to cardiovascular diseases. *Prev. Med.*, 4:20–36.

44. Stolley, P. D., Kuller, L. H., Nefzger, M. D., Tonacia, S., Lilienfeld, A. M., Miller, G. D., and Diamond, E. L. (1977): Three area epidemiological study of geographic differences in stroke mortality. II. Results. *Stroke*, 8:551–557.

45. U.S. Department of Health, Education and Welfare (1974): *The Framingham Study, Section 30*, United States Government Printing Office, Washington, D.C., Publication No. (NIH) 74–599.

46. Vessey, M. P., and Doll, R. (1969): Investigation of relation between use of oral contraceptives and thromboembolic disease. A further report. *Br. Med. J.*, 2:651–657.

47. Veterans Administration Cooperative Study in Antihypertensive Agents (1967): Effects of treatment on morbidity in hypertension: results in patients with diastolic blood pressures averaging 115 through 129 mm Hg. *JAMA*, 202:1028–1034.

48. Veterans Administration Cooperative Study on Antihypertensive Agents (1970): Effects of treatment on morbidity in hypertension—results in patients with diastolic blood pressure averaging 90-114 monthly. *JAMA*, 213:1143–1152.

49. Veterans Administration Cooperative Study on Antihypertensive Agents (1972): Effects of treatment on morbidity in hypertension. III. Influence of age, diastolic pressure, and prior cardiovascular disease; further analysis of side effects. *Circulation*, 45:991–1004.
50. Whisnant, J. P., Matsumoto, N., and Elveback, L. R. (1973): Transient cerebral ischaemic attacks in a community—Rochester, Minnesota, 1955 through 1969. *Mayo Clin. Proc.*, 48:194–198.
51. Whisnant, J. P. (1974): Epidemiology of stroke: emphasis on transient cerebral ischaemic attacks and hypertension. *Stroke*, 5:68–70.
52. Wolf, P. A., Dawber, T. R., and Kannel, W. B. (1973): Epidemiologic assessment of the stroke candidate: the Framingham study. *Neurology*, 23:418.
53. Wolf, P. A., Kannel, W. B., and Dawber, T. R. (1978): Prospective investigations: The Framingham study and the epidemiology of stroke. In: *Advances in Neurology, Vol. 19, Neurological Epidemiology: Principles and Clinical Applications*, edited by B. S. Schoenberg, pp. 107–120. Raven Press, New York.
54. Wolf, P. A., Dawber, T. R., and Kannel, W. B. (1978): Heart disease as a precursor of stroke. In: *Advances in Neurology, Vol. 19, Neurological Epidemiology: Principles and Clinical Applications*, edited by B. S. Schoenberg, pp. 567–577. Raven Press, New York.
55. Worth, R. M., Kato, H., Rhoads, G. G., Kagan, A., and Syme, S. L. (1975): Epidemiologic studies of coronary heart disease and stroke in Japanese men living in Japan, Hawaii and California: mortality. *Am. J. Epidemiol.*, 102:481–490.

Advances in Stroke Therapy, edited by
F. C. Rose. Raven Press, New York © 1982.

The Natural History of Ischaemic Cerebrovascular Disease as Background to Therapeutic Approaches

Jørgen Marquardsen

Department of Neurology, Aalborg Hospital, DK 9000 Aalborg, Denmark

It is customary to describe the natural history of stroke as a sequence of clinical events starting at the time of the ictus. It should be realised, however, that a stroke is not an acute disease in itself, but rather an acute manifestation of a chronic, progressive vascular disease. Accordingly, many of the clinical factors that influence the long-term prognosis are in fact identical with the risk factors that were present long before the stroke and were partly responsible for its occurrence. Treatment of such factors is an important part of both primary and secondary prevention. Thus from both the pathogenetic and prognostic points of view, it will be appropriate to discuss various aspects of the natural history in the section devoted to "risk factors".

CLASSIFICATION OF CEREBROVASCULAR DISEASE

The study of epidemiological features and the natural history of stroke is greatly handicapped by the fact that cerebrovascular disease, unlike ischaemic heart disase, comprises several types of brain lesion which, although pathogenetically different, are often clinically indistinguishable. As recommended by Pickering (10), at least the following three categories of cerebrovascular disease should be considered separately:

1. *Aneurysmal disease* comprises berry aneurysms on the arteries of the circle of Willis and its branches, and results in subarachnoid haemorrhage. This entity differs so much from other types of stroke that perhaps it should be removed from the category of cerebrovascular disease in the diagnostic coding system, as suggested by Kurtzke (5).

2. *Nodular arteriosclerosis—or atherosclerosis*—affects the large arteries in the neck (carotid and vertebral), heart, and legs. The stenotic or occlusive lesions of this type can result in intracranial arterial occlusion, either by direct propagation of a thrombus or by discharge of emboli, the result being cerebral infarction or transient cerebral ischaemia. Cerebrovascular disease belonging to this category shows the same geographical distribution and male preponderance as ischaemic heart disease. Elevation of blood lipids and abnormalities of platelet function may be more important risk factors than hypertension.

117

3. *Disease of the small intracerebral arteries* produces either microaneurysms leading to intracerebral haemorrhage, or microocclusion producing small, deep, "lacunar" infarcts (3,12). The dominating risk factor in this category is hypertension.

It would be a great advantage if all cerebrovascular accidents could be readily allocated to one of these pathogenetic categories but, in clinical practice, the application of the classification is hampered by the frequent coexistence of extracranial and intracranial arterial disease. In cases of cerebral infarction without angiographically demonstrable arterial occlusion, for example, it is often difficult to decide whether the stroke was caused by an embolic occlusion with subsequent recanalization (category 2 in the above classification), or by thrombotic small-vessel disease (category 3). Moreover, when ischaemic stroke is a complication of arteriosclerotic/hypertensive heart disease, the mechanism can be either haemodynamic disturbances or embolism from a mural thrombus.

In order to overcome the above difficulties, several attempts have been made to base the clinical classification of ischaemic stroke not only on the cerebral symptoms and signs, but also on such factors as previous transient ischemic attack (TIA), evidence of extracranial arteriosclerotic disease (myocardial infarction, intermittent claudication), detectable sources of emboli, angiographic findings, and CT scan. In a stroke registry in Harvard (8), for example, the following three types of ischaemic stroke were considered: a) Large artery thrombosis, characterized by stepwise or stuttering onset, often preceded by TIA in the same vascular territory, evidence of large vessel disease, angiographic occlusion of major vessels. b) Lacunes: clinical lacunar syndrome (e.g. "pure motor hemiplegia"), normal angiogram, CT scan normal or showing small, deep infarct. c) Embolism: sudden or fluctuating onset, usually without preceding TIA, cardiac source or large vessel arterial source, angiographic branch occlusion (often transient) of intracranial artery, CT scan showing haemorrhagic infarction.

The prognostic implications of such a grouping of ischaemic stroke according to pathogenesis are not yet known, but the present chapter attempts to give an account of the natural history of ischaemic cerebrovascular disease—particularly of the long-term prognosis—with a background of pathogenetic considerations.

IMMEDIATE PROGNOSIS FOR LIFE

The importance of stroke as a cause of death often has been emphasized. In the WHO Stroke Registration Study (1) based on stroke registers operating in various parts of the world, the 3-week fatality rate for all centres combined was 30%. Despite wide variations in age distribution of the registered patients and availability of medical facilities, the fatality rates found in different communities were surprisingly similar, the highest and lowest rates being 43% and 26%, respectively.

It is generally accepted that the risk of a fatal outcome is 3 to 4 times higher for intracerebral haemorrhage than for cerebral infarctions. However, the main determinant of whether or not a stroke becomes fatal is not the pathoanatomic type of the lesion but the extent of brainstem dysfunction produced by either direct involvement or indirect involvement by transtentorial herniation resulting from hemispheric haemorrhage or oedema. This means that the clinical signs known to be of grave prognostic import—in particular impairment of consciousness, pupillary changes, respiratory abnormalities—are the same for haemorrhagic or ischaemic stroke as for nonvascular cerebral lesions.

Deaths from cerebral haemorrhage tend to occur earlier than those from cerebral infarction, the reason being that patients in the former category usually die from the cerebral lesion itself, whereas many patients with infarction succumb to secondary, extracranial complications. In about 20% of all strokes, death occurs suddenly (i.e. within 24 hr of onset). Nearly all sudden deaths are caused by intracranial bleeding; in the rare cases of "instantaneous" stroke death, the lesion responsible is almost invariably a subarachnoid haemorrhage (9).

FUNCTIONAL PROGNOSIS

In the WHO Stroke Study (1) comprising 8,754 cases of cerebrovascular accident, all surviving patients were followed for a minimum of 1 year. At time of onset, 71% of patients had hemiplegia or paraplegia. After 3 weeks, hemiplegia was still present in 67% of those surviving at that time and after 1 year in 46% of the survivors (or 20% of the original series). Of the one-year survivors observed in the European centres, only 14% were back in gainful work; 60% were independent in self-care, and only 9% were totally dependent.

Owing to the much lower incidence and higher fatality rate of haemorrhagic stroke as compared with ischaemic stroke, all representative series of stroke survivors consist mainly of cases of cerebral infarction. According to the pathogenetic classification referred to above, atherosclerotic large-vessel disease often results in extensive cortical and subcortical infarcts. The clinical picture of such patients, who are often normotensive, is characterized by hemiplegia accompanied by dysphasia, dyspraxia, neglect, or other gnostic disturbances. The prognosis for recovery is unfavourable in this group (11). By contrast, patients with deep, lacunar infarcts caused by hypertensive small-vessel disease usually present with pure motor hemiplegia (4) without sensory impairment or disturbances of higher nervous function; such patients can be expected to make good recoveries.

Regardless of the pathogenetic background outlined above, the main factor deciding the functional prognosis is the extent and the site of the cerebral lesion as reflected in a multitude of neurological signs whose prognostic significance has been assessed in many papers [for a review, see Marquardsen (6)]. Risk factors such as hypertension or heart disease exert only a modest influence on the prognosis for recovery.

LONG-TERM PROGNOSIS

Many follow-up studies, performed in various countries, have demonstrated that the late mortality of survivors from stroke is much higher than that of the corresponding general population. This is apparent from Fig. 1, which is based on a

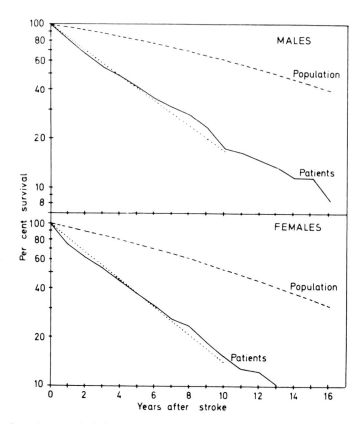

FIG. 1. Long-term survival after stroke (150 males and 257 females) compared with the survival of the Danish population, matched for age and sex. *Dotted lines* represent the average annual probability of dying. Logarithmic scale. (From ref. 6.)

follow-up of 407 patients with stroke, admitted to Frederiksberg Hospital, Copenhagen, in the period 1940 to 1952 (6). It is seen, for example, that the median survival time was less than 4 years for the patients, but over 10 years in the general population, matched for age and sex. Further, the slope of the survival curve is nearly constant throughout the period of observation. As the graphs were drawn on a semilogarithmic scale, this means that the annual death rate—or probability of dying—remains constant, regardless of the length of time that has passed since the stroke. Thus, the mortality experience of stroke patients can be expressed as the average annual probability of dying, which in the series in question was 0.16 for males, 0.18 for females. In other words, the number of survivors decreased at a constant annual rate of 16% and 18%, respectively.

In Fig. 2 (top), the survival data from the Danish study are compared with those based on 701 cases of presumed nonembolic cerebral infarction that were diagnosed and observed in Rochester, Minnesota from 1955 to 1969 (15). Considering that the two series are samples of quite different populations, selected according to

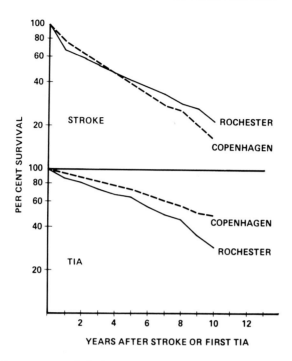

FIG. 2. Top: Long-term survival after stroke, as observed in Copenhagen (ref. 6) and in Rochester, Minnesota (ref. 15). **Bottom:** Long-term survival after TIA, as observed in Copenhagen (ref. 13) and in Rochester, Minnesota (ref. 15). Logarithmic scale.

different criteria, the survival curves are strikingly similar, the only difference being a slightly higher annual death rate in the Danish series. These findings do not lend support to the belief, expressed by some authors, that the excess mortality of stroke patients tend to decrease after a period of 5 to 6 years, thus suggesting a "cessation of activity" of cerebrovascular disease. On the contrary, the graphs shown in Fig. 2 are compatible with the view that a stroke, at least of the ischaemic type, is merely an incident in the progressive course of a generalized vascular disease that is responsible for the excess mortality. This applies to the bulk of ischaemic strokes due to arteriosclerotic and/or hypertensive vascular disease, but not necessarily to infarcts caused by treatable blood disorders, oral contraception, and other such factors.

The influence of preexisting vascular disease on survival after stroke is illustrated by Fig. 3, which shows the unfavourable prognosis of patients with a history of heart failure (i.e. dyspnoea on slight exertion and/or oedema). The difference between patients with, and those without, heart symptoms is particularly noticeable in the first 3 years after stroke. Furthermore, high blood pressure, as recorded during the inital hospital stay, is another bad prognostic sign, particularly in younger men (Fig. 4). Elderly women, on the other hand, seem to be relatively immune to the effects of hypertension.

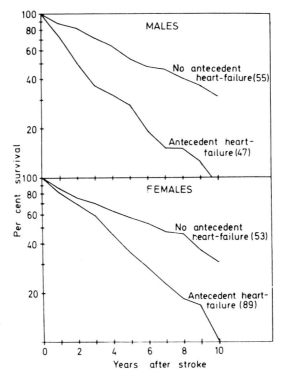

FIG. 3.   Survival of stroke patients with and without a history of heart failure. (From ref. 6.)

In the Frederiksberg series, 23% of deaths were caused by recurrent stroke, but about 40% by heart disease. Again, this emphasizes the importance of extracranial vascular disease in cases of stroke.

A more recent series of patients with cerebral infarction admitted to Frederiksberg Hospital was the basis of a study of late survival with respect to angiographic findings in the acute or subacute phase. Almost identical survival curves were found for patients with intracranial arterial occlusion (usually of the middle cerebral artery) and for those with diffuse arteriosclerotic lesions without occlusion, the average annual probability of dying (a.a.p.d) being 0.22 or 0.21, respectively. Conversely, patients with occlusion of the internal carotid artery had a slightly better survival rate mainly in the first 3 years after stroke (a.a.p.d.: 0.17). This difference may reflect the fact that patients with carotid occlusion as compared with the remaining patients had lower blood pressure levels but higher frequencies of previous TIA and intermittent claudication. Contrary to expectation, a correlation between angiographic findings and cause of death could not be demonstrated in this series.

Factors other than hypertension and heart disease such as diabetes mellitus, elevated blood lipids (mainly in youngish males), increased blood viscosity, are recognized as risk factors for atherothrombotic brain infarction. The influence of such factors on the late survival after stroke has not yet been fully evaluated.

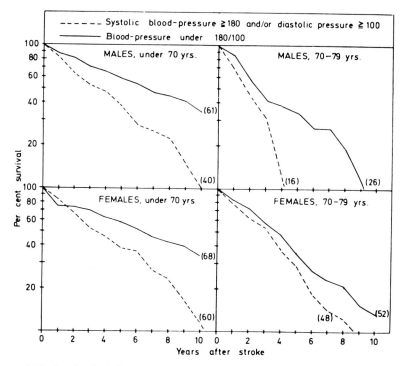

FIG. 4. Survival after stroke, by height of blood pressure. (From ref. 6.)

Recurrences

In the original Frederiksberg series, 8 to 10 new strokes occured per 100 observed patient-years, the annual rate being almost constant over the entire observation period, indicating uninterrupted propagation of the underlying vascular disease. It seems logical to conclude that every stroke patient who survives long enough is likely to have another cerebrovascular accident. Owing to the high risk of death from other causes, only about one-third of patients will actually live to suffer a recurrence.

In survivors from cerebral infarction, the recurrent stroke is usually of the same pathological type and affects the same hemisphere as the initial episode. In the presence of very high blood pressure, however, the recurrence may be a cerebral haemorrhage, often developing in the contralateral hemisphere. Thus, it is possible that to some extent, an arterial occlusion can protect the ipsilateral hemisphere from harmful effects of high blood pressure.

The same risk factors that are inversely related to long-term survival are also associated with an increased risk of recurrence. In the Frederiksberg series, the recurrence rate was found to rise steadily with the blood pressure level: Recurrences were over four times as frequent in patients with diastolic blood pressure over 120 mm than in those whose pressures were under 100 mm. Auricular fibrillation or other ECG abnormalities were associated with a twofold risk of recurrence. Of the Frederiksberg patients subjected to angiography, those with carotid artery occlusion seemed to have a lower recurrence rate than the remaining patients, but the difference was not quite significant. On the other hand, in a series of young stroke patients, the risk of recurrence was particularly high in cases of premature atherosclerosis (14).

Many studies of patients in the acute phase of thrombosis have demonstrated abnormalities of coagulation, fibrinolysis, or platelet activity, but the question of cause and effect is still open. There is little doubt that thrombotic episodes can be triggered by some sort of temporary "hypercoagulable state." In view of the form of the survival curves discussed above, such short-term risk factors do not appear to be of primary importance in the long-term prognosis after stroke.

TRANSIENT ISCHAEMIC ATTACKS

TIA is an important precursor of stroke. Moreover, although characterized by focal cerebral symptoms of less than 24 hr duration, TIA cannot be sharply distinguished from mild strokes with reversible neurological deficit. Hence, the long-term prognosis of TIA should be considered in any account of the natural history of stroke.

According to many reports, 10 to 35% of TIA patients will develop a stroke within an interval of 3 to 4 years after the initial TIA (16,17). Time intervals between the initial TIA and the subsequent stroke range from hours to many years, but the risk of stroke seems to be greater soon after the onset of TIA than later: In a series of patients followed for many years, Cartlidge et al. (2) found that over one-third of patients who had a stroke had their first stroke within 6 months of the onset of TIA.

Survival after TIA was recently studied in a series of 243 cases of TIA diagnosed in four neurological departments in Copenhagen (13). The prevalence of extracranial vascular disease in this group was very similar to that observed in the above-mentioned series of cerebral infarcts from the same geographical area. Figure 5 shows that the survival of the patients was significantly reduced as compared with that of the corresponding general population. In Fig. 6, the ratio of observed to expected survival is plotted on a semilogarithmic scale producing an almost straight line, the slope of which is a measure of the excess mortality. The numerical expression of the slope—in this series being 0.04—will facilitate comparisons of the survival of TIA patients selected from different populations. It should be noted that the excess mortality was not higher in the first year of observation than later. It is therefore impossible to define any interval of time after which the excess mortality is likely to decline.

Most, but not all, investigators have found that carotid TIAs carry a poorer prognosis for life than do vertebrobasilar attacks. Further unfavourable prognostic factors are associated heart disease or intermittent claudication, and a history of arterial hypertension.

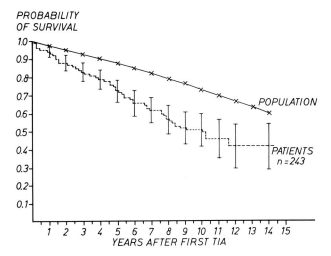

FIG. 5. Long-term survival after first TIA compared with the survival of the Danish population, matched for age and sex. *Vertical lines* represent ± 2 SD. (From ref. 13.)

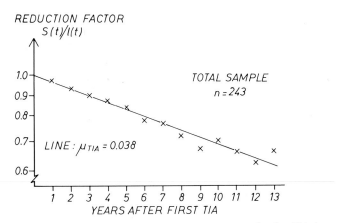

FIG. 6. Ratios of observed to expected survival in successive years after first TIA. Logarithmic scale. (From ref. 13.)

In Fig. 2 (bottom), the survival of the patients in the Danish TIA series is compared with that observed in 198 TIA patients in Rochester, Minnesota. Owing to a higher mean age, the American patients had lower survival rates than their Danish counterparts; otherwise, the curves are seen to be quite similar, both being rectilinear. A comparison of the upper and lower halves of Fig. 2 indicates that patients with TIA had a much better prognosis for life than those with completed stroke. The median survival time was less than 4 years in the stroke series. The corresponding average annual death rates were 6 and 17%, respectively. The difference is not a result of the disability found in many stroke survivors: even patients whose post-stroke disability was negligible had a higher mortality than TIA patients of similar age.

The causes of death observed in the decreased TIA patients were strikingly similar to those found in the Frederiksberg stroke series (6): Cerebrovascular accidents were responsible for 20% of deaths in the TIA series and for 23% in the stroke series; for heart disease, the percentages were 38 and 40, respectively.

It should be mentioned that considerable sex differences exist in the pathogenesis of TIA. In a Swedish study of TIA patients under the age of 55 (7) nearly all the men had arteriosclerosis of the extracranial arteries, and 47% had abnormal blood lipids. In the female group the main factor was abnormality of the coagulation system.

SUMMARY AND CONCLUSIONS

In the acute phase of stroke, regardless of its pathoanatomic type, the prognosis for life depends mainly on the extent of direct or indirect brainstem involvement. The primary aim of therapy is to prevent transtentorial herniation through treatment of cerebral oedema, evacuation of clots, etc.

The prognosis for functional recovery and rehabilitation depends mainly on the extent of cerebral (in particular cortical) damage. Even with the same degree of motor deficit, the chances of recovery are much better after deep, lacunar lesions than after hemispheric infarcts caused by large vessel atherosclerotic disease. Any medical or surgical measure that might increase collateral blood flow can improve the outlook.

The long-term survival rate after stroke is characterized by an annual death rate that, regardless of the time elapsed since the stroke, is much higher than that of the general population. The cause of death is most often vascular, heart disease being a more frequent cause than recurrent stroke. Factors of ominous prognostic significance are the same as the well known risk factors for stroke (hypertension, heart disease, etc.). The risk of recurrent stroke, like the risk of death, remains constant over the years after stroke.

These findings indicate that, even after apparent recovery from stroke, the progression of the underlying vascular disease will continue. This means that treatment of risk factors is as important after stroke as before.

The prognostic influence of the pathogenetic type of cerebral infarction (large-vessel arterio-sclerosis, embolism, lacunar disease) remains to be properly evaluated.

The long-term mortality of TIA patients, although lower than that of stroke victims, is higher than that of the general population. The survival curve presents the same characteristics as that found in stroke series. Moreover, the predisposing factors, the causes of death, and the factors influencing the long-term prognosis are almost identical. It seems probable, therefore, that most cases of TIA have the same pathogenetic background as the common types of ischaemic stroke, the difference being that TIA is an earlier manifestation of the underlying disease than cerebral infarction; this would explain the longer survival of TIA patients.

The treatment of risk factors is obviously as important after TIA as after ischaemic stroke. The constant excess mortality over the years following the onset of TIA makes it very difficult to decide on the discontinuation of prophylactic therapy after any particular length of time.

REFERENCES

1. Aho, K., Harmsen, P., Hatano, S., Marquardsen, J., Smirnov, V. E., and Strasser, T. (1980): Cerebrovascular disease in the community: Results of a WHO collaborative study. *Bull. WHO*, 58:113–130.
2. Cartlidge, N. E. F., Whisnant, J. P., and Elveback, L. R. (1977): Carotid and vertebral-basilar transient cerebral ischemic attacks. *Mayo Clin. Proc.*, 52:117–120.
3. Fisher, C. M. (1969): The arterial lesions underlying lacunes. *Acta Neuropathol. (Berlin)*, 12:1–15.
4. Fisher, C. M., and Curry, H. B. (1965): Pure motor hemiplegie of vascular origin. *Arch. Neurol.*, 13:30–44.
5. Kurtzke, J. F. (1969): *Epidemiology of Cerebrovascular Disease*, p. 106 ff. Springer-Verlag, Berlin, Heidelberg, New York.
6. Marquardsen, J. (1969): *The Natural History of Cerebrovascular Disease*, pp. 43, 95, 131. Munksgaard, Copenhagen.
7. Mettinger, K. L., and Söderström, C. E. (1978): Pathogenetic profile of TIA before 55. *J. Neurol. Sci.*, 36:341–348.
8. Mohr, J. P., Caplan, L. R., Melski, J. W., Goldstein, R. J., Duncan, G. W., Kistler, J. P., Pessin, M. S., and Bleich, H. L. (1978): The Harvard Cooperative Stroke Registry: *Neurology*, 28:754–762.
9. Phillips, L. H., Whisnant, J. B., and Reagan, T. J. (1977): Sudden death from stroke. *Stroke*, 8:392–395.
10. Pickering, G. (1966): Cerebral vascular disease. *Acta Med. Scand.* (Suppl.), 445:423–425.
11. Prineas, J., and Marshall, J. (1966): Hypertension and cerebral infarction. *Br. Med. J.*, 1:14–17.
12. Russel, R. R. (1975): How does blood pressure cause stroke? *Lancet*, ii:1283–1285.
13. Simonsen, N., Christiansen, H. D., Heltberg, A., Marquardsen, J., Pedersen, H. E., and Sørensen, P. S. (1981): Long-term prognosis after transient ischemic attacks. *Acta Neurol. Scand.*, 63:156–168.
14. Snyder, B. D., and Ramirez-Lassepas, M. (1980): Cerebral infarction in young adults. *Stroke*, 11:149–153.
15. Whisnant, J. P. (1976): A population study of stroke and TIA: Rochester, Minnesota. In: *Stroke*, edited by F. J. Gillingham, C. Mawdsley, and A. E. Williams, pp. 21–39. Churchill Livingstone. Edinburgh, London, New York.
16. Whisnant, J. P., Matsumoto, N., and Elveback, L. R. (1973): Transient cerebral ischemic attacks in a community. *Mayo Clin. Proc.*, 48:194–198.
17. Ziegler, D. K., and Hassanein, R. S. (1973): Prognosis in patients with transient ischemic attacks. *Stroke*, 4:666–673.

Advances in Stroke Therapy, edited by
F. C. Rose. Raven Press, New York © 1982.

The Search for a Thrombotic Tendency in Stroke

G. P. Mulley, *S. Heptinstall, *P. M. Taylor, and *J. R. A. Mitchell

*Department of Health Care of the Elderly, Sherwood Hospital, Nottingham, NG5 1PD; and *Department of Medicine, University Hospital, Queens Medical Centre, Nottingham NG7 2UH, England*

Serendipity apart, if we are to develop effective prophylactic therapy for stroke, we must understand the underlying pathological processes involved. Over the past 50 years, there have been major changes in our understanding of the pathogenesis of stroke which have led to the investigation of therapeutic agents that may be useful in stroke prevention. It is now accepted that most cerebral infarcts are due to extracranial arterial disease and cardiac embolism. What is the composition of these thrombi, and how might we prevent their occurrence?

Thrombus forming in heart chambers is composed of many strands of fibrin lying among elements of formed blood. The proportion of fibrin in a thrombus increases in inverse proportion to the rate of blood flow. Thrombus forming in a fibrillating atrium is soft, dark red, and gelatinous—the so-called red thrombus. Anticoagulants that modify fibrin formation are therefore potentially of considerable therapeutic importance. The Framingham survey showed that asymptomatic people with idiopathic atrial fibrillation (AF) were five times more likely to develop stroke than those in sinus rhythm; it would thus seem prudent to anticoagulate people in AF. However, AF may be a marker of widespread vascular disease, and stroke may occur because of haemorrhage, carotid thrombosis, mural thrombus overlying myocardial infarction, or reduced cerebral blood flow. To anticoagulate prophylactically all patients in AF is potentially hazardous: since the majority are old, and Charcot-Bouchard aneurysms are age-related, they are at increased risk of cerebral haemorrhage. Ideally before instituting anticoagulant therapy we should identify those patients with AF who have intraatrial thrombus. Unfortunately we cannot yet detect all atrial thrombi by noninvasive techniques.

Thrombus arising on the atheromatous surface of an extracranial vessel consists of aggregates of blood platelets with peripheral leukocytes and fibrin. The thrombus is firm and pale—a white thrombus. Although we are as yet unable to prevent or reverse atheroma, we do have drugs (such as aspirin, dipyridamole, and sulphinpyrazone) that modify platelet behaviour. If we could identify those people at particular risk of developing platelet thrombi, we could then administer prophylactic antiplatelet drugs in the hope of preventing thrombotic events.

PLATELET BEHAVIOUR AND THROMBOSIS

Arterial thrombus formation is influenced by three factors: the vessel wall, the flow of blood, and the blood itself. The blood constituents are the most easily studied and, of these, platelets stand out as being the most likely contributors to the thrombotic mass.

Studies of platelets in the test tube have revealed aspects of platelet behaviour that may operate in thrombus formation. First, platelets adhere to foreign surfaces. Of particular interest is their ability to adhere to the subendothelial layer of blood vessels that is exposed when blood vessels are injured. Certainly, exposed sub-endothelium is important in the haemostatic process; perhaps it also plays a part in thrombogenesis. Second, platelets also can be induced to aggregate. Aggregation can occur spontaneously or in response to one of a variety of aggregating agents such as adenosine diphosphate (ADP), adrenalin, collagen, or thrombin. It can be either reversible or irreversible, and the changes in light absorbance that occur when a suspension of platelets to which an aggregating agent has been added is stirred suggests that aggregation can occur in two phases. Third, once platelets have become adherent to a foreign surface or have been induced to aggregate, they can undergo a release reaction in which the contents of intracellular storage granules are discharged from the cells. Some of the materials that are released (e.g., ADP, serotonin, and catecholamines) are themselves aggregating agents and so propagate the signal. This release of stored materials is at least partially responsible for the second phase of aggregation that is sometimes observed. Fourth, as well as releasing stored aggregating agents, platelets can synthesise proaggregatory prostaglandins and thromboxanes. The release reaction and the synthesis of these materials are often interrelated. Thus aspirin, an inhibitor of prostaglandin and thromboxane synthesis, prevents both the ADP-induced release reaction and the second phase of aggregation that stems from it.

PLATELET BEHAVIOUR IN STROKE

There are several ways of trying to discover whether platelet behaviour is associated with the development of thromboembolic stroke. First, tests of platelet reactivity could be performed on a large population and the subjects followed up for many years to see if any relationship exists between platelet behaviour and the tendency to develop stroke. A higher yield of stroke cases would be obtained if the study was limited to patients with risk factors for stroke such as hypertension. Second, we could study patients with so-called transient ischaemic attacks (TIA). However, TIA is a symptom, not a diagnosis, and may be caused or mimicked by a large number of disorders. Moreover, a history of preceding TIA is obtained only in a minority of stroke patients. The third approach is to study patients who already have had a stroke. This is a useful starting point: If we cannot differentiate between platelet behaviour in normal people and those who have sustained a stroke, it is unlikely that the platelet test we are using will be helpful in identifying people susceptible to cerebrovascular disease.

There are many ways of studying platelet behaviour including measurement of adhesion of platelets to glass, tests of aggregation in response to a variety of stimuli, measurement of platelet constituents extruded during the release reaction, studies of physical properties of platelets such as electrophoretic mobility, and determinations of the length of time that platelets survive in the circulation. To date, the majority of reports of platelet behaviour in completed stroke have involved studies of platelet adhesiveness and the ability of platelets to aggregate.

PLATELET ADHESION STUDIES

A simple way to test platelet stickiness is to measure the number of platelets that adhere to glass when blood or platelet-rich plasma is placed in a rotating glass bulb or passed through a glass bead column. In their pioneering study of platelets in neurological disease, Nathanson and Savitsky (11) found high values of adherence in patients with a variety of neurological disease. In 60 patients with multiple sclerosis, those with clinical fluctuations and exacerbations had increased platelet adhesion whereas the platelets taken from those whose condition was considered stationary were within the normal range. However, platelets from 10 patients with stroke were found to behave normally. The authors did not record the type of stroke nor did they state the interval between onset of stroke and time of platelet test.

Danta (4) studied platelet adhesiveness in stroke patients within 48 hr of stroke and repeated the tests serially for 6 weeks. He compared these 10 patients with 172 patients with established stroke and with 65 controls. He found that patients with stroke have platelets that are significantly more adhesive to glass than platelets from control subjects, irrespective of the length of time that had elapsed since the stroke occurred. The increased adhesiveness was noted within 1 day of stroke and did not alter within the first 6 weeks of onset. There was no change in hyperadhesiveness within 6 months in those patients with established stroke. Danta suggested that platelet adhesiveness was unlikely to be a direct consequence of stroke, but that it may have preceded or coincided with the event. However, in a subsequent study with Acheson and Hutchinson (1), Danta could not find any association between increased platelet adhesiveness after stroke and frequency of stroke, degree of disability, or duration of symptoms and concluded that increased adhesiveness appears to be an epiphenomenon that bears no obvious relation to stroke and does not reflect prognosis.

A later study of young Indian men with stroke (16) confirmed that platelet adhesiveness in acute stroke is significantly higher than adhesiveness in a control group.

PLATELET AGGREGATION STUDIES

Platelet aggregation can occur in stirred anticoagulated whole blood or in platelet-rich plasma, both spontaneously and in response to stimulation by a variety of agents. In platelet-rich plasma, aggregation can be measured photometrically: the amount of light transmitted through a platelet suspension increases as the platelets clump together. Materials such as ADP tend to induce aggregation that is either reversible (shortly after the aggregation has been induced the platelets disaggregate again) or irreversible, depending on the concentration of ADP used. At an intermediate concentration of ADP, aggregation can occur in two phases, primary aggregation being followed by a secondary response. The latter is known to be associated with both prostaglandin and thromboxane synthesis and the release reaction.

In an attempt to measure "circulating" aggregates, fresh whole blood has been subjected to screen filtration under pressure (8). Another technique has involved collecting blood into formalin and EDTA (18). Whether these techniques actually measure circulating platelet aggregates or merely reflect the degree of spontaneous activation during blood collection remains to be determined.

Let us first analyse those studies of platelet aggregation that have been carried out shortly after a stroke has occurred. Kalendovsky and colleagues (7) studied four people under 40 years of age who had repeated strokes. Using the screen filtration method, they found that there was increased aggregability after the onset of symptoms. Follow-up showed that the platelet abnormality persisted.

Petrova et al. (14) assessed platelet behaviour by measuring both spontaneous aggregation and ADP-induced aggregation in 20 healthy controls and 120 stroke patients. One-fourth of the stroke patients came to necropsy and the rest were diagnosed as having haemorrhagic or ischaemic stroke on clinical grounds. Clinical diagnosis of stroke is notoriously inaccurate, and the findings therefore must be interpreted cautiously. It was found that in occlusive stroke, spontaneous aggregation occurred in 60% of cases, the increased activity being most marked in the first 5 days. By contrast, spontaneous aggregation did not occur in the haemorrhagic group or the control group. Second-phase aggregation was observed in all patients with occlusive stroke but in only 3 of the 43 patients with cerebral haemorrhage. The authors postulate that the increased platelet behaviour after occlusive stroke may be due to the release of thromboplastin rich tissue from damaged brain and suggest that ADP-induced aggregation may serve as a test for differentiating haemorrhagic and occlusive stroke.

In the study of Dougherty et al. (5), 53 patients with cerebral infarction (the majority of whom had diagnostic procedures, including computerized tomography (CT) scan) whose mean age was 60 were compared with 29 patients with transient stroke and a group of neurological controls. The control group unfortunately included patients with brain tumor and multiple sclerosis—conditions associated with abnormal platelet behaviour (11). Aggregation was assessed using the technique described by Wu and Hoak (18). It was found that the hyperaggregability in the acute phase returned to normal within 6 weeks; there was little difference in platelet behaviour between transient and completed stroke and there was considerable overlap in the results from the three groups, indicating that although the test may be useful in comparing groups of patients, it is of little value in discriminating between individuals.

Other studies have measured aggregation in the recovery phase of stroke; in none has the nature of the stroke been accurately established. Danta (3) used the optical density method in 97 patients to assess ADP-induced aggregation at least 3 months post stroke. Compared with 13 young, healthy volunteers and 40 patients with miscellaneous conditions, the stroke patients required a lower average concentration of ADP to stimulate second-phase aggregation. Using the same technique, Sano et al. (15) studied Japanese subjects. In 10 stroke patients over the age of 50 years, Sano found the sensitivity of platelets to ADP was higher in the acute than in the convalescent period. Indeed, after the acute phase, the platelet behaviour was indistinguishable from that found in healthy male controls. Whereas Danta had found no trend in platelet aggregation with increasing age in his stroke patients, the Japanese workers noted that there was age-related increase in sensitivity to ADP-induced aggregation in the control group.

Neri Serneri et al. (13) found both increased adhesion to glass and increased sensitivity to ADP-induced aggregation in patients with chronic cerebrovascular disease compared with age-matched controls. They also found considerable overlap between the results from the stroke and the control group.

In a comparison of platelet aggregation with transient and completed strokes in 18 patients aged 60 or under with 21 similar patients over 60, Couch and Hassanein (2) found that platelets from the young stroke patients aggregated more readily than controls. However, the aggregation was similar in older patients, whether or not they had sustained a stroke. These workers also found no differences in aggregability when measured within the first month and again after a year.

Lou et al. (9) compared 11 stroke patients under the age of 50 with 40 age-matched controls. The platelet studies were done on average 22 months after the onset of the stroke, none being done within the first 8 months. Using the optical density method to measure ADP-induced aggregation, they found that young stroke survivors have platelets that can be more easily aggregated than controls.

Ten Cate et al. (17) found spontaneous platelet aggregation in 50 of 130 patients with cerebrovascular insufficiency, ages 21 to 82 years. The spontaneous aggregation was normal in all 80 controls. These workers also found that all those with spontaneous aggregation showed a low threshold for ADP-induced second phase aggregation.

Kobayashi et al. (8), measuring aggregability by the screen filtration pressure method, found that aggregation was higher in stroke patients and hypotensive patients than in healthy elderly controls. They also noted a difference in aggregation between clinically diagnosed thrombotic and haemorrhagic patients, but this ceased to be apparent 30 days after the stroke. In patients judged to have had thrombotic stroke, the aggregation gradually declined with time. There was no change in aggregation with increasing age.

In a study of spontaneous aggregation in 52 patients under the age of 55 years who appeared to have had an ischaemic stroke 6 to 16 weeks earlier, Mettinger et al. (10) found no differences between patients and controls.

STUDIES OF THE PLATELET RELEASE REACTION

Second-phase aggregation is associated with the release of materials from platelets, some of which are platelet aggregating agents. These include ADP and serotonin. It is possible to label the intracellular pool of serotonin by incubating platelets with radiolabeled serotonin. When platelets are then stimulated sufficiently for the release reaction to occur, the amount of labeled serotonin that is released serves as a measure of the extent of the release reaction. The proportion of intracellular radiolabeled serotonin that is released is expressed as a percentage of that taken up into the platelets (6). It is reasonable to assume that the more active platelets would release larger proportions of radioactive serotonin in response to a given concentration of aggregating agent.

We have studied the extent of ADP-induced release reaction in 108 stroke patients and 54 controls. Briefly, our findings are as follows:

First, there was no significant difference in the extent of tritiated serotonin release between patients who had recently sustained a stroke and the control group. Second, in 43 of the stroke patients whose diagnosis was determined either by CT scan or necropsy, there were marked differences in release between haemorrhagic and thromboembolic groups. Patients who had sustained an intracerebral haemorrhage or a subarachnoid haemorrhage had platelets that released only small amounts of labeled serotonin whereas those with occlusive disease displayed a wide range of values. Finally, in those patients whose platelets released only small amounts of serotonin when tested immediately after stroke, the extent of the release reaction remained low. In contrast, in the majority of patients with a high release in the acute phase, the extent of the release reaction tended to be lower a year later.

INTERPRETATION OF TESTS OF PLATELET
BEHAVIOUR IN STROKE

We cannot draw any firm conclusions from these studies of platelet behaviour in stroke. Different workers have used different tests; those who have examined platelet aggregation have used different techniques. Studies of spontaneous aggregation cannot be compared directly with those of ADP-induced aggregation or aggregation by the screen-filtration method. Few workers have determined the type of stroke by necropsy or CT. The interval between onset of stroke and platelet test has varied from a few days to many months. Some have limited their studies to young patients, others to older patients. In some cases, age-matched controls have been used: some include young healthy volunteers, while some use no control group. There may be racial differences in platelet behaviour and we cannot assume that results obtained in the United Kingdom will be the same as those obtained in Japan or Russia. Nonetheless, some data do emerge from these studies:

1. Young people who have sustained a stroke subsequently tend to have increased platelet activity.

2. Abnormal post stroke platelet behaviour does not remain abnormal but the time taken for the platelets to return to normal levels is unclear.

3. Many studies (but not all) suggest that there is an increase in platelet activity with increasing age in normal people.

4. Platelet abnormalities in acute stroke bear no relation to subsequent morbidity or mortality.

5. Values obtained from measurements of platelet aggregation and the extent of the platelet release reaction in the acute phase appear to differ from values obtained in haemorrhagic stroke. We do not know whether this is a reflection of the nature of the lesion, whether it is an age-related phenomenon, or whether there is another explanation. There may be scope here for using platelet tests in stroke diagnosis. We must bear in mind the possibility that determination of platelet hypoactivity may be as important as tests of hyperactivity in community surveys of people at risk from cerebrovascular disease.

6. Tests of platelet behaviour are not specific in stroke and studies of adhesion and aggregation, and the release reaction suggests that these tests cannot be recommended for community screening.

REFERENCES

1. Acheson, J., Danta, G., and Hutchinson, E. C. (1972): Platelet adhesiveness in patients with cerebral vascular disease. *Atherosclerosis*, 15:125–127.
2. Couch, J. R., and Hassanein, R. S. (1976): Platelet aggregation, stroke and TIA in middle-aged and elderly patients. *Neurology*, 26:888–895.
3. Danta, G. (1970): Second phase platelet aggregation induced by adenosine diphosphate in patients with cerebral vascular disease and in control subjects. *Thromb. Diath. Haem.*, 23:159–169.
4. Danta, G. (1970): Platelet adhesiveness in cerebrovascular disease. *Atherosclerosis*, 11:223–233.
5. Dougherty, J. H. Jr., Levy, D. E., and Weksler, B. B. (1977): Platelet activation in acute cerebral ischaemia. Serial measurements of platelet function in cerebrovascular disease. *Lancet*, i:821–824.
6. Heptinstall, S., and Mulley, G. P. (1977): Adenosine diphosphate induced platelet aggregation and release reaction in heparinized platelet rich plasma and the influence of added Citrate. *Br. J. Haematol.*, 36:565–571.
7. Kalendovsky, Z., Austin, J., and Steele, P. (1975): Increased platelet aggregability in young patients with stroke: diagnosis and therapy. *Arch. Neurol.*, 32:13–21.
8. Kobayashi, I., Fujita, T., and Yamazaki, H. (1976): Platelet aggregability measured by screen filtration method in cerebrovascular disease. *Stroke*, 7:406–409.
9. Lou, H. C., Dalsgård Nielsen, J., Bomhold, A., and Gormsen, J. (1977): Platelet hyperaggregability in young patients with completed stroke. *Acta Neurol. Scand.*, 56:326–334.
10. Mettinger, K. L., Hyman, D., Kjellin, K. G., Sideń, Å., and Söderström, C. E. (1979): Factor VIII related antigen, antithrombin III, spontaneous platelet aggregation and plasminogen activator in ischaemic cerebrovascular. A study of stroke before 55. *J. Neurol. Sci.*, 41:31–38.
11. Millac, P. (1967): Platelet stickiness in patients with intracranial tumours. *Br. Med. J.*, 4:25–26.
12. Nathanson, M., and Savitsky, J. P. (1954): Platelet adhesive index studies in multiple sclerosis and other neurological disorders. *Bull. N.Y. Acad. Med.*, 28:462–468.
13. Neri Serneri, G. G., Silvestrini, E., Gensini, G. F., and Abbate-Gensini, R. (1974): Platelet hyperreactivity and decreased survival in chronic cerebrovascular patients. Chronic defibrination syndrome? In: *Platelet Aggregation in the Pathogenesis of Cerebrovascular Disease*, edited by A. Agnoli and C. Fazio, pp. 136–150. Springer-Verlag, Berlin.

14. Petrova, T. R., Pavlishchuk, S. A., and Grigoriev, G. L. (1975): Phase analysis of platelet aggregation in acute disturbances of cerebral circulation. *Cor Vasa*, 17:102–111.
15. Sano, T., Boxer, M. G. J., Boxer, L. A., and Yokoyama, M. (1971): Platelet sensitivity to aggregation in normal and diseased groups. *Thromb. Diath. Haem.*, 25:524–531.
16. Sharma, S. C., Vijayan, G. P., Suri, M. L., and Seth, H. N. (1977): Platelet adhesiveness in young patients with ischaemic stroke. *J. Clin. Pathol.*, 30:649–652.
17. Ten Cate, J. W., Vos, J., Oosterhuis, H., Prenger, D., and Jenkins, C. S. P. (1978): Spontaneous platelet aggregation in cerebrovascular disease. *Thromb. Diath. Haem.*, 39:223–229.
18. Wu, K. K., and Hoak, J. C. (1975): Increased platelet aggregates in patients with transient ischaemic attacks. *Stroke*, 6:521–524.

Advances in Stroke Therapy, edited by
F. C. Rose. Raven Press, New York © 1982.

Antithrombotic Drugs and the Prevention of Stroke After Transient Ischaemic Attacks

Charles Warlow

Clinical Reader in Neurology and Honorary Consultant Neurologist, University Department of Clinical Neurology, The Radcliffe Infirmary, Oxford OX2 6HE, England

When evaluating the evidence for and against therapy in patients with transient ischaemic attacks (TIA) there are five general principles to be considered:

1. Historical controls, particularly a so-called natural history in the literature, are unacceptable, and prospective random allocation to treatment strategies is absolutely essential. It is impossible to find a control group in the literature, or even in one's own experience, that can be satisfactorily matched with a treated group with respect to the prognostic variables that are known, leaving aside those that remain to be discovered. The outcome in a group of TIA patients must depend on many prognostic variables including age, sex, prevalence of hypertension, extent of arterial disease, the presence of ischaemic heart disease, and the duration and accuracy of follow-up. It is perhaps not surprising, therefore, that the answer to the questions, "What is the risk of stroke after TIA"? and "What is the mortality after TIA"? varies enormously depending on which study is considered. Furthermore, no study has addressed the problem of the risk of myocardial infarction (MI) which is the most frequent cause of death in these patients (15). In general, trials based on historical controls tend to overestimate the effects of treatment, or find effects that do not exist (11).

2. If the effect of a treatment is modest, and potential treatments of TIA probably are rather modest, trials must be large to have a reasonable chance of reliably detecting such a result. Even a 25% reduction in risk of stroke would be of importance, since TIAs are common (about 0.3 per 1,000 population per annum) (16) and the risk of stroke and/or death substantial (about 10% per annum) (2,5). To have an 80% chance of detecting such a risk reduction, at the conventional level of significance ($p < 0.05$), approximately 2,000 patients need to be randomised in a trial lasting 4 to 5 years (15).

3. Unless total mortality is the only end-point of interest, blindness of both patient and observer is highly desirable, and if it can be arranged it should be. Even so-called 'hard' end-points such as stroke and MI can be misdiagnosed frequently enough to ruin an analysis if the observer is systematically biased for or against the treatment being evaluated. Furthermore, stroke has to be distinguished from

TIA by the duration of the neurological disability (usually 24 hr) and the patient, observer, or both, may very easily overestimate or underestimate the duration of an event lasting between a few hours and a few days. Blindness is not only reassuring to the observer (and any clinical audit committee) when assessing a possible end-point, but also confounds the critical suspicion that systematic diagnostic bias has occurred.

4. Cessation, or reduction in frequency of TIA is usually a minor and subsidiary objective of treatment since a) they are usually infrequent, and rarely a serious problem since by definition they leave no permanent disability; b) treatment preventing small emboli, believed to be the usual cause of TIA, may not necessarily prevent large emboli or occlusive thrombosis, believed to be the cause of subsequent stroke, and c) treatment which reduces the frequency of TIA could increase the risk of stroke, and trials using stroke as an end-point instead of the rather trivial end-point of TIA are essential (for example, anticoagulants even if they reduce the risk of TIA may increase the risk of cerebral haemorrhage so much that they are not worth using unless the risk of cerebral infarction is substantially reduced).

5. TIA is a clinical diagnosis that embraces more than one pathogenetic mechanism. Most TIA are probably due to atherothromboembolism, some are due to embolism or the heart and, in some, no embolic source from any kind of underlying disease can be identified (6). It is rather unlikely that a single treatment will be useful for all TIA patients but, unless major pathogenetic subgroups can be identified reliably, a trial of treatment in all TIA patients may fail to show a benefit even if that treatment is useful in one of the pathogenetic subgroups. If a conservative angiographic policy is being pursued and if cardiac evaluation is incomplete, then it is very difficult, if not impossible, to subdivide TIA patients by suspected underlying pathology, with the exception of clinically obvious and major potential cardiac sources of embolism (for example, mitral stenosis with atrial fibrillation).

ANTICOAGULANTS

There have been five randomised trials of anticoagulation in TIA patients (2,3,4,9,14) and none of short-term or emergency anticoagulation. These trials were all far too small since the largest contained 60 patients and even in aggregate there were only 227 patients (see point 2 above). Sometimes, stroke caused by cerebral haemorrhage was not included in the analysis, and in some trials, the anticoagulation was stopped early and strokes occurring later were not mentioned or included in the analysis even though strokes occurring in the control patients throughout the trial were included. In all the trials added together, there was a total of 26 strokes that were evenly distributed between the anticoagulated and control groups. It is quite impossible to conclude that anticoagulation is either effective or ineffective in reducing the risk of stroke. Unless there is a revival in interest in this form of treatment, there never will be an adequate trial, and we will never know whether this potentially useful treatment has been discarded in error.

ANTIPLATELET DRUGS

Aspirin

Currently, the most promising antiplatelet drug, and certainly the one that we are most familiar with, is aspirin. The Canadian Co-operative Study Group trial of aspirin in threatened stroke (5) revealed a 31% risk-reduction in stroke and/or death attributable to aspirin, 325 mg q.d.s. However, the 95% confidence limits of this result would have embraced a zero risk reduction and, even with nearly 600 patients, the trial may have been too small to identify a rather modest treatment effect with certainty, if this effect is really true. The greater benefit in males, and the greater risk of stroke in females taking aspirin compared to those not taking aspirin, was a surprising finding that requires examination in further trials before the conclusion can be made that aspirin is appropriate for men, but contraindicated for women. This trial was somewhat complicated by the two-by-two factorial design that allowed a simultaneous examination of the effect of another antiplatelet drug, sulphinpyrazone. Although not statistically significant, there was a trend towards synergism between aspirin and sulphinpyrazone, and the overall effect of aspirin was not reflected in the group taking aspirin only; 26 strokes and/or deaths occurred compared with 27.2 expected on the null hypothesis that the outcome in all four groups would be the same. This might have been a chance effect in a group of patients that was not particularly large but is something of an embarrassment to those who are convinced that aspirin is an effective drug. There have been two other trials that were too small to draw meaningful and reliable conclusions (7,8,12).

By itself, the Canadian trial is not enough to recommend that all TIA patients, or perhaps all male TIA patients, should be given aspirin 325 mg q.d.s. for life. Therefore, another, larger trial is underway in the United Kingdom (the UK-TIA Aspirin Trial) (13) in which approximately 2,000 patients are being allocated randomly to aspirin 600 mg b.d., 300 mg daily, and placebo. The lower dose has been included since there is some evidence that a low, infrequent dose of aspirin may be more, or as effective, as an antithrombotic agent. Unfortunately, how low and how infrequent this dose needs to be is debatable and, in the end, only clinical trials will answer this question.

Sulphinpyrazone

Sulphinpyrazone was tested in the Canadian trial but reduced the risk of stroke only by a statistically insignificant 10%. By itself, it is probably not worth pursuing but in combination with aspirin, there might be a synergistic effect that could be usefully explored in further trials.

Dipyridamole

Alone, dipyridamole is unlikely to be a useful antithrombotic drug but in combination with aspirin, there is theoretical evidence that the antihaemostatic effect of aspirin is enhanced. Unfortunately, the theory was not borne out in practice in a large trial after myocardial infarction (10) and so far, no trial in TIA patients has been completed, although several are underway.

CONCLUSIONS

At the moment there is no compelling reason to use any antithrombotic drug in TIA patients, although in a patient with frequent and frightening attacks it may be worth at least a short-term trial of anticoagulation or aspirin to see if the attacks can be stopped. If it is felt that a TIA patient must be offered something, even if nothing is definitely useful, I would favour aspirin 600 mg b.d. However, my own opinion is that further trials are essential and in my own practice patients are entered into the UK-TIA Aspirin Trial. If too many physicians insist on using aspirin despite the lack of evidence favouring its efficacy and too few burden themselves with clinical trials, we shall never know which treatments are useful and, in a few years, we will have abandoned aspirin in favour of some new and more fashionable treatment. Perhaps it is only the treatments that change while our inability to evaluate them remains the same.

REFERENCES

1. Baker, R. N., Broward, J. A., Fisher, C. M., Groch, S. N., Heyman, A., Karp, H. R., McDevitt, E., Scheinberg, P., Schwartz, W., and Toole, J. F. (1962): Anticoagulant therapy in cerebral infarction. Report on co-operative study. *Neurology*, 12:823–829.
2. Baker, R. N., Ramseyer, J. C., and Schwartz, W. S. (1968): Prognosis in patients with transient cerebral ischaemic attacks. *Neurology*, 18:1157–1165.
3. Baker, R. N., Schwartz, W. S., and Rose, A. S. (1966): Transient ischaemic strokes. A report of a study of anticoagulant therapy. *Neurology*, 16:841–847.
4. Bradshaw, P., and Brennan, S. (1975): Trial of long-term anticoagulant therapy in the treatment of small stroke associated with a normal carotid angiogram. *J. Neurol. Neurosurg. Psychiat.*, 38:642–647.
5. Canadian Co-operative Study Group (1978): A randomized trial of aspirin and sulphinpyrazone in threatened stroke. *N. Engl. J. Med.*, 299:53–59.
6. De Bono, D. P., and Warlow, C. P. (1981): Potential sources of emboli in patients with presumed transient cerebral or retinal ischaemia. *Lancet*, i:343–346.
7. Fields, W. S., Lemak, N. A., Frankowski, R. F., and Hardy, R. J. (1977): Controlled trials of aspirin in cerebral ischaemia. *Stroke*, 8:301–315.
8. Fields, W. S., Lemak, N. A., Frankowski, R. F., and Hardy, R. J. (1978): Controlled trial of aspirin in cerebral ischaemia. Part II—Surgical Group. *Stroke*, 9:309–318.
9. Pearce, J. M. S., Gubbay, S. S., and Walton, J. N. (1965): Long-term anticoagulant therapy in transient cerebral ischaemic attacks. *Lancet*, i:6–9.
10. Persantine-Aspirin Reinfarction Study Research Group. (1980): Persantine and aspirin in coronary heart disease. *Circulation*, 62:449–461.
11. Peto, R. (1978): 'Clinical Trial Methodology'. *Biomedicine, (Special issue)* 28:24–36.
12. Reuther, R., and Dorndorf, W. (1978): Aspirin in patients with cerebral ischaemia and normal angiograms or non-surgical lesions. The results of a double-blind trial. In: *Acetylsalicylic Acid in Cerebral Ischaemia and Coronary Heart Disease*, edited by K. Breddin, W. Dorndorf, D. Loew, and R. Marx, pp. 97–106. F. K. Schattauer Verlag, Stuttgart.
13. UK-TIA Study Group. (1979): Design and protocol of the UK-TIA Aspirin Study. In: *Drug Treatment and Prevention in Cerebrovascular Disorders*, edited by G. Tognoni and S. Garattini, pp. 387–394. Elsevier, Amsterdam.
14. Veterans Administration. (1961): An evaluation of anticoagulant therapy in the treatment of cerebrovascular disease. *Neurology*, 11:132–138.

15. Warlow, C. P. (1981): Transient ischaemic attacks. In: *Recent Advances in Clinical Neurology, Volume 3*, edited by W. B. Matthews and G. H. Glaser. Churchill Livingstone, Edinburgh.
16. Whisnant, J. P., Matsumoto, N., and Elveback, L. R. (1973): Transient cerebral ischaemic attacks in a community. Rochester, Minnesota—1955 through 1969. *Mayo Clin. Proc.*, 48:194–198.

Advances in Stroke Therapy, edited by
F. C. Rose. Raven Press, New York © 1982.

European Stroke Prevention Study**

*A. Lowenthal, **T. J. Steiner, and **F. Clifford Rose

*Department of Neurology, Independent Umiversity of Antwerp, B-2610 Wilrijk, Belgium;
and **Stroke Unit, Department of Neurology, Charing Cross Hospital,
London W6 8RF, England*

In 1976, in recognition of the need for further therapeutic advances in prevention of stroke in those with cerebrovascular disease, proposals were discussed in the Department of Neurology, Charing Cross Hospital, for a new, major, clinical trial of antiplatelet medication. The initial protocol was developed and then piloted at Charing Cross and Hillingdon Hospitals. The study would be double-blind, randomised, placebo controlled, and assess the combination of aspirin (ASA), 1.0 g daily, and dipyridamole (Persantin), 225 mg daily. The end-points would be death and stroke.

Following a meeting at Charing Cross Hospital in 1979 of all physicians who intended to participate, the study was launched on a multicentre, multinational basis. A second meeting in Antwerp in 1981 discussed modifications of the protocol in the light of the broadened experience. The study takes place after others in the same field whose areas of success or failure were then known.

The proposals upon which the protocol was finally based can be summarised as follows:

a. Cerebrovascular disease is defined as a degenerative disorder of arteries that supply the brain. It leads to central nervous system lesions that are ischaemic or haemorrhagic and associated with the clinically recognised condition of "stroke," where the acute onset of lasting neurological deficit results. The European study recognises the clear pathological distinction between cerebrovascular lesions that are primarily haemorrhagic and those primarily ischaemic, even though there may be aetiological overlap. The study concerns only the prevention of ischaemic cerebral infarction. By virtue of the progressive nature of cerebrovascular disease, certain patients may be recognised as "stroke-prone" before the onset of stroke. It is in these patients that prophylactic therapy of proven value is desirable. Those with a previous history of transient cerebral ischaemic attack (TIA), reversible ischaemic neurological deficit (RIND), or ischaemic cerebral infarction are specifically at risk of cerebral infarction in the future, the degree of risk falling with time at least for the first few months following the previous episode.

b. The diagnosis of TIA, RIND, or cerebral infarction is made clinically. The study protocol recognises both the desirability and the impracticality of excluding

143

in every case, by computerized axial tomography (CAT) scan, intracerebral haemorrhage and space occupying lesions presenting with stroke-like syndromes. The study documentation therefore asks for as thorough an investigative assessment of all relevant systems as can be obtained reasonably if CAT scanning is not available. Cerebral angiography is required only where clinically appropriate, which may be in a high proportion of cases potentially eligible for the study, since the indications for consideration of arterial reconstruction are similar to those for trial entry. Where angiography is carried out, an aetiologically based diagnosis may be possible with a high degree of confidence but those in whom surgical correction is undertaken become ineligible for the study.

Clinical signs do not necessarily parallel the results of investigations: Transient symptoms presenting as a TIA may be associated with CAT scan evidence of significant infarction. Clinical subdivision of the patients at entry into TIA, RIND, and infarct groups will nonetheless be maintained for classification of results.

c. Patients are admitted within 3 months of the qualifying ischaemic episode and assessed thereafter at least every 3 months for 2 years. Apart from the record of end-points, the usual attention is paid to recurrences of TIA or RIND, other changes in clinical condition of the patient, side effects, intercurrent illness, and other medication newly introduced.

d. Assessment of results will be affected by numerous factors: the variable natural history of the disease and its clinical characteristics even when aetiological uniformity has been aimed for, the nature, size, and number of lesions and their site, metabolic influences and those of other systemic disorders, genetic, racial, environmental, and social characteristics. This implies that a large number of patients must participate.

e. For this reason, the study will admit at least 2,500 patients over a period of 3 to 5 years at 14 European centres. Such a study, carried out double-blind and stratified, requires a relatively complex but important coordinating structure. Interpretation of the outcome will be managed by an independent statistician but ultimate control rests with a steering committee whose members are the heads of the participating departments of neurology.

PARTICIPATING CENTRES

GREAT BRITAIN

F. Clifford Rose
(Chairman, Steering Committee)
Physician-in-Charge
and T. J. Steiner
Lecturer in Experimental Neurology
Department of Neurology
Charing Cross Hospital (Fulham)
Fulham Palace Road
London W6 8RF

J. D. Carroll
Royal Surrey County Hospital
Farnham Road
Guilford
Surrey GU2 5LX

D. Park
Consultant Neurologist
Southend General Hospital
Cricclewell Chase
Westcliff-on-Sea
Essex SS0 0RZ

D. J. Fisher
Consultant Physician
Cardiff Royal Infirmary
Newport Road,
Cardiff CR2 1SZ

B. S. C. Sastry
West Wing
Cardiff Royal Infirmary
Newport Road,
Cardiff CR2 1SZ

EIRE

R. J. Galvin
Consultant Neurologist
Cork Regional Hospital
Wilton
Cork
Eire

N. Callaghan
Consultant Neurologist
Cork Regional Hospital
Wilton
Cork
Eire

BELGIUM

A. Lowenthal
(Chairman, Coordinating Centre)
and A. Boogers
Independent University of Antwerp
Universiteitsplein 1
B-2610 Wilrijk

G. Franck
Hôpital de Bavière
Neurologie-Electroencéphalographie
Bd de la Constitution 66
4020 Liege

C. H. Laterre
Cliniques Universitaires St-Luc
Service de Neurologie
Avenue Hippocrate 10
1200 Bruxelles

HOLLAND

J. W. Ten Cate
Wilhelmina Gasthuis
Afdeling Hematologie
Eerste Helmersstraat 104
Amsterdam

J. Vos
Sint Lucas Ziekenhuis
Afdeling Neurologie
Jan Tooropstraat 164
1061 AE Amsterdam

FINLAND

P. Riekkinen
Professor and Chairman
Department of Neurology
University of Kuopio
P.O. Box 138
SF-70101 Kuopio 10

DENMARK

The Neurological Department F,
3rd Floor
Aarhus Municipal Hospital
DK-8000 Aarhus C.

Advances in Stroke Therapy, edited by
F. C. Rose. Raven Press, New York © 1982.

A Long-Term Randomized Trial of Antiaggregant Drugs in Threatened Stroke

A. Rascol, B. Guiraud-Chaumeil, B. Boneu,
J. David, and M. Clanet

Service de Neurologie—CHU Toulouse Purpan, Toulouse, France

The purpose of this chapter is to present the results of a randomized trial aiming at the prevention of stroke and vascular death by antiaggregant drugs in patients who have had either a transient ischemic attack (TIA) or a minor stroke. In such conditions, French patients and physicians customarily resorted to long-term treatment with drugs like papaverine or hydergine. In 1972, after the publication of some results on the positive effects of aspirin, we decided to try to answer the question: "Does the addition of antiaggregant drugs to hydergine reduce the risk of major stroke and death in this kind of patient?" and set up the randomized trial presented here.

METHOD

In this randomized trial, we compared the evolution, for at least 3 years, of three groups of patients, each of which received different treatments:

Group I: Hydergine per os 4.5 mg/day
Group II: Hydergine 4.5 mg + Aspirin 1 g/day
Group III: Hydergine 4.5 + Aspirin 1 g/day + Dipyridamole 150 mg/day

Because of the question asked, no placebo group was necessary. The trial was not double blind due to the length of the follow up; it did not seem ethical to leave both patients and their family physicians unaware of the treatment they were to follow for as long as 3 to 6 years.

It was a single-center trial. Four neurologists took part in the recruitment, two being responsible for the follow-up. All the biological examinations took place in the same laboratory. A secretary and a computer center coordinated the trial.

The number of patients required for the study was estimated on the basis of the information available in the literature in 1972 regarding the occurrence of stroke after TIA. It is well known how unreliable, and even divergent, are the data (2,10). A fairly reasonable estimate of a major stroke following a TIA or a minor stroke is approximately 20% over 3 years. This estimate is quite close to that of the Mayo

Clinic (11,12) and to that, more recently, of Fields (22% at 42 months) (6). The statisticians thought it necessary to have 100 patients (followed for 3 years) in each group but, taking into account the potential drop-out, we decided to carry out our study with 450 patients (150 × 3).

We included patients who had one or more focal TIAs or minor strokes, vertebrobasilar as well as carotid, within 3 months of the inclusion date. Isolated vertigo, loss of consciousness, transient global amnesia, and epileptic seizures were excluded as were strokes of infectious, inflammatory, haematological, and migraineous etiology. Also excluded were patients with evident cardiac embolism (a small percentage of patients with cardiac dysrhythmia was included in all three groups when the etiological diagnosis of cardiac embolism or atheromatous arterial disease was not definite), congestive heart failure, long-term treatment with anticoagulants, aspirin or antiinflammatory drugs, and surgical cases.

Cerebral angiography was not mandatory and the finding of a surgically accessible arterial stenosis did not necessarily lead to an operation. The study was randomized on a preestablished chance table to one of the three treatments.

Risk factors were systematically noted and medically treated when possible. Follow-up was carried out by two of us for each patient through a standardized examination, both clinical and with special investigations every 4 months for at least 3 years.

Compliance to treatment was assessed in different ways. Patients bought "hydergine" and "claragine," every purchase being controlled by "Sécurité Sociale" reimbursement. The "Persantin-Aspirin" treatment was given every control examination and controlled by pill-count. The efficiency of antiaggregating drugs was assessed by platelet aggregation tests performed at each control examination. No drug estimation of the blood was made.

During follow-up, patients were excluded who did not carefully follow the treatment instructions or supervision rules, had a therapeutic accident, or developed severe chronic disease.

"End of trial" patients were those who died because of vascular death (cerebral or extracerebral) and those who had a cerebral infarct, irrespective of the neurological deficit. Recurrent TIAs were not considered as end of trial, but were numbered.

The therapeutic results were analyzed using Kaplan-Meier's actuarial method. Classical statistical methods were used to assess the homogeneity of the three groups and to analyze the group of patients who had systematically followed the rules set up for the trial, as well as patients who had been excluded.

RESULTS

Four hundred and forty patients (181 TIA, 259 minor strokes) were included between June 1973 and July 1976. The trial came to an end August 1, 1979.
- 247 patients (56.2%) had their accident in the carotid artery
- 134 patients (31.2%) had their accident in the vertebrobasilar territory

• in 59 patients (13.2%), it was difficult to determine precisely the territory

The main characteristics of included patients are presented in Table 1. Analysis reveals that the three groups are homogeneous for the type of accident that induced inclusion, age, sex, risk factors, and number of angiographies.

The greater number of male patients can be explained by the way in which patients were recruited for 2 years: Males were collected in both clinics and wards whereas females were collected in clinics only.

The following data illustrates the diversity of types of lesions found in 256 patients with angiography:

• normal: 49 cases
• lesions located on vertebrobasilar arteries: 64 cases
• (isolated 43, associated with carotid artery lesions 21)
• On carotid arteries: 143 cases
  —- Of these 143 carotid artery lesions:
      intracranial branch occlusions: 59
      intracranial internal carotid artery lesions: 11
      extracranial carotid artery occlusions: 18
      extracranial carotid artery stenosis:

TABLE 1. Main characteristics of included patients

	Hydergine	Hydergine + aspirin	Hydergine + aspirin + dipyridamole
Number	155	147	138
TIA	45%	37%	40%
RIA	55%	63%	60%
Mean age (years)	63(± 9)	62.2(± 9.8)	62(±9.7)
Less than 40 years	0	1.36%	0.72%
40–54 years	21.29%	18.37%	21.74%
55–64 years	29.03%	40.13%	21.74%
65 years +	49.68%	40.13%	41.30%
Men	85.81%	85.71%	83.33%
Women	14.19%	14.29%	16.67%
Arteriography	53.50%	61.90%	59.40%
Hypertension			
Systolic ≤160	49.68%	51.02%	47.83%
Diastolic ≤ 95	10.30%	10.40%	8.30%
Coronary insufficiency	9.68%	10.20%	10.87%
Paroxysmal arythmia	0.64%	2.04%	1.45%
Continuous arythmia	8.38%	5.44%	3.62%
Myocardial infarction	7. %	2.70%	8.70%
Hyperglycemia 3.60 N 6.10 mmol/l	10.30%	10.40%	8.30%
Hyperuricemia 150 N 476 μmol/l	29.03%	27.21%	28.26%
Hypercholesterolemia 3.35 N 6.50 mmol/l	8.39%	14.29%	14.49%
Hypertriglyceridemia 0.35 N 1.70 mmol/l	11.61%	14.97%	12.32%

— $\geq 85\%:15$
— between 25 and 85%:10
— $\leq 25\%:30$

The results of our follow-up study, based on Kaplan-Meier's method, are shown in Tables 1, 2, and 3.

Table 1 shows the evolution after 3 years of each of the three groups, on the single basis of the outcome as a major stroke. No significant difference was found between the three groups, and there are only 6 to 7% major strokes after 3 years.

During the initial period (the first year) when the risk of recurrence is highest (as indicated by the Mayo Clinic study); there is an insignificant difference between lines corresponding to groups II and III (with antiaggregant drugs) and the line corresponding to group I (exclusively hydergine), but this difference is not statistically significant.

Table 2 shows similar results when major and minor strokes are added together.

Table 3 shows the same results when strokes and vascular deaths are added together.

Direct analysis distinguishes two populations: First, there were 299 patients who followed systematically the rules set for the trial. This group shows evidence of the very same profile as the whole population included in the study. Of these, 15 had a new TIA, 27 (or 9%) had a stroke, of which six were minor and 21 (or 7%) were major.

Of these 27 strokes, 7 (or 25%) occurred in an arterial territory different from the one that led to inclusion (Table 2). Thirteen died due to vascular cause (or

TABLE 2. Topography of next TIA and restroke

	TIA 15	Minor stroke 6	Major stroke 21
Good concordance	12	5	15
No concordance	3	1	6

TABLE 3. Excluded patients

	Hydergine N = 63	Hydergine + aspirin N = 45	Hydergine + aspirin + dipyridamol N = 33	Total N = 141
Wrong diagnosis	9	7	7	23
Associated diseases	7	10	6	23
Lost to follow-up	3	8	3	14
Failure to take study medication	44	20	17	81

4.3%). In the second group, we found 141 patients who had been excluded (Table 3), 81 due to poor compliance. However, we were able to check their outcome at the end of 3 years, and 16 (or 19.3%) had a stroke, 7 (or 8.6%) died due to vascular cause.

We were particularly interested in the evolution of lesions of the internal carotid artery (Table 4). Of 15 patients with a tight stenosis regularly followed for more than 3 years, only 2 had a stroke.

The side effects of therapy were carefully noted and are shown in Table 5. (Patients with evidence of a peptic ulcer were excluded.)

DISCUSSION

The answer to our initial question is that addition of antiaggregating drugs to Hydergine did not modify substantially the outcome of cerebral infarct or vascular death in our population.

TABLE 4. Evolution of lesions of internal carotid artery

		With recurrence	Without recurrence	Other disease	Lost to follow-up
Occlusion					
Good follow-up	14	0	11	3	0
Bad follow-up	4	2	1	1	
Stenosis ≥ 85%					
Good follow-up	15	2	11	2	0
Bad follow-up	0	0	0	0	0
Stenosis 25 to 85%					
Good follow-up	8	0	7	1	0
Bad follow-up	2	0	2	0	0
Atheromatous plaques ≤25%					
Good follow-up	22	3	18	1	0
Bad follow-up	8	1	3	2	2

TABLE 5. Therapeutic side effects

Drug	Reaction	Number patients
Hydergine	Indigestion	1
Hydergine + Aspirin	Indigestion	3
	Melena	1
	Hemorrhage	1
Hydergine + Aspirin + Dipyridamole	Indigestion	4 (aspirin)
	Skin allergy	1 (dipyridamole)
Total		11

Our results are very close to the results of Fields (7,8) who found no significant reduction in the risk of stroke or death and differ from the positive findings by the Canadian Group (4,5). Furthermore in our study no difference was found between the sexes. It is difficult and dangerous to compare these different studies, as the questions posed are not strictly the same and, despite similar inclusion criteria, differences can appear in the patients, e.g., surgically accessible carotid lesions represent 63% of patients with ischemia in the territory supplied by the carotid artery in the Canadian Study, while we had only 25%.

It could be argued that the aspirin dose was too high, taking into account papers published since 1973 (3) on prostacyclin and the suggestion that "lower" doses of aspirin would have a better antithrombotic effect, but, as far as we know, no clinical study has yet been published regarding these findings.

It could also be argued that our population was not homogeneous. We did carefully exclude patients with nonatheromatous stroke but, among atheromatous strokes, we are aware that there are different physiopathologic mechanisms. It was impossible for us in 1973 to distinguish homogeneous groups with accuracy on the basis of physiopathological types, but hope that randomization divided them evenly between the three groups.

At the end of the 3 year follow-up, we found only a relatively small percentage of recurrent stroke as compared to that found in the literature. Whether these results depend upon hydergine or antiaggregating drugs is unclear, but it seems most likely that continuous control of risk factors throughout follow-up plays a prominent part in this positive result, which is of relevance in choosing between surgical and pharmacological treatments.

REFERENCES

1. Barnett, H. J. M., Gent, M., Sackett, D. L., and Taylor, D. W. (1980): Randomized trial of therapy with platelet antiaggregants for threatened stroke. 2: Observations on the pathogenesis and natural history of threatened stroke. *CMA J.*, 122:535–539.
2. Brust, J. C. M. (1977): Transient ischemic attacks: natural history and anticoagulation. *Neurology (Minneap.)*, 27:701–707.
3. Burch, J. W., Stanford, N., and Majerns, P. W. (1978): Inhibition of platelet prostaglandin synthetase by oral aspirin. *J. Clin. Invest.*, 61:314–319.
4. The Canadian Cooperative Stroke Study Group. (1980): Randomized trial of therapy with platelet antiaggregants for threatened stroke. *CMA J.*, 122:293–296.
5. The Canadian Cooperative Study Group. (1979): A randomized trial of Aspirin and sulfinpyrazone in threatened stroke. *N. Engl. J. Med.*, 299:53–59.
6. Fields, W. S. (1981): Traitement chirurgical ou medical dans l'ischémie transitoire? *Rev. Neurol.*, 137:305–318.
7. Fields, W. S., Lamak, A. N., Frankowski, R. F., and Hardy, R. J. (1978): Controlled trial aspirin in cerebral ischemia. Part II: Surgical group. *Stroke*, 9:309–319.
8. Fields, W. S., Lemak, A. N., Frankowski, R. F., Hardy, R. J. (1977): Controlled trial aspirin in cerebral ischemia. *Stroke*, 8:301–316.
9. Jaffe, E. A., and Weksler, B. B. (1979): Recovery of endolbeliol cell protacyclin production after inhibition by low doses of aspirin. *J. Clin. Invest.*, 63:532–535.
10. Laugie, B. (1978): Histoire naturelle des accidents ischémiques transitoires. *Thèse Toulouse. Revue de la Littérature.* p. 133.
11. Whisnant, J. P., Matsumoto, N., and Elveback, L. R. (1973): A.I.T. in a community. Rochester 1955 through 1969. *Mayo Clin. Proc.*, 48:194–198.

12. Whisnant, J. P., Matsumoto, N. and Elveback, L. R. (1973): The effect of anticaogulant therapy on the prognosis of patients with cerebral ischemic attacks in a community. Rochester, Minnesota 1955 through 1969. *Mayo Clin. Proc.*, 48:845–848.

Advances in Stroke Therapy, edited by
F. C. Rose. Raven Press, New York © 1982.

Use of Sulphinpyrazone in the Prevention of Restroke and Stroke in Man

M. Gawel and F. Clifford Rose

*Stroke Unit, Department of Neurology, Charing Cross Hospital,
London W6 8RF, England*

The studies of Burns et al. (3) showed that a thio derivative of phenylbutazone was metabolised in man to a sulphoxide, sulphinpyrazone, that was found to have potent uricosuric properties, and was introduced for the treatment of chronic gout. Sulphinpyrazone is metabolised in man by the introduction of the hydroxyl group in the para position of the benzene ring (4); this hydroxy derivative is rapidly metabolised and excreted, and also has uricosuric properties. A thioether metabolite was later isolated (14).

Dieterle et al. (6) studied the absorption, transformation, and elimination of sulphinpyrazone in human male volunteers. They found that absorption from the gastrointestinal tract was rapid and complete, the plasma concentrations of the unchanged drug reaching maximum values after about 1 or 2 hr. The half-life in the two subjects, calculated from the decline by 3 and 8 hr, was 2.7 and 2.2 hr. There were four specifically determined metabolites: the sulphone, the parahydroxy compound, the full hydroxy compound and the thioether compound. A large proportion was excreted as the unchanged drug in the volunteers; about 8.2 and 8.8% was present as the parahydroxy metabolite, 2.7 and 3% as the sulphone metabolite; and .6 and .8% as the full hydroxy metabolite. Thus 95% of the total radioactivity was recovered within 4 days, 85% from the urine and 10% from the faeces.

For a long time, sulphinpyrazone was used as uricosuric agent but in 1965, it was shown to inhibit platelet function by Smyth et al. (17). Sulphinpyrazone inhibits platelet release with collagen and adrenalin, prolongs bleeding time in human volunteers in chronic dosage, and inhibits MDH production (16). It also has been shown to prolong the reduced platelet survival seen in some patients with gout, prosthetic heart valves, coronary heart disease, rheumatic valvulitis, and recurrent venous thrombosis (19–22). The thioether metabolite is responsible for most antiplatelet activity (15) and, although the actual mechanism of the inhibitory effect on platelet function is not completely known, it is thought to be due to inhibition of thromboxane synthetase. This effect is reversible and can be removed by washing and resuspending the platelets, suggesting that the effect of sulphinpyrazone, unlike that of aspirin, is reversible. The effect of sulphinpyrazone on platelet function lasts only as long as the drug is present in the circulation.

PREVIOUS STUDIES

Historically, sulphinpyrazone was among the first antiplatelet drugs to be used in the treatment of thromboembolic phenomena and more specifically, in the prevention of strokes following transient ischaemic attacks as well as restroke. Evans (8) showed a reduction in frequency of attacks of amaurosis fugax in a small double-blind, crossover study. Blakely and Gent (2) showed that sulphinpyrazone appeared to reduce the frequency of death from vascular causes in patients in a geriatric home, but the cause of death was not defined by autopsy, and there have been other criticisms of this study. The findings initiated a number of other studies of sulphinpyrazone, both singly and in combination with other drugs, in the prevention of stroke following transient ischaemic attacks (TIAs) and in the prevention of restroke.

Sulphinpyrazone also has been used in the prevention of other thromboembolic events such as recurrent venous thrombosis (12), where the reduced platelet survival found in these patients is prolonged by the use of this treatment. Similarly Kaegi (12), using two prospective double-blind studies, showed that sulphinpyrazone reduces the frequency of shunt thrombosis in patients with arteriovenous shunts used for chronic haemodialysis; in this group, the benefit was more marked in men than in women. Steel et al. (18) found that sulphinpyrazone also prolongs the shortened survival time found in patients following aortic valve replacement and made the observation that all of the patients with Starr Edwards valves and a history of postoperative thromboembolism had shortened platelet survival, although many patients without a history of thromboembolism also had a shortened platelet survival. They made the assumption that these patients may be at risk and that the measurement of platelet survival was a valid technique to detect such at risk population.

The use of sulphinpyrazone in TIAs was reported by Steel et al. (18), who studied 25 patients whose episodes of cerebral ischaemia were in the carotid artery distribution; three had transient monocular blindness. There were 21 men and 4 women. Nine of the patients had had carotid arteriography that demonstrated occlusive arteriosclerosis of the carotid artery in all. Platelet survival half-time was measured using chromium labeling and was shortened in all patients, the average being 2.5 days which was significantly different from the norm of 3.7 days ($p < 0.001$). Sulphinpyrazone treatment significantly increased platelet survival time in these patients from 2.4 to 2.8 days and in four patients, the platelet survival time was rendered completely normal. In 10 of the 19 patients treated with sulphinpyrazone, there were no more episodes, an effect that has been maintained. No patient on treatment had a stroke while, of the six patients who did not get sulphinpyrazone, two had a stroke, one had a reduction in frequency of TIAs, and there was no change in frequency in the other three. The clinical effect of the sulphinpyrazone could be predicted from the alteration in platelet survival time; of 10 patients with a marked reduction in frequency of ischaemic attacks, there was an increase in platelet survival time in seven, four of whom were normal. This encouraging trial suggested that platelet survival could be used to detect patients at risk for TIA, and that platelet survival could be altered with sulphinpyrazone treatment with consequent clinical benefit.

MULTICENTRE TRIALS IN PREVENTION OF STROKE

Two trials were initiated to assess the clinical benefit of antithrombotic therapy in the prevention of stroke. The first was coordinated in the United States by Fields (9), begun in 1972 and continuing for 37 months. There were 178 patients with carotid TIAs who were randomly allocated to aspirin or placebo to determine the incidence of subsequent TIAs, cerebral or retinal infarction, and death. The results were disappointing in that significant differences in favour of the aspirin group were found only when all the end-points were grouped together. If TIA was excluded as an end-point, there was no statistically significant difference between the aspirin and placebo treatments.

The second trial, which assessed the effects of antithrombotic therapy on occurrence of TIAs or stroke, was a collaborative study organised by Barnett (5) in Canada and published in 1978. In this trial, 585 patients with threatened stroke were followed in a randomised, clinical trial for an average of 26 months to determine whether aspirin or sulphinpyrazone, either separately or in combination, influenced the subsequent occurrence of TIA, stroke, or death. Eighty-five subjects developed a stroke, 42 of whom died. Aspirin reduced the risk of continuing ischaemic attacks, stroke, or death when taken together by 19% and also reduced the risk for stroke or death by 31%. This effect was most marked in the men, where the risk reduction was 48% for stroke and death ($p < .005$), but there was no significant change among women. In the group given sulphinpyrazone alone, there was no reduction in TIA and a small and not significant reduction in the risk of stroke or death. The conclusions made from this study were that there was no synergistic effect between aspirin and sulphinpyrazone, but reexamining the data suggests that there may well be a tendency for synergism, since the differential results always show a trend in favour of the combined medication. In this study, there was a significant number of patients with what would now be called residual ischaemic neurological deficits, i.e., minor strokes. Whether these should be considered TIAs, i.e., patients with recovery within 24 hr, is a matter for debate and has been discussed in detail by Kurtzke (13). Perhaps the clinical distinction is not so important, since we are interested in prevention of stroke in patients clearly at risk.

One criticism of both the Canadian and American studies as well as other studies of antithrombotic therapy in TIAs, including a very recent one from Argentina (11), is that TIAs are grouped together as end-points with stroke or death. There is no evidence at present that the frequency of TIAs is clearly related to the subsequent development of stroke or that the pathogenesis of transient cerebral ischaemia is always identical to that of stroke. The two events are linked epidemiologically but there may be a different pathophysiological substrate. Another trial of sulphinpyrazone in the treatment of TIAs was reported by Hassan et al. (10), but patients who had had a stroke were excluded from further analysis, so that this trial does not help in assessing the drug in the prevention of stroke.

THE CHARING CROSS STUDY

Because of the preceding considerations, we were prompted to carry out a double-blind trial of sulphinpyrazone and placebo in the prevention of restroke in a group of patients who had had cerebral infarction as shown either by computerized tomography (CT scan), angiography, or gamma scanning, and who were not candidates for surgical intervention. The patients were stratified according to age, sex, number of strokes, and history of smoking. The active group was given sulphinpyrazone (Anturan) 200 mg tablets four times a day, while the control group had identical placebo tablets. Patients were entered several weeks after onset of stroke to ensure that any concurrent problems had settled and that improvement was reaching a plateau. There were 30 patients on placebo medication and 25 patients on active medication. The average age in the Anturan group was 67.7 ± 8.8 years. During the trial, both groups showed good improvement in their general state apart from those who achieved end-points. There were five end-points in the active group all of which were nonfatal stroke while in the placebo group, there were seven end-points, two of which were myocardial infarctions leading to death, the others being nonfatal strokes. During the trial, levels of beta thromboglobulin (BTG), a platelet release reaction-specific protein, were measured in both groups and later, fibrinopeptide A and BB1-42 were also assayed. The former is a measure of fibrinogen activation and the latter is a measure of plasmin activity; the levels of both the BTG and fibrinopeptides in the two groups were not statistically different. We found no evidence of any effect on BTG levels in the Anturan treated group. The trial was stopped on January 1, 1981 after an average follow-up time of 1.5 years for an analysis of results. Although the patient numbers were small, we found very little evidence of any influence of sulphinpyrazone on this particular aspect of platelet function or on the occurrence of restroke, the incidence being identical in the two groups, although there were two myocardial infarctions in the placebo group.

DISCUSSION

It may be argued that the numbers in the Charing Cross Study were so small that any benefit would have been obscured, but the patients were very carefully examined and followed up at regular intervals so that any minor changes such as TIAs or minimal deterioration would have been noted; this is important since not all restroke is manifested by a massive increase in disability. A recent paper (1) by Blakely examined 1,260 geriatric patients who had recovered from the acute effects of stroke and were identified in chronic care hospitals. Stroke had been attributed to thrombosis in 794 patients but those with acetonaemia, hyperuricaemia, anaemia, gout, bleeding diathesis, active peptic ulcer, malignancy, severe disability, poor immediate prognosis, and who were on antiplatelet or anticoagulant therapy were excluded. Eventually 290 patients consented and were randomly allocated sulphinpyrazone 800 mg daily, or placebo. Patients were followed double-blind until December, 1978. Randomisation was stratified for age, sex, normal or abnormal ECG, and interval of more or less than 6 months since onset of stroke. Over the course of the study, 107 ceased to take medication, 52 in the treatment and 55 in the placebo group; all but 6 were followed to the end of the study. There were 53 deaths, 25 in the treated and 28 in the placebo group, and 44 of the patients had stopped taking the study medication at the time of death. The overall mortality rates did not suggest that sulphinpyrazone improved survival after recovery from presumed thrombotic stroke.

The evidence regarding the efficacy of Anturan seems at first sight conflicting, since some studies suggest that sulphinpyrazone has a beneficial effect whereas the more recent assessment by Blakely and our study are against this view, but closer examination may clarify the issue. The trials performed by Barnett and the trials of platelet survival in TIAs were looking at platelet-related phenomena, i.e. TIAs and measurements of platelet behaviour such as platelet survival. Apart from the study on platelet survival in patients with TIAs, there is at present no clear evidence that there is any chronic platelet abnormality between episodes of TIAs, and certainly, our results, using BTG as a marker, would support this view. The study of Dougherty et al. (7) suggested that there may be transient platelet activation during the ischaemic phase, but this may be secondary to cerebral ischaemia. With increasing realisation of the effects of cardiac and atheroembolic factors in the aetiology of transient cerebral ischaemia and stroke, it may be that the platelet does not necessarily play a central role.

The findings of platelet emboli in the circulation may be due to platelet activation secondary to an episode of ischaemia. Even if platelets are activated and are primary in causing transient cerebral ischaemic attacks there is a difference between transient cerebral ischaemia and stroke. In our study of acute strokes examining BTG and fibrinopeptide levels, we found that there was no activation of platelets as measured by BTG following acute, cerebral infarction. There was an activation of fibrinopeptide A, and B, indicating an activation of the thrombin and plasmin system. Thus it may be possible to prevent TIAs in patients and yet not influence their likelihood of getting a stroke, except in a number of especially susceptible individuals.

We have found some indirect evidence for this in one patient who had TIAs in 1975 with normal carotid angiography and who was placed on aspirin therapy. Over the next 5 years, his TIAs never recurred, but noninvasive assessment of his carotid system showed that a 50% stenosis had developed while on aspirin therapy. Clearly this stenosis could have progressed further and could have caused carotid occlusion, and yet this man has been on active therapy with complete cessation of TIAs. Further evidence for the necessity for differentiating between TIAs and stroke is provided by the two huge trials of antithrombotic therapy where, only by lumping end-points, were any significant changes found. This is perhaps overstating the case, but the question of the involvement of platelets and other coagulation factors in the aetiology of both TIA and stroke needs to be evaluated further.

REFERENCES

1. Blakely, J. A. (1979): From: *7th International Congress on Thrombosis and Haemostasis*, Stuttgart.
2. Blakely, J. A., and Gent, M. (1977): Platelets, drugs and longevity in a geriatric population. In: *Platelets, Drugs and Thrombosis*, edited by J. Hirsch, J. F. Cade, A. S. Gallus, et al., pp. 284–291. S. Karger, Basel.
3. Burns, J. J., Yu, T. F., Ritterbrand, A., Perei, J. M., Gutman, A. B., and Brodie, B. B. (1957): A potent new uricosuric agent, the sulfoxide metabolite of the phenylbutazone analogue. *J. Pharmacol. Exp. Ther.*, 119:418–426.
4. Dayton, P. G., Sicam, L. E., Landrau, M., and Burns, J. J. (1961): Metabolism of sulfinpyrazone (Anturane) and other thio analogues of phenylbutazone in man. *J. Pharmacol. Exp. Ther.*, 132, 3:287–290.
5. The Canadian Cooperative Study Group. (1978): A randomized trail of aspirin and sulfinpyrazone in threatened stroke. *N. Engl. J. Med.*, 299:53–58.
6. Dieterle, W., Faigle, J. W., Mory, H., Richter, W. J., and Theobald, W. (1975): Biotransformation and pharmacokinetics of sulfinpyrazone (Anturan) in man. *Eur. J. Clin. Pharmacol.*, 9:135–145.
7. Dougherty, J. H. Jr., Levy, D. E., and Weksler, B. B. (1977): Platelet activation in acute cerebral ischaemia. *Lancet*, i:821–824.
8. Evans, G. (1972): Effect of drugs that suppress platelet surface interaction on incidence of amaurosis fugax and transient cerebral ischemia. *Surg. Forum (USA)*, 23:239–241.
9. Fields, W. S., Lemak, N. A., Frankowski, R. F., and Hardy, R. J. (1977): Controlled trial of aspirin in cerebral ischaemia. *Stroke*, 8:3:301–315.
10. Hassan, M. N., Parsonage, M. J., and Russell, J. G. (1977): Sulphinpyrazone in the treatment of transient ischaemic attacks. In: *Thromboembolism—A New Approach to Therapy*. Edited by J. R. A. Mitchell and J. G. Domenet, pp. 143–151. Academic Press, New York.
11. Herskovits, E., Famulari, A., Tamaroff, L., Gonzalez, A. M., Matera, V., Vazquez, A., Smud, R., Fraiman, H., and Vila, J. (1981): Randomised trial of pentoxifylline versus acetylsalicylic acid plus dipyridamole in preventing transient ischaemic attacks. *Lancet*, 1:966–967.
12. Kaegi, A., Pineo, G. F., Shimizu, A., Trivedi, H., Hirsh, J., and Gent, M. (1974): Arteriovenous-shunt thrombosis. *N. Engl. J. Med.*, 290:304–306.
13. Kurtzke, J. F. (1979): Critique of the Canadian "TIA" study. In: *Cerebrovascular Diseases*, edited by T. R. Price and E. Nelson. Raven Press, New York.
14. Lecaillon, J. B., and Souppart, C. (1976): Quantitative assay of sulphinpyrazone in plasma and urine by high-performance liquid chromatography. *J. Chromatography*, 121:227–234.
15. Maguire, E. D., Pay, G. F., Turney, J., Wallis, R. B., Weston, M. J., White, A. M., Williams, L. C., and Feidhlim Woods, H. (1981): The effects two different dosage regimens of sulphin-pyrazone on platelet function ex vivo and blood chemistry in man. *Haemostasis*, 10:153–164.
16. Pay, G. F., Wallis, R. B., and Zelashci, D. (1981): The effect of sulphinpyrazone and its metab-olites on platelet function in vitro and ex vivo. *Haemostasis*, 10:165–175.
17. Smythe, H. A., Ogryzlo, M. A., Murphy, E. A., and Mustard, J. F. (1965): The effect of sulfin-pyrazone (Anturan) on platelet economy and blood coagulation in man. *Can. Med. Assoc. J.*, 92:818–821.
18. Steele, P., Carroll, J., Overfield, D., and Genton, E. (1977): Effect of sulfinpyrazone on platelet survival time in patients with transient cerebral ischemic attacks. 8:3:396–397.
19. Steele, P. P., Weily, H. S., Davies, H., and Genton, E. (1974): Platelet survival in patients with rheumatic heart disease. *N. Engl. J. Med.*, 290:537.
20. Steele, P. P., Weily, H. S., and Genton, E. (1973): Platelet survival and adhesiveness in recurrent venous thrombosis. *N. Engl. J. Med.*, 288:1148–1152.
21. Weily, H. S., and Genton, E. (1970): Altered platelet function in patients with prosthetic mitral valves. Effects of sulfinpyrazone therapy. *Circulation*, 42:967–972.
22. Weily, H. S., Steele, P. P., Davies, H., Pappas, G., and Genton, E. (1974): Platelet survival in patients with substitute heart valves. *N. Engl. J. Med.*, 290:534–537.

Advances in Stroke Therapy, edited by
F. C. Rose. Raven Press, New York © 1982.

Combined Medical and Surgical Single-Centre Approach to Management of Carotid Territory Cerebral Infarction

*T. J. Steiner and †R. M. Greenhalgh

*Department of Neurology, Charing Cross Hospital; and †*Professorial Department of Surgery, Charing Cross Hospital Medical School, London, England*

Probably just under two new cases of stroke occur each year in England and Wales for every 1,000 of the population. The figure of 1.86 most usually quoted is based on statistics derived in Oxford nearly 20 years ago (1), though a later Bristol survey produced a similar finding (16). Other estimates have been both higher and lower, but in all cases the figures are averages reflecting variations between subpopulations, with age the major determining factor, and therefore regional differences are to be expected. From the West London catchment of Charing Cross Hospital, currently declining between 146,000 and 127,000 according to Regional Health Authority statistics, a 3-year survey of Accident and Emergency Department admissions recorded a mean of 226 acute stroke cases brought in each year. This figure is subject to errors arising from imperfect record keeping and retrieval and uncertain first diagnosis, but is not likely to be an overestimate. It is about 30% lower than figures derived from Regional Health Authority discharge statistics, which are compiled also from incomplete records but should be diagnostically more sound, except that the classification system (I.C.D., 8th Revision) is not used in a way that distinguishes between incident and prevalent (new and old) conditions. The number of admissions for acute stroke approaches the expected total incidence in the population served ($1.86 \times 146 = 271$; $\times 127 = 236$); Carlisle, as an example said to be typical, reported in contrast a 60% admission rate (9). The difference reflects in part a high referral rate from London general practitioners together with an observed readiness of patients to present directly to Casualty, in part a teaching hospital drainage from beyond its strict geographical catchment, and in part a greater than average incidence arising from the relatively high proportion of elderly people in the population served. To some extent, therefore, stroke cases admitted to Charing Cross Hospital may not be an entirely similar group to other hospital series.

Of all strokes, it is still being said that 90% are ischaemic rather than hemorrhagic (e.g., 11), although computerized tomography (CT) scanning of our own admissions suggests this is a significant overestimate. Other individual series also have reported a much higher proportion of haemorrhages (e.g., 15). Unless all available stroke cases are investigated adequately to confirm the pathological diagnosis, information of this sort will never become available. This is one good reason for attempting to adopt a unified, interdepartmental policy for the management of this very hetero-geneous condition which may present first to physicians or to surgeons. Other reasons for unified management concern improvements in care that can be achieved by defining strictly the strategy to be followed, whoever first sees the patient, so that group outcome may be the subject of continuous audit. In such a context, and probably only thus, can medical and surgical treatments be compared, for the variable influences operating in the alternative multi-centre approach are so nu-merous they may defeat the objectives of the study.

DIAGNOSIS

The management policy briefly can be laid down in terms of three principles. Clinical diagnosis, the starting point (see Fig. 1), is made by the neurologist. Those in whom the diagnosis may be carotid territory stroke are investigated by CT scan. This is now unequivocally the mainstay of diagnostic confirmation (e.g., 12,15), though on occasion other tests for this purpose may be useful or necessary (8). Angiography is rarely to be employed as a diagnostic test. The first principle then is that *management depends upon the pathological diagnosis*. Hence the objective of diagnostic investigation is to select for combined management those with carotid territory ischaemia as the presenting process, and to separate them (Fig. 1) from cerebral haemorrhage, vertebrobasilar ischaemia, tumours presenting with stroke-like syndromes, and processes resulting in cerebral atrophy.

PREDISPOSITION AND ASSOCIATED FACTORS

It is routine to search for related and possibly causative or aggravating conditions. Knowledge of these is important to any study of stroke outcome but, more im-mediately, may be of particular significance in individual patients. Hypertension and hyperviscosity syndromes such as polycythaemia, if found, are controlled. Atrial fibrillation and other cardiac dysrhythmias are treated where necessary. So are diabetes mellitus, occurring in over 40% of these patients (17), cardiac ischaemia and/or enlargement, valvular disease or disorders, hyperlipidaemias, and syphilis, all of which are identified or excluded by adequate investigation. Smoking is discouraged. Beyond this, these factors may not influence overall management any more than does advanced age per se. Though each case is judged on its merits, and it is appropriate to assess surgical risk individually, none of these factors lessens the probability of there being carotid arterial disease. If there is, with symptoms related to the territory of distribution, it is difficult to presume lack of causality even with the additional presence, for instance, of atrial fibrillation.

ASSESSMENT AND STRATIFICATION

At the basis of further management is the second of the three principles: *Man-agement of moderate or severe stroke is directed first at promoting recovery, but*

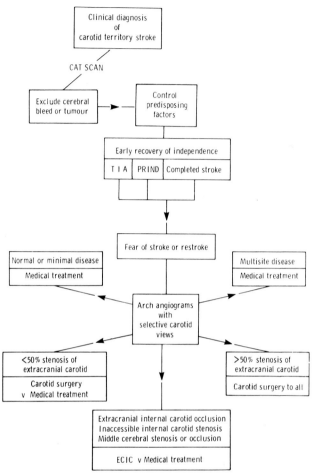

FIG. 1. Basis of the combined medical and surgical approach to management of carotid territory cerebral infarction.

the major objective in managing mild stroke, which should be energetically pursued, is to prevent additional episodes for fear that they may not be mild. This latter aim is not different from the aim of management of transient ischaemic attack (TIA) or prolonged, reversible, ischaemic neurological deficit (PRIND), from which a patient recovers completely, and there may be an intermediate group of strokes where both aims are appropriate from the outset. Furthermore, in this highly variable disease, it must be recognised that patients can change from one category to another during management. While applying generally, these objectives also may need to be adapted in the presence of severe or greater disability from other causes.

Though either purpose to some extent may be served by medical or surgical means, prophylaxis is better promoted than recovery by currently available surgical techniques and, consequently, it is to mild stroke that this combined approach is mainly applied. Mild stroke in this scheme is defined as "such that the patient remains fully independent and fit enough for unsupported living at home, or becomes so within six weeks of the stroke onset." Patients remaining independent throughout are stratified for treatment purposes early, usually within the first week, and are therefore managed exactly as those with TIA. All others are reassessed at 6 weeks, and stratification is undertaken then in the remaining mild strokes. This timing is not wholly arbitrary, deriving from the known dangers of early surgical revascularisation following extensive cerebral infarction (4,5,7,20) even though surgery eventually undertaken in embolic infarction may not involve any element of revascularisation. It is one of several instances where the management policy is constrained by balancing the possible risks of intervention against the likely outcome, if determined solely by natural history.

According to the third principle, *stratification depends upon full cerebral angiography: arch aortography with selective catheterisation and injection of both carotids and two-plane intracranial and extracranial views.* Carotid angiography may be carried out in ways other than this but, however done, it carries a very significant morbidity and mortality. These are variously reported, the figures depending not only upon the centre, the operator, the method, and the patients selected, but also (and perhaps mainly) on how morbidity is assessed: in particular, whether prospectively or retrospectively. Harrison (14) quoted combined figures between 0.5 and 2.5%, which results in a significant charge against whatever subsequent treatment is adopted and is sufficient to cause some patients to withhold consent even though, without treatment, the risk of restroke is substantially higher (e.g., 19).

Patients who, for whatever reason, are not subjected to angiography, cannot be considered for surgery and therapeutic possibilities are thereby limited. Noninvasive tests cannot be substituted yet for angiography with even nearly adequate resolution, and therefore our policy is to reserve these (CPA, OPG, MAVIS) for asymptomatic patients, whom we manage conservatively but always follow-up. Those who have angiography are stratified into 4 main categories (Fig. 1):

A. No apparent disease.
B. Localised extracranial carotid disease only, graded as follows:
   1. Minimal disease
   2. Disease with irregularity but not stenosis, or with less than 50% stenosis
   3. Disease with stenosis exceeding 50%
   4. Extracranial carotid occlusion
C. Localised intracranial disease only: carotid or middle cerebral disease with stenosis or occlusion.
D. Multiple-site disease: multiple (tandem) lesions within one carotid and its distribution, or generalised cerebral arterial disease.

MANAGEMENT

Treatment is determined by stratification. It is always medical for: 1. those not having angiography, 2. those in categories A and B1 (minimal or no disease), who have no lesions that usefully could be corrected, 3. those in category D (inoperable multisite disease), in whom multiple tandem lesions are not amenable to endarterectomy; bypass is not practicable where there is generalised disease and not helpful in treating embolic sources.

Medical treatment consists of whatever is thought most appropriate in the circumstances and may include therapy aimed at inhibiting platelet aggregation, even though this is of uncertain value (Warlow, *this volume*).

Treatment is always surgical for category B3 disease. Carotid stenosis greater than 50%, since it already approaches occlusion, can be expected to proceed towards that event; at some intermediate point, it begins to interfere significantly with flow (2,3,6). Carotid endarterectomy can be curative (though not always permanently), but is associated with twin intraoperative dangers of embolisation and cerebral ischaemia (perhaps in an already compromised zone), the latter occasioned if the carotid trunk is clamped without adequate protection by shunting. Combined mortality and morbidity from this operation can be high (14) but need not exceed 1% (18).

Grade 2 disease in category B may be ulcerating or early stenotic lesions and may or may not represent sources of emboli. Reliable angiographic interpretation is most difficult with disease of this sort (10). Neither this nor grade 4 disease has been shown to benefit from surgery: the cooperative carotid endarterectomy trial (13) was inconclusive (11). Surgical benefit in category C (intracranial) disease is equally unproven, and Barnett's trial of extracranial to intracranial bypass is still recruiting. If medical treatment had been proved helpful, surgery need not be contemplated. However, this is not the case, which is probably why carotid endarterectomy is widely practised in the absence of unequivocal indications and why extracranial to intracranial (EC/IC) bypass is rapidly following. EC/IC bypass has a lower theoretical morbidity than carotid endarterectomy, which makes it easy to recommend for localised intracranial carotid or middle cerebral disease before any value is established.

The benefits accruing from both operations for these medical conditions need careful scrutiny in new comparative trials. It is doubtful, however, that Fields' study (13) ever can be repeated, and Barnett's multinational EC/IC bypass trial may be grouping together so many disparate centres with different techniques, strategies, operators, and patient populations, that the averaged outcome may not be applicable to any one centre. At Charing Cross, patients in category B2 (localised extracranial carotid disease with less than 50% stenosis) are randomly allocated either to medical treatment or carotid endarterectomy, matched according to age, sex, and side affected. Patients in categories B4 (extracranial carotid occlusion) or C (localised intracranial disease) are similarly randomised between medical treatment and EC/IC bypass. Patients in either category may have antiplatelet agents or any other medical therapy, whether surgically or medically treated, and physical therapy is available to all. The *only* difference between groups is that medical patients do not have surgery. Despite the slow recruitment which is the necessary penalty, this cooperative management policy within a single centre may be the only realistic way to compare surgery with no surgery, which is the real aim. Like all surgical trials, at best it can only show what is possible, and its applicability may not extend to all other centres.

TRANSIENT ISCHAEMIC ATTACKS

The policy does not distinguish between TIA (or PRIND) and mild stroke for purposes of stratification, for both conditions indicate a stroke-prone patient in whom arterial disease may be a cause, and treatment is aimed to prevent major stroke. Prevention of recurrent TIA is not seen as a useful aim in itself, since we cannot conclude that this will prevent stroke; treatment achieving only this effect may merely interfere with the recognised association between the two conditions.

The acute abdomen is a good surgical analogy: The patient may be grateful for analgesia that calms his main symptoms, but to offer this without due investigation is unwise treatment; by the same token, just giving TIA sufferers antiplatelet medication ought to be deplored. If TIAs stop, at best the underlying and uninvestigated main problem—threatening stroke—is liable to be forgotten.

SUMMARY

A cooperative management policy between neurologists and vascular surgeons aims to rationalise the treatment of carotid territory ischaemic stroke in which both medical and surgical approaches may play a part. After confirmation of the diagnosis and control of predisposing factors, mild stroke patients are managed in the same way as those with TIA or PRIND. Following arch and carotid angiography, they are stratified (Fig. 1) according to site and severity of carotid disease into categories for which surgery appears appropriate, for which it is inappropriate, and for which its role is uncertain. The last group is randomised between medical and surgical treatments and, in due course, the role of each in a single centre will be assessed.

REFERENCES

1. Acheson, R. M., and Fairbairn, A. S. (1970): Burden of cerebrovascular disease in the Oxford area in 1963 and 1964. *Br. Med. J.*, 2:621–626.
2. Ackerman, Robert H. (1980): Non-invasive carotid evaluation. *Stroke*, 11:675–678.
3. Alter, M., Kieffer, S., Resch, J., and Ansari, K. (1972): Cerebral infarction. Clinical and angiographic correlations. *Neurol. (Minneap.)*, 22:590–602.
4. Bauer, R. B., Meyer, J. S., Fields, W. S., Remington, R., MacDonald, M. C., and Callen, P. (1969): Joint study of extracranial arterial occlusion. III. Progress report of controlled study of long-term survival in patients with and without operations. *J.A.M.A.*, 208:509–518.
5. Blaisdell, W. F., Clauss, R. H., Galbraith, J. G., Imparato, A. M., and Wylie, E. J. (1969): Joint study of extracranial arterial occlusion. IV. A review of surgical considerations. *J.A.M.A.*, 209:1889–1895.
6. Brice, J. G., Dowsett, D. J., and Lowe, R. D. (1964): Haemodynamic effects of carotid artery stenosis. *Br. Med. J.*, 2:1363–1366.
7. Bruetman, M. E., Fields, W. S., Crawford, E. S., and De Bakey, M. E. (1963): Cerebral haemorrhage in carotid artery surgery. *Arch. Neurol.*, 9:458–467.
8. Buonanno, F., and Toole, J. F. (1981): Management of patients with established ("completed") cerebral infarction. *Stroke*, 12:7–16.

9. Chin, P. L., Angunawela, R., Mitchell, D., and Horne, J. (1981): Stroke register in Carlisle: a preliminary report. In: *Clinical Neuroepidemiology*, edited by F. Clifford Rose, pp. 131–143. Pitman Medical, Tunbridge Wells, England.
10. Croft, R. J. (1981): Pitfalls of carotid arteriography. *Hospital Update*, 7:784–786.
11. Croft, R. J., Harrison, M. J. G., Marston, A., Chapple, C., and Thakkar, R. (1981): Surgery for stroke. *J.R. Soc. Med.*, 74:330–332.
12. Davis, K. R., Taveras, J. M., New, P. F. J., Schnur, J. A., and Roberson, G. H. (1975): Cerebral infarction diagnosis by computerized tomography. Analysis and evaluation of findings. *Am. J. Roentgenol. Rad. Ther. Nucl. Med.*, 124:643–660.
13. Fields, W. S., Maslenikov, V., Meyer, J. S., Hass, W. K., Remington, R. D., and MacDonald, M. (1970): Joint study of extracranial arterial occlusion. V. Progress report of prognosis following surgery or nonsurgical treatment for transient cerebral ischemic attacks and cervical carotid artery lesions. *J.A.M.A.*, 211:1993–2003.
14. Harrison, M. J. G. (1980): Surgery for ischaemic stroke. *Br. J. Hosp. Med.*, 24:108–112.
15. Kinkel, W. R., and Jacobs, L. (1976): Computerized axial transverse tomography in cerebrovascular disease. *Neurol. (Minneap.)*, 26:924–930.
16. Langton Hewer, H. R., Day, R. E., and McDonald, I. (1972): Incidence and cause of non-transient vascular hemiplegia in the community. Royal College of Physicians. *Report of the Geriatric Committee Working Group on Strokes*.
17. Steiner, T. J., and Clifford Rose, F. (1981): Diabetes in cerebrovascular disease. In: *Hormones and Vascular Disease*, edited by R. M. Greenhalgh, pp. 152–165. Pitman Medical, Tunbridge Wells, England.
18. Thompson, J. E., and Talkington, C. M. (1976): Carotid endarterectomy. *Ann. Surg,*, 184:1–15.
19. Wolf, P. A., Dawber, T. R., Thomas, H. E., Colton, T., and Kannel, W. B. (1977): Epidemiology of stroke. In: *Stroke: Advances in Neurology, Vol. 16*, edited by R. A. Thompson and J. R. Green, pp. 5–19. Raven Press, New York.
20. Wylie, E. J., Hein, M. F., and Adams, J. E. (1964): Intracranial hemorrhage following revascularization for treatment of acute stroke. *J. Neurosurg.*, 21:212–215.

Advances in Stroke Therapy, edited by
F. C. Rose. Raven Press, New York © 1982.

The Present Place of Carotid Surgery in Stroke Prevention

H. H. G. Eastcott

St. Mary's Hospital, London, England

More than a quarter of a century has passed since we reported the first case of repeated transient hemiplegic attacks to be cured by carotid artery reconstruction (5). The patient's subsequent course was satisfactory; she suffered no further cerebrovascular symptoms and died of old age in 1974. Why was her case so successful? In retrospect, quite unawares, we chose what has now come to be realised as the perfect set of indications: a short history of many repeated attacks of blindness in the left eye with accompanying paralysis of the right half of the body lasting between 10 and 30 min and shown on angiography to be associated with a narrowed left internal carotid sinus. The lesion was resected, and the healthy cut ends of the common and internal carotids were anastomosed, the total clamp time being 20 min, the patient having been cooled to 28°C.

Why have there not been hundreds of similar patients in the experience of each vascular surgeon in this country? Last year I wrote to 18 of the most active British vascular surgeons asking about their work load in several of the common clinical conditions that require arterial surgery. Their replies revealed that they were, on the average, operating upon 100 patients with lower limb arteriosclerotic occlusive disease each year, and that the trend was a rising one. Table 1 shows the contrast between this and their reported activity in the correction of the equally common occlusive lesions of the neck arteries; only eight surgeons were operating on more than 10 such patients per year. Almost all said that they would be prepared to do more of these operations if requested. Techniques are similar and the facilities

TABLE 1. *18 U.K. vascular surgeons, 1980*

Yearly carotid endarterectomies	
> 20	5
10–20	3
< 10	4
"Few"	3[a]
"None"	2[a]
No answer	1

[a]"Restricted referrals."

required are generally available. The difference must surely be in the tolerance to ischaemia in the tissues supplied: a minor technical problem in the lower limb arterioplasty seldom brings harm to the extremity, but the same difficulty in the carotid procedure may cause a stroke, often irreversible, and sometimes fatal. Tables 2 and 3 list the experience of eleven vascular surgeons in a Middle West community hospital environment (6). During the 7 years of the review, 227 operations were performed (an average of just under 3 per year per surgeon). The combined postoperative stroke mortality rate of well over 20% is at least 5 times as high as that which has been reported from centres of expertise (Table 4).

CAROTID ENDARTERECTOMY: WHERE ARE THE RISKS?

As in the whole of surgery, when the outcome of an operation is poor, the fault may lie either with the patient or the surgeon, or quite often both.

TABLE 2. *Carotid endarterectomy in two community hospitals*

Preop. state	Patients	Postop. stroke	Death
Asymptomatic	11	18.2%	0
TIA	73	17.8%	5.5%
Established stroke	99	15.2%	9.1%

From ref. 6.

TABLE 3. *Carotid endarterectomy in two community hospitals*

227 operations by 11 surgeons
Stroke or death in 48 (21.1%)
  If shunt used: (159) 28.3%
  No shunt used: (45) 20.0%
Complication rate steady during all years
  1970–1977

From ref. 6.

TABLE 4. *Results of operation (percentages)*

Reference	Death	Permanent defect	Satisfactory at late follow-up
Fields et al. (1970)	3.5	7.7	46.6
De Weese et al. (1973)	1.0	6.0	89.9
Thompson et al. (1973)	2.3	1.5	81.0
Eastcott (1976)	1.7	2.8	90.0
Bouchier-Hayes and Mac Gowan (1979)	7.0	8.3	76.0

From ref. 6.

Patient-Related Problems

Patient-related problems (16) include the severity of the neurological picture, the extent of the angiological disease, and the general medical condition (Table 5). Upon these will depend whether the stroke risk is as low as 1% when all three factors are favourable, or as high as 10% when they are not. Some of these handicaps are unalterable, but hypertension, as in the medically treated patient, can be controlled with real benefit, particularly in the early postoperative period (19) when carotid baroceptor activity may be impaired by operative damage to the sinus branch of the glossopharyngeal, or by narrowing of the repaired carotid, which likewise reduces the efferent impulses to the controlling vasomotor centre. Intracerebral haemorrhage may exacerbate an infarct that was previously asymptomatic, and a patient, who had awakened after endarterectomy neurologically intact, becomes hemiplegic a few hours later. Close nursing supervision in a well staffed recovery or intensive care unit is therefore essential, and hypotensive medication must be ready, prescribed with the clear instruction that the drug should be given at a certain level of hypertension depending upon the previously steady readings, but in any event, if the systolic pressure exceeds 200 mm Hg.

The presence of unsuspected cerebral infarction should nowadays be investigated by computer assisted tomography (CAT) of the head, which may help to decide in favour of a conservative regimen, e.g., when there has been a recent history of a rather prolonged, though supposedly transient, ischaemic episode. This investigation is now routine in our unit at St. Mary's Hospital. When it was unheeded in a recent, severe progressing bilateral case, the outcome of operation was another fatal stroke.

Technical Errors

Technical errors, as we have seen, are related to the experience and understanding of the operating team. A refined and scrupulous level of care is essential; from the nurse we expect deft and immediate cooperation and attention to the need for avoiding delays, especially while the carotid is clamped, when a dropped instrument or missing suture may cost several minutes. The anaesthetist should be experienced in cardiovascular work, with a scrupulous and constant watch for the maintenance

TABLE 5. *Patient risk grouping[a]*

1. Neurologically stable, medically fit, favourable angiograms:
   Operative stroke risk: 1%
2. As in group 1, but with unfavourable angiograms:
   Operative stroke risk: 2%.
3. Neurologically stable, but medically unfit, whatever
   the angiographic features:
   Operative morbidity: 7%
4. Neurologically unstable, whatever rest of the picture:
   Operative stroke risk: 10%.

[a]Sundt et al., 1977.
From ref. 4a.

of good peripheral perfusion and for any cardiac irregularity or worsening of the ECG.

The surgeon should remember that this is the finest and most exacting operation of all peripheral vascular procedures; it should be programmed to be first on the day's list before the heavier and longer cases. We have mentioned carotid baroceptor difficulties: They can be minimised by careful dissection between the carotids and by the injection of a small quantity of 1% xylocaine around the nerve area if the anaesthetist should report vasomotor or cardiac disturbances, especially any clearly coincident fall in blood pressure.

Operative Embolism

Operative embolism is now considered to be the most important cause of peri-operative stroke. It is probably of much greater importance than the duration of carotid clamping, or the measured pressure in the clamped internal carotid (stump pressure). Careful, gentle operative manipulation of the exposed carotid bifurcation is essential in every case, in particular any that have shown recent neurological activity or whose angiograms indicate ulceration or raised irregularity signifying the probability of unstable thrombus in contact with the fast moving stream within the internal carotid. My practice now is to postpone dissection of the bifurcation until after the internal carotid has been isolated and controlled, well above the lesion (Fig. 1). This practice has proved effective in the prevention of foot emboli during aortic surgery and it is also advised in carotid endarterectomy (15).

Inadequate Repair

Inadequate repair may lead to early carotid occlusion either by thrombosis or prolapse and dissection of an arterial plaque. Patch grafting should be considered when the arteriotomy seems likely to be narrowed or at all distorted or irregular with primary closure. Operative arteriography is not as well suited to this purpose

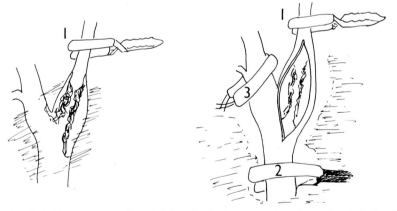

FIG. 1. Protective sequence of carotid clamping for the prevention of operative embolism from the thrombotic bifurcation lesion.

as it is in limb arterioplasty, but a sterile, hand-held ultrasound imaging probe, already reported satisfactory in detecting residual common duct stones and pancreatic calculi (10), also has been found effective in demonstrating defects in the lumen of the sutured carotid. In the author's opinion, if a patch is required, the saphenous vein at ankle level is the most suitable material, for not only is dacron fabric a more thrombogenic material, but its poor compliance with the already thinned, endarterectomised internal carotid will tend to cause false aneurysm, with further stroke risk from thrombus in the sac.

SHOULD A SHUNT BE USED?

As with most surgical procedures, particularly those in which technical failure carries a serious penalty, opinion is divided between those who routinely use an indwelling carotid shunt to maintain hemisphere supply during the endarterectomy and repair (18), those who never use one (2), and others who judge each case on its merits in this matter (22). The act of inserting the shunt may damage the carotid, either by setting up a dissection plane out of sight, higher in the carotid than the arteriotomy, or by the inadvertent dislodging of thrombus from either the internal or the common carotid. In the latter event, the loose material actually may be seen passing upwards within the shunt, in which event, it is best to have the first assistant ready with an artery forceps with which to clamp the shunt and stop the embolus from reaching the intetherenal carotid.

Yet, since the purpose of a shunt is to maintain cerebral blood flow during carotid clamping, it will be useful to know the actual level of the stump pressure before deciding to dispense with this precaution. Most surgeons feel that any patient whose clamped internal carotid pressure is less than 40 mm Hg is at risk of suffering from an inadequate cross flow into the affected hemisphere during the arterioplasty unless a shunt is inserted. The author also uses shunt protection under three other circumstances:

1. In the presence of an occluded opposite carotid (14),
2. Where there is a residual neurological defect (8),
3. In cases where patching is required.

NONCEREBRAL COMPLICATIONS

Noncerebral complications are mostly minor and transient and relate to the local motor and cutaneous nerves. The cervical branch of the facial and anterior cutaneous nerves of the neck will be affected more often if the incision is placed along the anterior border of the sternomastoid muscle than when an oblique skin crease line is followed. This however gives a poorer exposure at the upper and lower limits of the field where such restriction may be important with a high-placed lesion, or when a shunt must be inserted. The vagus may be bruised in dissecting it from the common carotid, usually after direct carotid arteriography more than a few days before, or in the case of a recurrent carotid stenosis with previous scarring adherence of the carotid. A weakness of the voice results. Temporary weakness of the ipsilateral half of the tongue can complicate local retraction needed during a high carotid endarterectomy. Normally, all these effects are transient and should clear up within a few weeks, for actual division of these nerves should be rare indeed (12).

NEW POSTOPERATIVE STROKE

The incidence of postoperative stroke, the prevention of which is the sole objective of the operation, varies considerably between different medical centres (Tables 2–4). In the most experienced hands, the operative major stroke rate should not exceed 3%. When higher figures are cited from such sources, it will usually be found that all new defects, many of them transient, have been included.

When this condition is recognised immediately on recovery from anaesthesia, it is good practice to return the patient to the operating theatre and review the carotid repair. Sometimes an early thrombosis can be corrected in this way before any irreversible neurological damage has been sustained. A positive, supraorbital Doppler test (arrest of the signals on temporal compression) supports the clinical diagnosis of carotid occlusive stroke, although of course an embolic detachment could have preceded the final closure of the repair.

OPERATIVE MORTALITY

A major infarct in the affected hemisphere can be fatal especially when there has been a preexisting defect; in fact, most deaths in the early years of this type of surgery were from this cause (21). Once it was realised that dense stroke is an absolute contraindication to carotid endarterectomy, the cause of death shifted away from the brain to the heart. We now realise that carotid patients with active ischaemic heart disease are at a specially high risk (3). Careful operative and anaesthetic management should minimise this risk, but the patient with angina or a recent myocardial infarct may be exposed to a mortality risk of 4 or 5%. Clearly such figures should be soberly considered, just as those of new postoperative stroke must be, against the known background of the untreated or the medically treated disease when any cardiac or completed-stroke patient is under assessment for carotid repair.

MANAGEMENT OF THE PATIENT WITH MULTIFOCAL OCCLUSIVE DISEASE

When carotid, cardiac, and peripheral arterial lesions are all judged to be active, the problem of priorities may be acute. In general, the more pressing peripheral emergencies such as leakage from an abdominal aortic aneurysm, or impending lower limb loss from acute embolism, will require first attention. The combined problem of active, symptomatic carotid, and coronary disease already has been mentioned as a most dangerous area in cardiovascular surgery, and one in which the surgeon must be guided by the apparent relative clinical severity of the two conditions in deciding which should be operated upon first. In cases of left main coronary or triple vessel disease, it is now considered advisable to operate on both areas at the same session, usually beginning with the carotid to ensure good cerebral perfusion during the subsequent cardiopulmonary bypass.

SIGNIFICANCE OF CAROTID BRUITS IN CARDIOVASCULAR SURGERY

The general review of such patients before operation should include carotid auscultation. If a bruit is heard, the patient and his relatives should be questioned as to whether amaurosis fugax or other fleeting symptoms such as hand numbness or speech difficulty have been noticed. A surprising number of cases may thus be transferred from the asymptomatic to the active group. Often it will be decided to correct the carotid condition before proceeding to the major peripheral operation but, in the absence of symptoms, there is evidence to support the safety of ignoring the carotid condition (7) although most centres would now assess the cerebrovascular state by a full set of noninvasive vascular laboratory tests.

SHOULD ASYMPTOMATIC CAROTID STENOSIS BE CORRECTED?

The condition of carotid stenosis must first be defined. Three types can be recognised:

1. The contralateral carotid in a previously operated case now symptom free. Opinion here is divided. Many would operate, for the reason that history is likely to repeat itself unless the presymptomatic lesion is removed (18). Others take the view that stroke from this cause is rare, with fewer than 3% of patients undergoing carotid endarterectomy eventually requiring contralateral operation (9).

2. The peripheral vascular patient under initial investigation or subsequent follow-up. This has already been discussed.

3. The truly incidental finding. With a few notable exceptions, most surgeons feel that such a patient normally should not go further than the noninvasive vascular laboratory but that, if those tests revealed severe or bilateral stenosis, an arch aortogram is advised. A small number of highly expert surgeons are sufficently confident in the safety of their methods to advise operation. If we combine the figures of the three main proponents of this policy, reported at a conference in Marseilles in October 1979 (17), we find that with a total of 493 patients operated upon for asymptomatic carotid stenosis, there was one postoperative death (0.2%) and eight late strokes (1.6%). Comparable figures for nonoperated patients are difficult to obtain, but stroke without warning transient ischaemic attacks (TIAs) has been recorded as occurring in between 12 and 30% of such patients (20). It seems therefore that, in some special centres, safe operation may be advised.

RECURRENT CAROTID STENOSIS

Recurrent carotid stenosis is much rarer than recurrent obstruction after limb artery endarterectomy, no doubt because of the short segment involved and the constant high flow rate. Young, hypertensive, and hyperlipidaemic patients seem to be at risk and comprise a significant proportion of the 3.6% of 361 followed up operations (4). Transient cerebral attacks occurred in 28 of 114 patients in another series in which the incidence of major stroke, as in most other series, was low at 1.75% (13).

CONCLUSION

Though we know more about the outcome of surgery than the natural course of the disease for which it is performed (since inevitably a large number of cases escape recognition), it safely can be stated that, in the hands of highly experienced vascular surgeons, carotid endarterectomy for transient cerebral ischaemic attacks carries a much lower combined stroke and mortality risk than that which follows nonsurgical treatment, perhaps 3 or 4% (early and late after operation) compared with 23 to 45% at 1 to 5 years in the conservative group (11). The detection of early, asymptomatic disease by noninvasive screening methods is advancing rapidly (1), and the benefits of operation when undertaken by the most experienced teams also are beginning to be accepted.

REFERENCES

1. Annotation (1981): Carotid stenosis. *Lancet*, i:535.
2. Baker, W. H., Dorner, D. B., and Barnes, R. W. (1977): Carotid endarterectomy: is a shunt necessary? *Surgery*, 82:321.
3. Bernhard, V. M., Johnson, W. D., and Peterson, J. J. (1972): Carotid artery stenosis. Association with coronary artery disease. *Arch. Surg.*, 105:837.
4. Cossman, D., Callow, A. D., Stein, A., and Matsumoto, G. (1978): Early restenosis after carotid endarterectomy.
4a. Eastcott, H. H. G. (1980): Carotid endarterectomy in the symptomless patient. The case against. In: *Artériopathies Cérébrales Extracraniennes Asymptomatique*, edited by R. Courbier, pp. 241–251. Oberval, Lyons.
5. Eastcott, H. H. G., Pickering, G. W., and Rob, C. G. (1954): Reconstruction of internal carotid artery in a patient with intermittent attacks of hemiplegia. *Lancet*, i:994.
6. Easton, J. D., and Sherman, D. G. (1977): Stroke and mortality rate in carotid endarterectomy. 228 consecutive operations. *Stroke*, 8:565.
7. Evans, W. E., and Cooperman, M. (1978): The significance of asymptomatic carotid bruits in preoperative patients. *Surgery*, 83:521.
8. Hertzer, N. R., Beven, E. G., Greenstreet, R. L., and Humphries, A. W. (1978): Internal carotid artery back pressure, intraoperative shunting, ulcerated atheroma and the incidence of stroke during carotid endarterectomy. *Surgery*, 83:306.
9. Johnson, N., Burnham, S. J., Flanigan, D. P., Goodreau, J. J., Yao, J. S. T., and Bergan, J. J. (1978): Carotid endarterectomy: a follow-up study of the contralateral non-operated artery. *Ann. Surg.*, 188:748.
10. Lane, R. J., and Glazer, G. (1980): Intra-operative B-mode ultrasound scanning of the extra-hepatic biliary system and pancreas. *Lancet*, ii:334.
11. Marshall, J. (1977): Management of cerebrovascular disease. *Medicine*, 34:2018.
12. Matsumoto, G. H., Cossman, D., and Callow, A. D. (1977): Hazards and safeguards during carotid endarterectomy. Technical considerations. *Am. J. Surg.*, 133:458.
13. Owens, M. L., Atkinson, J. B., and Wilson, S. E. (1980): Recurrent transient ischaemic attacks after carotid endarterectomy. *Am. J. Surg.*, 115:482–486.
14. Riles, T. S., Imparato, A. A., and Kopelman, I. (1980): Carotid artery stenosis with contralateral internal carotid artery occlusion. Long term results in 54 patients. *Surgery*, 87:363.
15. Starr, D. S., Lawrie, G. M., and Morris, G. C. (1979): Prevention of distal embolism during arterial reconstruction. *Arch. Surg.*, 114:412.

16. Sundt, T. M., Sandok, B. A., and Whisnant, J. P. (1975): Carotid endarterectomy complications and preoperative assessment of risk. *Mayo Clin. Proc.*, 50:301.
17. Thevenet, A., Thompson, J. E., and Wylie, E. J. (1980): In: *Artériopathies Cérébrales Extra-craniennes Asymptomatiques*, edited by R. Courbier. Oberval, Lyons.
18. Thompson, J. E., Patman, R. D., and Talkington, C. M. (1978): Carotid surgery for cerebrovascular insufficiency. In: *Current Problems in Surgery*, edited by M. M. Ravitch, pp. 1–68. Year Book Medical Publishers, Chicago.
19. Towne, J. B., and Bernhard, V. M. (1980): The relationship of postoperative hypertension to complications of carotid endarterectomy. *Surgery*, 88:575.
20. Wylie, E. J. (1980): Is an asymptomatic carotid stenosis a surgical lesion? In: *Artériopathies Cérébrales Extracraniennes Asymptomatiques*, edited by R. Courbier, pp. 231–240. Oberval, Lyons.
21. Wylie, E. J., Hein, M. F., and Adams, J. E. (1964): Intracranial haemorrhage following surgical revascularisation for treatment of acute strokes. *J. Neurosurgery*, 21:212.
22. Yao, J. S. T., and Bergan, J. J. (1979): Selective cerebral protection during carotid endarterectomy. In: *Progress in Stroke Research*, edited by R. M. Greenhalgh and F. C. Rose, pp. 367–374. Pitman Medical Publishing, Tunbridge Wells.

TABLE 2. *Potential methods of evaluating STA–MCA anastomosis in stroke prophylaxis*

Comparison of historical controls
Patients as own controls
By cessation of TIA
rCBF improvement
Neurological recovery
Clinical judgement
Randomization by imperfect methods
Randomization from secret prearranged tables

between patient populations that may be dissimilar, and does not allow for the annual decline of 5% per year in stroke that is currently being observed (11).

Patients as Their Own Controls

The use of the patients as their own controls is proposed, often, as an alternative method of evaluation. It produces an unsatisfactory denominator for credible evaluation of the procedure. If the cessation of TIA is to be accepted as an indication of successful treatment, the tendency for TIA to cease spontaneously would have to be disregarded (6). Improvement in the patient's rCBF cannot be accepted as an end-point since it may not be diminished preoperatively or, if it is its reduction may not be related to any of the symptoms. Some resolution of neurological symptoms and signs is expected as a sequel to ischemia so that an appraisal of clinical improvement is of no value in deciding upon benefit of the operation for the individual patients.

Clinical Judgement

Clinical judgement based on an experienced practitioner's "innate sense of what to expect" is not of any value. The presumption that good results are sensed by practitioners has little scientific credibility. Disputing the need to evaluate surgical procedures by rigidly designed and controlled studies, one writer has stated: "A system of intrinsic controls in the practice of surgery already exists. It is based on the referral of patients for surgical therapy by primary physicians who are not surgeons and are rewarded only by good therapeutic results. The referring physician is thus the surgeon's Food and Drug Administration" (4). Imperfections in the alternate systems must be corrected rather than accepting the inexactitudes of this conclusion. More believable methods than those implied by this statement must be utilized.

Randomization

Randomization is the control system required for evaluation of therapy for chronic disease with a limited number of end-points occurring over a long period of time. Balanced, predetermined randomization tables that are kept secret from the participants constitute the most acceptable design. This method is superior to an assignment of patients to treatment groups by alternating cases, by those admitted on even or odd days of the month, or by those with certain birth dates. All of these alternatives to secret randomization tables are subject to bias from conscious or unconscious manipulation.

THE COLLABORATIVE EC/IC BYPASS STUDY

Multicenter Clinical Trial

A multicenter clinical trial was designed to determine the possible benefit in stroke prevention for certain groups of patients who present with the clinical and radiological features described above. Utilizing a pooling of existing knowledge on the prognosis for TIA patients as a whole (since information is not available for the more specific groups), assuming a 4% operative morbidity and mortality, allowing for a 15% loss to follow-up or compliance, and basing the calculated sample-size requirements on a one-tailed test with $\alpha = 0.05$ and $\beta = 0.10$, the numbers required for a risk reduction varying from 30 to 80% and over both a 3 and a 5-year period are set out in Table 3.

Surgical Participation

Surgical participation in the study required that the neurosurgical participants agree to the randomization of all suitable patients, that each surgeon produced

TABLE 3. *Sample size required for each of the two treatment groups to show surgical benefits of varying size in reducing stroke and stroke recurrence*

Surgical benefit	Medical stroke rate[a]	Surgical stroke rate	Required sample size
80% over 3 years	16.8	3.4 + 4.0	197 + 15% = 227
70% over 3 years	16.8	5.0 + 4.0	314 + 15% = 361
60% over 3 years	16.8	6.7 + 4.0	545 + 15% = 627
50% over 3 years	16.8	8.4 + 4.0	1,100 + 15% = 1,265
80% over 5 years	23.6	4.7 + 4.0	100 + 15% = 115
70% over 5 years	23.6	7.1 + 4.0	152 + 15% = 175
60% over 5 years	23.6	9.4 + 4.0	247 + 15% = 284
50% over 5 years	23.6	11.8 + 4.0	442 + 15% = 509
40% over 5 years	23.6	14.2 + 4.0	955 + 15% = 1,098
30% over 5 years	23.6	16.5 + 4.0	3,109 + 15% = 3,575

Surgical benefit = the percentage reduction in the stroke rate among surgically treated patients as compared to medically treated patients.
Assuming a 2% operative mortality rate which must be counted against the surgical group plus a 2% operative nonfatal stroke rate.
Fifteen % have been added to the computed sample size to allow for dropouts.
Sample size calculations are based on a one-tailed test with $\alpha = 0.05$ and $\beta = 0.10$.
[a]An average stroke rate calculated from control patient populations in previous TIA studies.

radiological evidence of a minimum of an 80% patency rate in 10 consecutive patients who submitted to the procedure prior to joining the study, and an agreement that all procedures within the study were to be conducted by the accredited surgeon and not by associates or assistants.

Participating Centers

Participating centers have proliferated beyond the initial plan, since fewer cases met the entry criteria in most centers than had been set out in the original estimates. Thirty-six North American, 18 European, and 13 Japanese centers have been entering cases.

PROGRESS OF COLLABORATIVE STUDY

The progress of the study has been monitored closely at the Central Office in London, Ontario and at the Methods Center in Hamilton, Ontario. By the end of April 1981, a total of 1,080 cases had been randomized, 594 from North America, 364 from Europe, and 122 from the Japanese centers. The North American and European centers have randomized a higher proportion of patients with internal carotid than middle cerebral artery lesions, while the reverse has been the case from the Japanese centers (Table 4).

Entry Characteristics

The entry characteristics in the patients assigned to the medical and surgical groups indicate that no serious distortions have arisen by virtue of the randomization process (Table 5). There is a distinct difference, however, between populations from North America and Europe compared with those from Japan in that, although the latter have the same incidence of hypertension at entry, there were half as many Japanese with diabetes, an 80% reduction in patients with a history of myocardial infarction and angina pectoris, and a total absence of patients with a history of intermittent claudication. Furthermore, as might be anticipated from the preponderance of patients entered because of symptoms due to middle cerebral contrasted to internal carotid artery disease, the neurological disability score was greater in the Japanese patients than in those entered from Europe and North America.

TABLE 4. *Randomized lesion by geographical region*

	Middle cerebral artery		Internal carotid artery	
	Occlusion	Stenosis	Occlusion	Stenosis
North America	6%	14%	64%	16%
Europe	13%	8%	64%	15%
Japan	26%	36%	21%	17%

TABLE 5. *Entry characteristics of treatment groups in collaborative EC/IC bypass study (North America, Europe, and Japan)*

		Medical	Surgical
Sex:	% Male	81%	80%
Race:	% White	82%	85%
Age (in years):	Mean mid 50%	57	57
Smoking history:	% Cigarette smoker	56%	54%
Employment status:	% Employed	55%	48%
Antiplatelet drugs:	ASA	30%	31%
	Other	9%	8%
Precipitating events:	Stroke	62%	61%
	TIA	38%	39%
Vascular exam:	Mean diastolic blood pressure	84	84
	Mean systolic blood pressure	142	143
	Mean heart rate	74	76
Medical problems:	Hypertension	50%	52%
	Diabetes	20%	16%
	Myocardial infarct	11%	11%
	Intermittent claudication	11%	16%
	Angina pectoris	10%	11%
	Congestive heart failure	1%	2%
	Cardiac surgery	2%	1%
	Other	22%	21%

Quality of Care

Measures have been taken to ensure quality of medical and surgical care, and adherence to high standards is kept under continuing surveillance in the Central Office and Methods Center. Risk factor management particularly control of hypertension is recorded on the three monthly follow-up forms. Complications following surgery including scalp flap necrosis, hematoma formation, as well as perioperative cardiac or pulmonary lesions, are scrutinized in an ongoing manner and have remained well within conventional and acceptable limits. Postoperative angiograms are required in each case, and the patency rate for the anastomoses, as reviewed by the Neuroradiologist-in-Chief at the Central Office, is 91%.

Crossover

The crossover of patients randomized to one category of therapy and electing on their own volition or by outside medical advice to seek treatment in the other category leaves open the possibility of a distorting influence on the final results. In dealing with informed patients, however, it always must be accepted that this may occur. In the study to date, 18 patients randomized to medical therapy have been in receipt of advice that led to surgery; in the same period, 18 patients randomized to surgical treatment have decided against the procedure. These patients are categorized as "withdrawals" but will be followed at regular intervals until the conclusion of the trial.

Alerting System

An "alerting system" that could lead to the premature stopping of the study has been devised. The ethical requirement is that a highly significant benefit or harm from the procedure will not be overlooked to the detriment of the patients who have been randomized into the trial. The details of this are to be published elsewhere. The basic need has been to devise a system of a large series of computer simulations involving a biostatistician who is entirely aloof from the progress of the patient entry and all other operational aspects of the study. The total accumulation of end-point data is assembled at 6-month intervals, ensuring that all follow-up information is complete. If two successive 6-monthly analyses utilizing this process indicate that there is an unequivocal result to be declared in one direction or the other, the study will be stopped prior to the originally planned termination.

Sample Size

Revised sample size calculations have been made to allow for several unexpected developments in the evolution of the trial. Firstly the "crossover" cases who did not adhere to the prescribed randomization category will be replaced by an equal number of conforming cases. Patients with internal carotid artery occlusion, probably a low-risk group, have contributed an unexpectedly high 40% of the population of patients randomized into the study. Since this is a considerably higher proportion than was anticipated originally, an additional 300 cases have been added to the goal of the study. Finally, the Japanese patients have exhibited several characteristics at variance to the other racial groups. These differences make it prudent that this cadre of patients be submitted to separate analysis. Although the basic lesion is arteriosclerotic in both the Japanese and Caucasian patients, it is predominantly in middle cerebral artery rather than internal carotid artery distribution in the entries from Japan. It is not known whether this anatomical change will be reflected in a different prognosis for the racial groups, nor is it known what the effect will be of lack of homogeneity between the two major racial groups in respect to heart disease and symptoms of peripheral vascular disease. Separate analyses leading to the accumulation of another 250 to 300 cases over the original plan appear to be the wisest course. Sample size increases do not alter the protocol so that it is not a maneuver that will do anything other than strengthen the ultimate value of the trial.

CONCLUSIONS

It is anticipated that this study will produce a definitive answer with respect to the value of the anastomosis between the superficial temporal artery and cortical branches of the middle cerebral artery in stroke prevention.

If the study proves that cerebral bypass surgery has a contribution to make in stroke prevention, it is anticipated that it will be indicated in a relatively small number of patients presenting with TIA or minor stroke.

Without the denominator of a control group in a randomized trial, the worth of the procedure is highly speculative.

A collaborative study has been designed, began entering cases in 1977, and will continue case entry until 1982. Half of the patients are submitted by random selection to the surgical procedure, while all receive "best medical care."

No attempt is being made to evaluate STA–MCA anastomoses in improving the neurological status of patients who have suffered cerebral infarction.

No attempt is being made to evaluate bypass procedures that might be carried out on the posterior circulation to reduce the risk of stroke in vertebral–basilar artery territory. At present, this must be regarded as an area of preliminary experimentation.

REFERENCES

1. Austin, G., Laffin, D., and Hayward, W. (1974): Physiologic factors in the selection of patients for superficial temporal artery-to-middle cerebral artery anastomosis. *Surgery*, 75:861–868.
2. Barnett, H. J. M. (1979): The Canadian Cooperative Study of platelet-suppressive drugs in transient cerebral ischemia. In: *Cerebrovascular Diseases*, edited by T. R. Price, and E. Nelson, pp. 221–236. Raven Press, New York.
3. Barnett, H. J. M. (1982): Extracranial to intracranial bypass surgery. In: *Transient Ischemic Attacks*, edited by P. J. Morris and C. Warlow. Marcel Dekker, New York.
4. Bonchek, L. I. (1979): Are randomized trials appropriate for evaluating new operations? *N. Engl. J. Med.*, 301:44–45.
5. Furlan, A. J., Whisnant, J. P., and Baker, H. L. (1980): Long-term prognosis after carotid occlusion. *Neurology*, 30:986–988.
6. Harrison, M. J. G., and Marshall, J. (1977): The finding of thrombus at carotid endarterectomy and its relationship to the timing of surgery. *Br. J. Surg.*, 64:511–512.
7. Hinton, R. C., Mohr, J. P., Ackerman, R. H., Adair, L. B., and Fisher, C. M. (1979): Symptomatic middle cerebral artery stenosis. *Ann. Neurol.*, 5:152–157.
8. Meguro, K., Barnett, H. J. M., and Fox, A. J. (1981): Intracranial internal carotid artery stenosis. *Can. J. Neuro. Sci.*, 8:195.
9. Mohr, J. P. (1978): Transient ischemic attacks and the prevention of strokes. *N. Engl. J. Med.*, 299:93–95.
10. Peerless, S. J., and McCormick, C. W. (Eds.) (1980): *Microsurgery for Cerebral Ischemia*. Springer-Verlag, New York.
11. Soltero, I., Liu, K., Cooper, R., Stamler, J., and Garside, D. (1978): Trends in mortality from cerebrovascular diseases in the United States, 1960 to 1975. *Stroke*, 9:549–555.
12. Willis, T. (Ed.) (1973): *The London Practice of Physick*. Milford House Inc., Boston. p. 443.

Advances in Stroke Therapy, edited by
F. C. Rose. Raven Press, New York © 1982.

The Measurement of Spasticity

Emyr Wyn Jones and Graham P. Mulley

*Department of Medicine, University Hospital, Queen's Medical Centre, Nottingham NG7
2UH, and Department of Health Care of the Elderly, Sherwood Hospital,
Nottingham, NG5 1PD England*

WHAT IS SPASTICITY?

Even though spasticity occurs in a wide variety of neurological conditions, a precise and universally acceptable definition is not available (16). The term spasticity is applied to disorders of motor control resulting from lesions that can occur at different levels of the neuraxis, affect several neuronal systems, produce different functional problems for the patient, and respond (if at all) to different types of therapy (27). Different disciplines have their own perspective on the phenomenon of spasticity.

The Clinical Viewpoint

The clinician sees spasticity as increased muscle "tone" or increased muscle resistance to passive stretch which is dependent on the rate of muscle stretch (20). It is part of the "upper motor neurone syndrome" which includes muscle weakness, enhanced tendon reflexes, clonus, and abnormal surface reflexes and which is found in patients with lesions of motor pathways within the central nervous system. In some spastic muscles, the increase in resistance is followed by sudden relaxation (the clasp knife effect), and this characteristic helps in the clinical distinction between hypertonicity due to upper motor neurone lesions (spasticity) and that due to extrapyramidal lesions (rigidity) in which the increased resistance to muscle stretch is uniform throughout the range of movement, and independent of rate of muscle stretch (lead pipe effect).

The Physiotherapy Viewpoint

The physiotherapist sees spasticity in terms of reversion to the movement patterns of the primitive reflexes seen in infancy: as "... hypertonicity which predominates in muscles in one or more primitive patterns of movement of the affected part(s). The dysfunction of the nervous system imposes a stereotyped pattern of total synergy on attempted willed movement" (11). Thus spasticity is seen to interfere with the quality of movement and to prevent normal postural reactions. Much of the work of physiotherapists in the treatment of stroke patients is nowadays aimed at breaking "patterns of spasticity" as it is felt that if the influences of the reflexes that produce spasticity are allowed to continue, then they become reinforced so that the abnormal postures become harder to break up during the later rehabilitation period (7). It is felt that spasticity is an unnecessary evil; the spastic patient who has great difficulty in moving his hypertonic limbs is liable to poor mobility and unsteadiness.

The Neurophysiology Viewpoint

The neurophysiologist sees spasticity in terms of the complex mechanisms of the muscle stretch reflex (Fig. 1). Muscle spindles are complex, fusiform sensory structures within muscles that serve to signal changes in muscle length (12). These stretch receptors transmit information to the spinal cord along group Ia and II afferent fibres. The incoming afferent volley affects the alpha motoneurones of the stretched muscle, which then reflexly contracts.

The tendon jerk is an example of a phasic stretch reflex, where it is thought that the afferent volley makes a direct monosynaptic connection with the alpha motoneurones. Sustained muscle stretch, however, produces a tonic stretch reflex, where the asynchronous afferent volleys produced by a stretching movement connect with the alpha motoneurone by polysynaptic pathways involving a number of interneurones.

The sensitivity of muscle spindle receptors may be adjusted by the action of gamma motoneurones, or fusiform efferent fibres. Fusimotor control of tension in intrafusal fibres adjusts the sensitivity of primary endings so that they can signal changes in muscle length regardless of the overall muscle length at that moment.

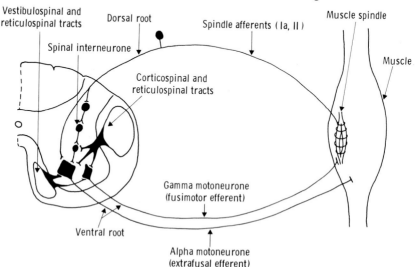

FIG. 1. A simplified diagram of a basic spinal reflex arc.

Without fusimotor activity, a muscle spindle would be sensitive only at one length of the muscle.

The spinal reflex mechanism is modified by messages traveling down the spinal cord from higher centres. These messages include inhibition by the descending corticospinal tracts and facilitation by the bulbospinal pathways. The character of spasticity therefore may differ in important respects according to the site of the lesion that causes it, and depending on the integrity or otherwise of various descending pathways that may influence and modify spinal neurones and reflex arcs. For example, following a cortical or capsular lesion, descending pathways such as the vestibulospinal, reticulospinal, and monoaminergic bulbospinal systems are still intact, and spasticity probably results from uncontrolled facilitatory activity in these pathways, and loss of descending inhibitory activity in the corticospinal pathways. In spinal transection, on the other hand, these pathways are all eliminated—spinal spasticity must therefore result from a different set of causes.

Lesions of the upper motoneurone anywhere from the cerebral cortex to the spinal cord may be accompanied by spasticity. In their course from cortex to alpha and gamma motoneurones, most fibres are interrupted by relays with neurones of the basal ganglia and brainstem nuclei and with interneurones at spinal level (though some monosynaptic corticospinal pathways do exist to motoneurones of muscles moving the fingers which accounts for the clinical observation that individual movements of the fingers are those most affected by lesions directly involving cerebral cortex).

Brainstem control of most primitive spinal reflexes is therefore not altered in cerebral spasticity so that dramatic changes in muscle tone can be effected by reducing the activity in the responsible bulbospinal pathways by manoeuvres such as altering head posture, turning the patient upside down, or using the opposite limb. Clinically the preservation of these primitive brainstem reflexes is manifested as the tonic labyrinthine reflexes, the symmetrical and asymmetrical tonic neck reflexes, and as stereotyped mass movements that accompany attempted voluntary movement (3). These also can be seen as "associated reactions" when the patient yawns, coughs, or carries out any movement under stress (5).

Summary

Spasticity is therefore not one particular disorder of motor control, but results from a variety of factors producing a range of clinical symptoms and signs that variously are interpreted by observers with differing interests and training. Although there is currently much interest in the physiology of spasticity, there has been little development in the basic understanding of the underlying mechanisms. We cannot yet explain the interesting empirical observations of physiotherapists in neurophysiological terms.

WHY MEASURE SPASTICITY?

Spasticity usually, but not always, occurs in the affected side of patients with stroke, and may adversely affect postural and functional recovery as well as lead to painful flexor spasms and long term complications such as contractures and joint instability. During treatment and rehabilitation of patients after strokes, a great deal of effort is directed towards the abolition of spasticity and to the removal or attenuation of factors thought to increase spasticity.

Physiotherapists use a variety of exercises and postural training to suppress primitive reflexes and enhance more mature "righting reflexes" in an attempt to delay and minimise the development of spastic synergy (7). Physical methods such as local cooling (14,17) and vibration (18) also are used in the belief that they reduce the discharge rate of the fusimotor efferent fibres, thus altering the sensitivity of the muscle spindles to stretch, and reducing spasticity.

The pharmaceutical industry has expended a great deal of time, effort, and money in the search for an effective and safe antispasmodic drug (6), and the fact that the search continues suggests that the drugs currently available have important limitations (diazepam causes drowsiness, dantrolene and baclofen produce unwanted weakness) (8).

Evaluation of these physical and pharmacological techniques of treating spasticity is often purely subjective and based on standard clinical scales such as the Ashworth scale (2) (Table 1) or the Oswestry scale (11). Such subjective methods of assessing a phenomenon as variable as spasticity are of necessity crude and unreliable, making evaluation of therapy difficult and open to error and bias. A need therefore exists for an objective and quantifiable method of measuring spasticity under standard conditions so that the effect of treatment may be evaluated accurately and more may be learned about the natural variability of spasticity and the factors that affect it.

HOW TO MEASURE SPASTICITY

The need for an objective measurement of spasticity has been recognized for many years (10) and many methods have been developed and evaluated but, to date, there is no universally acceptable, easily applicable method.

Investigators have tried to quantify different aspects of the spinal reflex in an attempt to find a method of measurement that correlates to a reasonable degree with the abnormal symptomatology and physical signs that the physician ordinarily sees, and of which their patients complain.

The Hoffmann or 'H' Reflex

Stimulation of a peripheral nerve with low intensity current results in excitation of the afferent nerve fibres arising from the muscle spindle, with exclusion of the

TABLE 1. *Spasticity: Ashworth scale*

0	Normal muscle tone
1	Slight increase in tone—"catch" when limb moved
2	More marked increase in tone but limb easily flexed
3	Considerable increase in tone
4	Limb rigid in flexion or extension

large efferent motor fibres that have higher thresholds. Therefore a response known as the 'H' reflex will be obtained via the spinal reflex arc and can be recorded by means of a surface electrode placed on the belly of the appropriate muscle. The H reflex has been shown to be transmitted by the monosynaptic spinal reflex pathway and therefore corresponds to the phasic stretch reflex elicited by tendon tapping. The latency of the H response is obviously longer than that of the direct response of the muscle to stimulation of its efferent motor fibres, known as the 'M' wave.

Measurement of the H reflex reflects the excitability of the monosynaptic pathway of the tendon jerk and has been used as a means of quantifying spasticity (24). Other workers (1) have used the ratio of the latencies of the H and M responses as a numerical measure of spasticity but the H reflex can be extremely variable in the same subject and cannot always be elicited. Also, although measurements of the H reflex and H:M ratio reflect the excitability of clinical tendon reflexes, they are a poor guide to the overall severity of spasticity in a given patient (19).

The 'F' Wave

The 'F' wave is another late response to stimulation of a peripheral nerve, differing from the H reflex in its behaviour on changing the strength of electrical stimulation. The origin of the F wave is uncertain—it may represent a spinal reflex response transmitted by slowly conducting afferent nerve fibres, and it is also likely that it is transmitted by a polysynaptic reflex pathway involving spinal interneurones. It therefore corresponds to the tonic stretch reflex elicited clinically by passive muscle stretch. A positive correlation has been found between the amplitude of F responses and the presence of spasticity (9), but this method only identified 60% of spastic patients and, as single fibre electromyography is necessary to clearly distinguish F waves from H reflexes (22,23), the method is too complex for everyday clinical use.

Measurements of H reflexes and F waves have not been used widely in clinical evaluation of spasticity, partly because the parameters being measured are removed from the clinical situation. Therefore methods have been devised that attempt to quantify the subjectively observed clinical manifestations of spasticity.

Phasic Stretch Reflex

The phasic stretch reflex has been measured (21,22) by eliciting the ankle jerk by applying a reproducible and uniform mechanical stimulus in the form of an electromagnetic hammer striking the patient's Achilles tendon. The hammer is driven by a rotational magnet excited by a constant current for a given time interval. Angular velocity, and hence angular momentum of the rubber head of the hammer, is proportional to the duration of the exciting current.

The strength of the hammer impact can be adjusted for each patient to provide stimulation above the threshold for eliciting the ankle jerk but below that needed for maximal response. This value is kept uniform for each patient and the foot is placed in the same position for each successive test so that the hammer strikes as closely as possible to the same place on the tendon.

The ankle reflex response is picked up by a transducer formed as a pedal with the vertical and horizontal positions of the patient's foot being fully adjustable to give proper relation between the ankle joint and pedal axis. The transducer is able to measure the ankle reflex either isotonically (angle measurement using an angle potentiometer coupled to the pedal axis) or isometrically (using a beam incorporating four strain gauges coupled in a full bridge giving a differential d.c. signal proportional to the torque).

The output signals from the angle potentiometer and the strain gauge bridge are fed back to an amplifier and then to an on-line analogue computer. This directly integrates the torque signal with the duration of the response and the angle of movement elicited by the same stimulus, giving a numerical reading proportional to the angular momentum of the reflex response. This reading is taken to represent the magnitude of the reflex.

This method is used to evaluate antispastic and antiparkinsonian therapy, and to document the effect of local cooling on spasticity. In order to separate the effects of cooling on the reflex response from the effects on the viscoelastic properties of the muscle, simultaneous electromyographic recordings are made from surface electrodes placed over the muscle bellies.

The method would appear to be successful in demonstrating changes in strength of phasic stretch reflex responses after oral and intravenous administration of the antispasmodic drug baclofen and after local cooling (15), but there is no report of these changes being associated with similar changes in clinical spasticity. The complexity of the apparatus required for carrying out these measurements of phasic stretch reflexes and the lack of obvious relationship between the results obtained and patient response seems to preclude its use for the routine evaluation of spasticity in the clinical situation.

Tonic Stretch Reflexes

Several workers have tried to measure spasticity by attempting to quantify the response of muscles to passive stretch, and an elaborate apparatus has been designed for this purpose. Passive stretch has been induced by applying a given weight for a given time (20), or by using electrical motors as torque generators to move a limb (25).

Muscle response has been recorded electromyographically (21) using surface electrodes placed over the muscle belly or alternatively, the actual resistance of the muscle to passive stretch has been recorded (4,26) and changes in this resistance taken as a measure of changes in spasticity. This latter method probably corresponds most closely to the common finding of increased muscle "tone" in spasticity.

Ideal System

Many considerations are involved in the design of an ideal system for recording muscle tone. Boshes et al. (4) list many of these requirements including:

1. Operation of the system should not be painful.

2. The system should not be complicated in operation or appearance and should not require darkening of the room or performance of other manoeuvres that might distract the patient.

3. The system must be accurate and capable of calibration and the results must be reproducible.

4. Tension of isolated muscle groups should be recorded in absolute units of force.

5. Tone should be measured during motion of an extremity in an horizontal plane (to neutralize the effects of gravity).

6. The procedure should be designed to eliminate voluntary tension and phasic reflexes in the muscles studied.

7. Tone must be measured during a constant velocity period of limb motion so that the mass of the limb will add no torque to that produced by muscle tension per se.

Webster (26) developed such a method of quantitating spasticity as a work function response to controlled rates of passive motion of the forearm or of the lower leg. Spasticity was defined as the work output in response to angular velocity input per 100 degree cycle of passive motion. The velocity-dependent nature of spasticity was utilised to derive a "spasticity index" obtained from the total work value at varying velocities. The method was used to assess the efficiency of anti-spastic agents, but difficulties were encountered with instability of long-term base-line levels of spasticity. The complexity of the machinery and the nonphysiological testing position precluded the use of the method as a clinically applicable means of measuring spasticity.

SUMMARY

Spasticity is a common finding in the affected limbs of patients with strokes, and the underlying mechanisms are complex and variable. Disparate views exist about the nature of spasticity, according to the training and speciality of the observer. Spasticity may affect adversely postural and functional recovery after strokes, and a great deal of effort is expended in trying to combat spasticity both physically and pharmacologically.

There is a need for a simple method of measuring spasticity in order to unify the various definitions of spasticity on a quantitative basis and to evaluate the natural variation in spasticity and the effects of various forms of therapy. Although many methods have been developed to quantitate different aspects of the spinal reflex in order to find a method of measurement that correlates to a reasonable degree with the clinical signs and symptoms of spasticity, none has yet been totally successful, and problems of complexity of instrumentation and clinical inapplicability have not been overcome.

Spasticity is so variable that problems of long-term, baseline stability of measurement are difficult to master. Many of the methods described are too cumbersome for repeated routine clinical use and too complex for easy application to stroke patients who are often too disabled both physically and mentally to comply for long periods with the demands that would be made on them.

In Nottingham, we have developed a portable machine (13) that accurately measures the resistance of the elbow joint to flexion and extension and provides us with objective measurements of spasticity. The machine has been used on the wards, in outpatient clinics, and in physiotherapy departments to monitor the progress of patients after strokes. The information gleaned from the measurement of spasticity is being used together with other, more functional assessments of progress, to help doctors and physiotherapists work out the best programme for each patient.

Although direct measurement of spasticity is an important goal, what actually matters to the patient is how well his hemiplegic side functions. Future studies of spasticity should include not only objective measures of resistance to stretch, but also more coarse-grained end-points relating to the patient's ability to perform everyday activities. If, as a result of our ministrations, the patient is at risk of falls, is unable to dress, walk, and go to the toilet independently or does not venture out of the house, we have not achieved very much.

REFERENCES

1. Angel, R. W., and Hoffmann, W. W. (1963): The H reflex in normal, spastic and rigid subjects. *Arch. Neurol.*, 8:591–596.
2. Ashworth, B. (1964): Preliminary trial of carisoprodol in multiple sclerosis. *Practitioner*, 192:540–542.
3. Bobath, B. (1971): Segmental static reactions. In: *Abnormal Postural Reflex Activity Caused by Brain Lesions* (2nd ed.), pp.20–56. William Heinemann, London.
4. Boshes, B., Wachs, H., Brumlik, J., and Mier, M. (1960): Studies of tone, tremor and speech in normal persons and parkinsonian patients. *Neurology*, 10:805–813.
5. Brunstrom, S. (1970): Motor behaviour in adult patients with hemiplegia. In: *Movement Therapy in Hemiplegia.* pp. 7–33. Harper and Row, New York.
6. Burke, D. J. (1975): An approach to the treatment of spasticity. *Drugs*, 10:112–120.
7. Dardier, E. (1980): Reflex activity, normal and abnormal. *The Early Stroke Patient, Positioning and Movement*, pp. 23–37. Bailliere Tindall, London.
8. Davidoff, R. A. (1978): Pharmacology of spasticity. *Neurology*, 28:46–51.
9. Eisen, A., and Odusote, K. (1979): Amplitude of the F wave: A potential means of documenting spasticity. *Neurology*, 29:1306–1313.
10. Fenn, W. O., and Garvey, P. H. (1934): The measurement of the elasticity and viscosity of skeletal muscle in normal and pathological cases: a study of so called "muscle tonus." *J. Clin. Invest.*, 13:383–361.
11. Goff, B. (1976): Grading of spasticity and its effect on voluntary movement. *Physiotherapy*, 62:385–361.
12. Hagbarth, K. E., Wallin, G., and Löfstedt, L. (1973): Muscle spindle responses to stretch in normal and spastic subjects. *Scand. J. Rehab. Med.*, 5:156–159.
13. Jones, E. W., Plant, G. R., Stuart, C. R., Mulley, G. P., and Johnson, F. (1982): Comments on design of an instrument to measure spasticity in the arm—S.A.M. *Eng. Med.*, 11:47–50.
14. Knutsson, E. (1970): On effects of local cooling upon motor functions in spastic paresis. *Prog. Phys. Ther.*, 1:124–131.
15. Knutsson, E., Lindbolm, U., and Martensson, A. (1973): Differences in effects in gamma and alpha spasticity induced by the GABA derivative baclofen (Lioresal). *Brain*, 96:29–46.
16. Landau, W. M. (1974): Spasticity: The fable of a neurological demon and the emperor's new therapy. *Arch. Neurol.*, 31:217–219.
17. Lee, J. M., and Warren, M. P. (1974): Ice, relaxation and exercise in reduction of muscle spasticity. *Physiotherapy*, 60:296–301.

18. Levine, M. G., Kabat, H., Knott, M., and Voss, D. E. (1954): Relaxation of spasticity by physiological techniques. *Arch. Phys. Med. Rehab.*, 34:214–223.
19. Matthews, W. B. (1966): Ratio of maximum H reflex to maximum M response as a measure of spasticity. *J. Neurol. Neurosurg. Psychiatr.*, 29:201–204.
20. Ogilvie, C. (1980): The Nervous System. In: *Chamberlain's Symptoms and Signs in Clinical Medicine. An Introduction to Medical Diagnosis*, (10th ed.), pp. 320–433. John Wright and Sons Ltd., Bristol.
21. Pedersen, E., Arlien-Soborg, P., and Mai, J. (1974): The mode of action of the GABA derivative baclofen in human spasticity. *Acta Neurol. Scand.*, 50:665–680.
22. Pedersen, E., Dietrichson, P., Gormsen, J., and Arlien-Soborg, P. (1974): Measurement of phasic and tonic stretch reflexes in antispastic and anti parkinsonian therapy. *Scand. J. Rehab. Med. (Suppl)*, 3:51–60.
23. Schiller, H. H., and Stalberg, E. (1978): F responses studied with single fibre EMG in normal subjects and spastic patients. *J. Neurol. Neurosurg. Psychiatr.*, 41:45–53.
24. Spira, R. (1976): Contribution of the H reflex to the study of spasticity in adolescents. *Physiotherapy*, 62:401–405.
25. Walsh, E. G., Lakie, M., Wright, G. W., and Tzementzio, S. A. (1980): Measurement of muscle tone using printed motors as torque generators. *Eng. Med.*, 9:167–171.
26. Webster, D. D. (1964): The dynamic quantitation of spasticity with automated integrals of passive motion resistance. *Clin. Pharmacol. Ther.*, 5:900–908.
27. Young, R. R., and Delwaide, P. J. (1981): Drug therapy, spasticity (first of two parts). *N. Engl. J. Med.*, 304:28–33.

Advances in Stroke Therapy, edited by
F. C. Rose. Raven Press, New York © 1982.

Studies in Hemiplegic Gait

P. -L. Chin, A. Rosie, M. Irving, and R. Smith

Department of Geriatric Medicine, Cumberland Infirmary, Carlisle, England

The aim of any rehabilitation service set up for hemiplegic patients is the restoration of independent self care and one of the basic requirements is that the patient should be able to walk. Purists may disagree with such a broad statement for it is undeniable that paraplegic patients and amputees can do wonders albeit from the compromised position of a wheelchair. However, most experienced workers in the field of hemiplegic rehabilitation would concur that the complexities of cerebral damage in the stroke patient precludes many achieving dextrous adapation to wheelchair life. The majority of hemiplegic patients resorting to the wheelchair to get about are dependent rather than independent for activities of daily living from the wheelchair.

When confronted with large numbers of patients for rehabilitation, as in stroke illness, pressure on bed space demands the discharge of patients as soon as they are safely able to manage in the environment in which they are to be resettled. It is perhaps not easy in such circumstances to pay too much attention to the details of even so basic a function as walking ability. On the other hand, in recent years several physical therapy techniques have been promoted in the rehabilitation of stroke patients (4,7,21,30), each purporting to give better results, but only Bodgardh (5) has resorted to objective measurements of gait parameters in the evaluation of results of her exercise programme.

Specific studies on hemiplegic locomotion (8,11,22,23,28) have been carried out in small groups of patients concentrating on different aspects of locomotion while large studies of the stroke population (1,12,24) concerning overall recovery give scant detail on the qualitative and quantitative aspects of walking ability.

In 1973 as part of a prospective study of stroke patients, an analysis of the various features of locomotion in hemiplegic patients was initiated in the Department of Geriatric Medicine, Carlisle. This was supported by a grant from the Research Committee of the Northern Regional Health Authority.

METHODS

In a study of walking disability following any physical or neurological insult, it is necessary to take into consideration other attendant pathologies, particularly in a condition such as hemiplegia, whose incidence is highest in the elderly (10,25,31,32). In such patients, multiple pathology is the rule rather than the exception and cardiovascular, locomotor, and other neurological disorders may complicate the issue. Conversely, the advance in diverse technology used in analysis of locomotion makes it impossible to encompass the whole spectrum of gait disorders (17). In general, studies in locomotion may be divided into two broad aspects: kinetic studies that are concerned with forces acting on joints, reaction forces at the foot; and kinematic studies that are concerned with aspects of walking ability such as step length, velocity, foot contact with the floor, as well as the angular movements of major joints in the lower limb, pelvis, and trunk.

Instrumentation for kinetic studies is both expensive and complicated and requires expert handling. At current prices, Grieve (17) has calculated that a fully equipped gait laboratory with technical backing excluding the accommodation and salaries of scientific and clinical investigators would cost approximately £100 per day. Budget and manpower constraints precluded studies of kinetic aspects of hemiplegic gait in our unit. Kinematics is the more "visual" aspect of locomotion familiar to clinicians. The requirements of instrumentation were that they should be relatively inexpensive yet robust and easily handled by clinical staff. Such instrumentation was not easily available commercially and so a major part of the project was engaged in designing and testing instrumentation for gait studies in strokes. Details of instrumentation are the subject of another report (9). Briefly, the methods used for observing gait patterns were as follows:

1. Visual and subjective account using a check list (7) designed specifically for hemiplegic gait.

2. Videotape records using two cameras simultaneously for frontal and side projections of subject. Videorecorder has capability of individual scan facility.

3. A high-speed camera—64 frames/sec with analysing projector allowing single frame and reverse frame facility.

4. Electrogoniometer incorporating a Bryant X-Y Plotter to produce gait cycle chart (16).

5. Temporal studies using a time-base recorder with foot switches and photo-electric cells to measure velocity over specified distance as well as frequency of steppage and step length.

6. Foot–floor contact sequence device incorporating pressure-sensitive insole and foot image display system to ascertain point of foot contact during early stance phase.

7. Vertical perception test using modified Witkin apparatus.

8. Evaluation of exoskeletal braces and functional electrical stimulator—Ljubjlana—as aids to ambulation.

Patients studied were those admitted to medical and geriatric wards at the Cumberland Infirmary and City General Hospital, Carlisle, from 1973 on. For purposes of studying clinical aspects in relation to ambulation, an initial clinical profile of all patients was recorded. This forms part of a long-term prospective study of cerebrovascular disease in Carlisle. The clinical profile of patients and assessment methods were based on data obtained from several authors (1,3,13,18,19,26).

In the absence of a standardized definition of walking competence in stroke patients, a preliminary study of ambulatory requirements of stroke patients in performance of activities of daily living was initiated. Discussion with relatives and patients showed that one of the most important basic tasks was the ability to get to the nearest toilet and move around inside the house. Isaacs (19) has also pointed out that this is a major daily activity of a patient.

Figure 1 shows the distribution of distances between a sitting room and a toilet in 50 "typical homes" in East Cumbria Health District. The homes visited ranged from modern bungalows to farm houses and large and small Victorian households where the toilet may be situated outside the main building. In such a survey it is obvious that distances vary widely, but in 80% of the houses visited 20 metres was found to be the mean distance between the nearest toilet and the sitting room. We

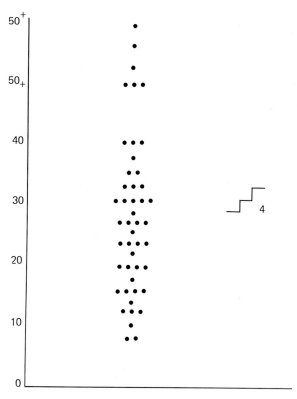

FIG. 1. Distance from sitting room to nearest toilet (metres) in 50 households.

therefore defined our walking competence as ability to rise from a chair and to walk at least 20 metres on a smooth surface with or without a walking aid but not requiring physical help.

RESULTS AND DISCUSSION

For continuity of theme and convenience, the results and discussion of observations for each particular section of the project are considered together.

Overall Recovery Patterns

A total of 620 patients were studied between 1971 and 1979. Classification of walking activity was based on the above definition, 1971 to 1973 retrospectively and from 1974 to 1979 prospectively. The age range of patients was from 35 to 92, 79% of patients being over the age of 65. There were no sex differences in achievement of walking competence. Table 1 shows the overall recovery pattern of the 620 patients who had survived the initial insult of the stroke. Thus, the overall recovery pattern cannot be taken to be a true reflection of the overall picture of stroke admissions to a hospital. A cut off point of three weeks was chosen arbitrarily because analysis of mortality of admissions in previous years had shown that on average, 30% of stroke admissions died within this period.

Of the 620 patients admitted, 52% were found to achieve the level of competence of walking defined above, and of these, only about one-third walked without any aids and could negotiate different terrain confidently. When this is considered in the context of the whole study population, the figure falls to 17% (103 patients).

The overall figure of 52% achieving ambulation is lower than that in other hospital series (1,24) that report achievement of walking ability in approximately 60% of their series (Table 2). However, in these reports, there was no definition of walking competence but it can be deduced that approximately 25 to 30% of patients recovered to walk "confidently."

More recently Garroway (14), studying rehabilitation of stroke patients in medical wards and a stroke unit, reported that 54% of survivors were mobile and walking.

TABLE 1. *Prognosis in 620 stroke patients—6 months at Cumberland Infirmary, 1971–1979*

Prognosis	No. patients	% Total
Ambulant—without physical help	322	52
Confident—walk on most terrains (32%)		
Independent self-care (32%)		
Safe ambulation with walking		
aid held in one or both upper limbs (68%)		
Wheelchair bound—only walk with physical help	106	17
Partially independent from wheelchair		
Bed bound or static chair bound, unable to manoeuvre wheelchair,	81	13
usually incontinent, mental impairment		
Died with two months of stroke, having survived	111	18
initial episode		

TABLE 2. *Functional recovery of stroke survivors (hospital-based studies)*

Study	No.	% Mobile/ walking	Type of study
Adams (2) Belfast	1,374	59	Geriatric adm.
Droller (12) Leeds	121	57	Geriatric adm.
Marquardsen (24) Copenhagen	404	68	Neurological unit
Chin (9) Carlisle	620	52	Medical and geriatric adm.
Garraway (14) Edinburgh	234	54	Medical and stroke unit

TABLE 3. *Functional recovery of stroke survivors (community studies)*

Study	No.	% Moblie/walking
Gresham (15) Framingham	119	80
Brocklehurst (6) Manchester	135	68
Chin (10) Carlisle	106	69

On the other hand, community studies covering all stroke incidences, show a higher proportion of survivors from stroke capable of walking (Table 3). Gresham (15) reported that 80% of 119 stroke survivors were mobile and walking. Brocklehurst (6), in a community study, reported that 68% of 135 were mobile. In a prospective register of stroke patients in 1978 to 1979 we found that 69% of 106 stroke patients who survived after 1 month were ambulant. This difference between community- and hospital-based studies is most probably due to the fact that community studies include a fair number of people who recover spontaneously from their stroke and never need hospital care.

Qualitative Aspects of Walking Ability

In the early stages of our project, it was thought that specific gait patterns could be identified easily. However, it became evident quite soon that (using visual analysis assisted by videotape recordings and cinematography) the majority of patients could not be categorised easily into specific gait patterns. One reason was that most patients were elderly in whom multiple pathology was the rule rather than the exception, and the presence of different locomotor and other pathologies precluded easy categorisation. In view of this and because we were interested in the overall recovery pattern of a stroke population, we simply resorted to classifying the gait patterns according to the type of walking aid used; this was found to be one of the major factors in alteration of gait pattern. Patients were divided into three major groups. Table 4 shows the walking ability of the 322 patients. Types

TABLE 4. *Walking ability in 322 patients*

Group I:	Ambulant without aids	32%
Group II:	Ambulant	48%
	(a) With cane or metal stick 42%	
	(b) With tripod or quadrupod 58%	
Group III:	Ambulant with pulpit-type walking frame	20%

of patients belonging to the different groups and their clinical and gait characteristics are the subject of another report. Over two-thirds of the patients required an aid of some sort to walk safely. Plotting the distribution of types of aids used against age groups we found that older stroke victims relied more on tripods and Zimmer frames. It was also evident that the type of walking aid used varied with time and inclination. Patients tended to move from one group to the other but for purposes of this study, the aid ascribed to the patient was that in which the patient felt most confident and preferred.

One hundred and three patients (32%) were able to walk without aid confidently. However, closer analysis of this group showed that 40% still had perceptible disturbance of gait such as intermittent scuffing of the ground, particularly when they were tired, a slight limp, and reduced or total loss of swinging movement of the hemiplegic upper limb. Some patients reported that the lack of arm movement during the walking cycle was not just a residual marker of the stroke but that loss of active movement in the hemiplegic upper limb was a distinct disadvantage when crossing rough and difficult terrain when their balance was compromised. Those who had normal upper limb swing felt quite confident even when their balance was disturbed when walking on rough ground.

Approximately one-half of those who were able to walk without aid could run, suggesting a persistence of some disturbance of balance mechanisms even when confident walking ability was achieved.

Characteristics of Posture and Movement Patterns During the Gait Cycle

Using videotape and high-speed cinematography, we analyzed the characteristics of posture and movement patterns during gait cycle in 257 patients whose major disability was from the stroke. These patients did not have any other locomotor or neurological disorder that might have clouded the issue. In this particular aspect of the study, we were interested in ascertaining the type of neurological deficit that determined different types of postures during the gait cycle. Table 5 shows the common abnormalities noted using a modified Brunnstrom gait chart designed specifically for hemiplegic patients. Some patients had a combination of various abnormalities in the stance and swing phase, and it was not possible to categorise the majority of patients into specific types of gait pattern. In 18% who had strong extensor synergy in the lower limb, a characteristic posture in early stance phase, in which the forefoot in equinovarus position was seen to hit the ground first with

TABLE 5. *Common abnormalities noted in 257 patients*

Stance phase	%	Swing phase	%
Hip: Forward tilt	45	Circumduction	22
Trendelenberg	9	Slow and stiff swing	20
Knee: Hyperextension	40	Stiff, held in extension	40
Slight flexion	15	Exaggerated flexion	6
Ankle: Toe contact first	65	Toe drag	70
or		and	
Whole sole down		Floor scuffing	

a short stance phase. In some, this was one-half that of the nonhemiplegic limb. In such patients, circumduction was seen commonly in the swing phase. Colaso (11) reported a study of gait patterns in 50 young hemiplegic patients walking without aid. He found that the commonest disability in this group of patients was the presence of a drop foot. The other most common characteristic was the presence of extensor synergistic patterns in the hemiplegic limb.

Knuttson's study (22) of motor control in the gait of 26 hemiparetic patients using interrupted light photography and electromyography showed that there were several different motor patterns of recovery. In other words observed abnormalities of lower limb behaviour visually or on videotape recordings are probably as different as the brain lesions causing them. On the other hand, the same abnormalities noted may be due to different mechanisms.

In the stance phase, it would appear that forward tilt of the trunk, hyperextension of the knee joint, and forefoot contact or whole sole contact of the ground at the ankle joint were the most common features observed. In the swing phase, circumduction and a slow swing of the hip with the knee held stiffly either in slight flexion or in extension resulting in dragging of the toes, were the main features. This section of our project, although difficult to quantify, was perhaps of most practical value. A study of the variations in gait pattern and posture in stroke patients enabled the rehabilitation team to reappraise causes of particular abnormalities during the swing or stance phase so that corrective measures could be taken. In some cases, scraping of the floor by the hemiplegic foot may be seen as due to a drop foot whereas the major problem was found to be lack of flexion at the hip or knee joint due either to motor weakness or marked extensor spasticity. Braces prescribed to control drop foot were ineffective in many instances.

In this context, we feel that a videotape system that allows for quick replay and sequential records of patients' performance is a useful tool for the physiotherapist. Methods of evaluating the effectiveness of video recordings in rehabilitation of stroke patients are fraught with problems of design and measurement. Nevertheless, it is our experience that by studying video recordings of patients, inapparent faults were identified and in some, these were easily remedied, particularly when patients could observe themselves on a video monitor.

Kinematic Studies

Most people walk with deceptive facility and the ability to cope with different terrains by altering of gait pattern and speed is taken for granted. The central nervous control of these complex changes depends on intact sensory feedback and modulation of the musculoskeletal system through central efferent outflow. The extent to which cerebral damage affects walking ability must necessarily depend on sites of damage and compensatory mechanisms of normal residual function. Thus, wide variations in different parameters of gait are to be expected. We investigated three temporal aspects of gait in stroke patients:

1. Cadence (the number of steps taken in 1 min) and velocity.

2. Step length of hemiplegic and nonhemiplegic legs.

3. Regularity of steppage.

Sixty-two patients were selected for the study of temporal aspects of gait. They were selected following visual observations and videotape studies to represent various groups of patients with similar gait features to indicate variation of temporal aspects of gait. For velocity and step length, estimation of the mean of three traverses between two photoelectric cells placed 3 m apart were calculated. Patients were tested at their free walking speed, i.e., at the pace at which they felt most comfortable. A few patients who had full recovery of balance mechanisms were also asked to walk at their fastest rate. Figure 2 shows the speed of walking with type of aid used. The range of walking speed over the whole group was 5 to 64 m/min. This shows a wide scatter. The mean of 20 normal patients studied for free walking was 59 m/min. It is seen in Fig. 1 that the mean of group 1, i.e., those who walk without aid, was 51 m/min which is slightly below the mean of normal, but approximates that of normal people at the lower range on the scattergram. Examination of those patients with similar walking speeds in the various groups, i.e., those walking with or without aid, showed that extensor synergistic pattern was the main determinant of their speed of walking. Most of these patients had equinovarus deformity in the erect posture.

Norton and her colleagues (27), in their study of correlation between gait speed and spasticity at the knee, measured subjects walking at their fastest. The range of the fastest walking speed in her group varied from 16 to 104 m.

Our method of measuring walking speed of patients assumes a steady forward progression, and any hesitation during the traverse increases the time. Therefore, this method of measurement of velocity has the inherent faults of any system that measures speed by relying on traverses through marked distances.

Steppage

Observation of tracings taken on patients using foot switches on a time-base recorder showed the irregularity of steppage, that is, the step length of both hemi-

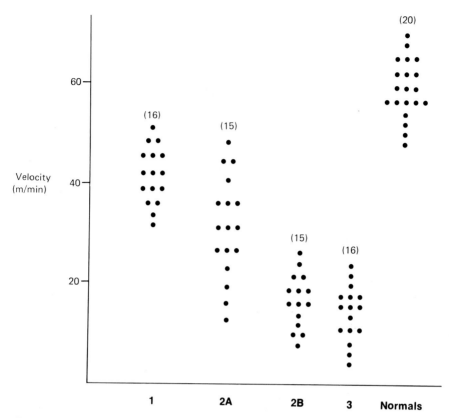

FIG. 2. Variation in walking speed with type of aid used. Group 1: Hemiplegics walking without aid (mean—51.0 m/min). Group 2A: Hemiplegics walking with cane (mean—38.5 m/min). Group 2B: Hemiplegics walking with tripod or quadrupod aids (mean—21.0 m/min). Group 3: Hemiplegics walking with pulpit walking frame (mean—16.8 m/min).

plegic and nonhemiplegic patients varied considerably, particularly in patients who required a tripod or pulpit type of walking frame. Once again, there were wide variations in step length ranging from 10 to 50% of step length between the two legs. Details of the steppage studies are being prepared for another report.

Summary

It may be said that wide variations in walking speed are found in stroke patients. As expected, the speed varied with the type of aid used. There was little difference between those who walked without aid from a group of normal patients paired for age and sex.

Goniometry

The study of angular movements of various joints during the stance and swing phases is another useful way of delineating abnormalities in gait patterns. The use of polarised light goniometry in studies of joint movements is discussed by Steiner et al. *(this volume)*. We have used a locally designated electrogoniometer with potentiometers mounted around the two major joints, the hip, and the knee. The outputs were relayed to an X–Y recorder plotting hip against knee angle (16). The gait abnormalities of 116 patients were investigated using electrogoniometry, and a summary of findings is reported. Figures 3 and 6 show the evolution of gait patterns in stroke patients. Progress or regress in walking ability reflected in the expansion or reduction in total area may be quite clearly illustrated on the "cardioid" diagram. These diagrams can be used as permanent records of one of the gait abnormalities seen in hemiplegics.

One of the interesting features of the study is that in 22 patients the diagram of the nonhemiplegic leg appeared to be similar to that drawn for the hemiplegic leg (Figs. 3, 4 and 5). Marks and Hirschberg (23), in kinetic studies of hemiparetic gait, showed that the loading curves obtained from some hemiplegic limbs and nonhemiplegic limbs were similar. They wondered whether the stiff knee effect of the paretic leg associated with a negative knee moment set up a mechanical situation that was transferred to the nonparetic limb. To test this hypothesis, they examined above-knee amputees in a similar manner. These patients had prosthetic devices

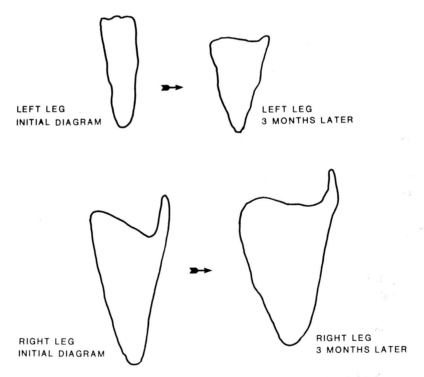

FIG. 3. Left hemiplegic showing improvement in gait pattern. Note widening of left leg diagram and shape more like right leg.

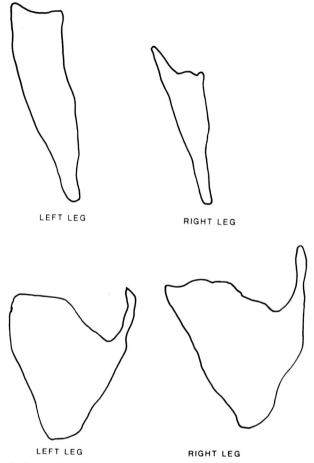

LEFT LEG　　　　RIGHT LEG

LEFT LEG　　　　RIGHT LEG

FIG. 4. **Top:** Patient N. M.—Right hemiplegic with marked extensor synergy in right leg. Note similarity of left leg diagram. **Bottom:** Patient K. S.—Left hemiplegic walking with cane. Note similarity between hemiplegic and nonhemiplegic leg.

that made it impossible for them to develop negative moments during the stance phase of the gait cycle. They found that the ground reactions in the normal limb in these patients were similar to those of normal subjects. Thus, mechanical constraints imposed by the paretic limb could not be entirely responsible for the observations. They concluded that although mechanical constraints may play a role in the production of bilateral patterns of motor abnormality in patients with unilateral brain lesion, it was conceivable that these changes could reflect the capabilities of the brain to undergo reorganisation or functional capacities in an attempt to compensate for deficiencies imposed by the pathological process. We do not have an explanation as yet for the similarity of Grieve charts in the hemiplegic and non-hemiplegic limbs drawn using electrogoniometry. We did consider whether mechanical constraints of the hemiplegic limb imposed on the nonhemiplegic limb

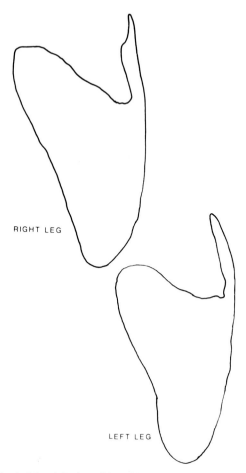

RIGHT LEG

LEFT LEG

FIG. 5. Patient C. H.—Left hemiplegic walking without aid. Note similarity of right and left legs.

induced it to behave goniometrically like the hemiplegic limb. We consider that if this was so, then in the group of patients who had similarities in the hemiplegic leg, such as those with extensor synergistic tie, there would be imposed similar mechanical constraints on the nonhemiplegic leg. Further, the Grieve chart of the nonhemiplegic leg in these patients would show close similarities. However, we found wide variations in the nonhemiplegic limb charts of this group of patients. These preliminary findings require further explanation. A separate project has been designed to study this aspect in greater detail.

SUMMARY

Of 620 patients admitted to Carlisle Hospitals over a ten-year period (1971–1979) who survived the acute insult of a stroke, 322 (52%) achieved the level of

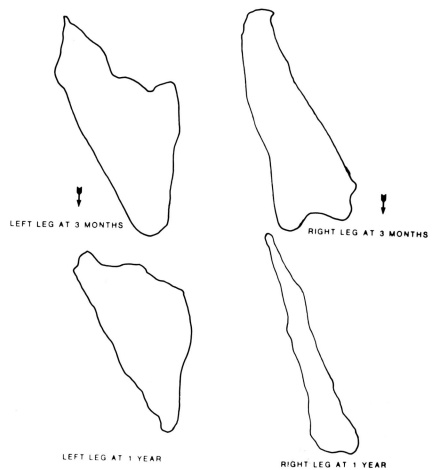

LEFT LEG AT 3 MONTHS

RIGHT LEG AT 3 MONTHS

LEFT LEG AT 1 YEAR

RIGHT LEG AT 1 YEAR

FIG. 6. Patient S. K.—Deterioration in gait pattern in right hemiplegic knee showing hyper-extension and extensor synergy in right leg. One year after the patient's stroke, his right leg became very spastic with little movement at the knee. Note the diagonal inclination of the diagram and that the left leg diagram is also abnormal. The shape of these diagrams is indicative of the spastic gait pattern found in 18% of patients.

walking competence defined as "ability to rise from a chair, walk at least 20 m on a smooth surface with or without a walking aid, but not requiring physical help."

Just under one-third were ambulant without using a walking aid. The characteristics of posture and movement patterns of the gait cycle in stroke patients are reported. Wide variations were found in speed of walking, step length, step frequency within the whole population studied and between identifiable groups categorised according to type of walking aid used. An electrogoniometer designed and built in our unit was used to plot hip against knee angles of the hemiplegic and normal leg. The diagrams produced proved extremely useful for charting the progress of patients, and served as permanent objective records of one of the gait abnormalities in hemiplegics.

ACKNOWLEDGMENTS

This project was supported by a grant from the Research Committee of the Northern Regional Health Authority. We would also like to acknowledge the generous donation of videotape equipment by the Carlisle Round Table in 1973.

REFERENCES

1. Adams, G. F., and Hurwitz, L. J. (1963): Mental barriers to recovery after strokes. *Lancet*, ii:533–537.
2. Adams, G. F. (1971): Clinical outlook for stroke patients. *Gerontol. Clin.*, 13:181–188.
3. Allison, R. S. (1962): *The Senile Brain*, pp. 79–93. London and Arnold Limited, London.
4. Bobath, B. (1960): *Adult Hemiplegia: Evaluation and Treatment*, p. 160. William Heinemann Medical Books, London.
5. Bodgardh, E., and Richards, C. (1974): Gait analysis and relearning of gait control in hemiplegic patients. In: *Proceedings of the 7th International Congress on Physical Therapy*, pp. 443–453. Fed. Physio, Oslo.
6. Brocklehurst, J. (1978): How much physiotherapy for stroke patients. *Br. Med. J.*, 1:1301–1307; 1696–1697.
7. Brunnstrom, S. (1964): *Movement Therapy in Hemiplegia: A Neurophysiological Approach*, pp. 101–128. Harper and Row, New York.
8. Brunnstrom, S. (1965): Walking preparation for adult patients with hemiplegia. *Phys. Ther.*, 45:17–25.
9. Chin, P. L., Rosie, A., Irving, M., and Smith, R. (1980): Final Report on Hemiplegic Gait Studies to the Research Department, Northern Regional Health Authority, Newcastle upon Tyne.
10. Chin, P. L., Angunawela, R., Watson, J., and Mitchell, D. (1979): Stroke register—Carlisle preliminary report. *Proc. Conf. Neuroepidemiology*, edited by F. C. Rose, pp. 131–148. Pitman Medical, London.
11. Colaso, M., and Jayant, J. (1971): Variations of gait patterns in adult hemiplegia. *Neurol. India*, 19:212–216.
12. Droller, H. (1965): The prognosis of hemiplegia. In: *Current Achievements in Geriatrics*, pp. 84–93. Pitman Medical, London.
13. Feldman, D. (1961): A comparison of functionally oriented medical care and formal rehabilitation in the management of patients with hemiplegia due to cerebrovascular disease. *J. Chron. Dis.*, 15:311–326.
14. Garraway, M., Akhtar, A. J., Prescott, R. J., and Hockey, L. (1980): Management of acute strokes in the elderly: Preliminary results of a controlled trial. *Br. Med. J.*, 280:1040–1043.
15. Gresham, G. E., et al. (1975): Residual disability in survivors of stroke—the Framingham study. *N. Engl. J. Med.*, 293:954–956.
16. Grieve, D. W. (1969): Assessment of gait. *J. Physiother.*, 55:452–460.
17. Grieve, D. W. (1980): Monitoring gait. *Br. J. Hosp. Med.*, 24:198.
18. Hurwitz, L. J. (1966): Sensory defects in hemiplegia. *Physiotherapy*, 52:338–342.
19. Isaacs, B. (1971): Identification of disability in the stroke patient. *Mod. Geriatr.*, 1:390–402.
20. Isaacs, B., and Marks, R. (1973): Determinants of outcome of stroke rehabilitation. *Age Ageing*, 2:139–149.
21. Knott, M., and Voss, D. E. (1968): *Proprioceptive Neuromuscular Facilitation: Patterns and Techniques*, pp. 26–89. Harper and Row, New York.
22. Knuttson, E., and Richards, C. (1979): Different types of disturbed motor control in gait of hemiparetic patients. *Brain*, 102:405–430.
23. Marks, M., and Hirschberg, G. G. (1958): Analysis of hemiplegic gait. *Ann. NY Acad. Sci.*, 74:59–77.
24. Marquardsen, J. (1969): *The Natural History of Acute Cerebrovascular Disease*, pp. 32–53. Munkgaard, Copenhagen.

25. Marquardsen, J. (1980): Stroke registration: Experiences from a WHO multicentre study. In: *Proc. Conf. Neuroepidemiology*, edited by F. C. Rose, pp. 105–111. Pitman Medical, London.
26. Meyer, J. S., and Basson, D. W. (1960): Apraxia of gait. *Brain*, 83:261–283.
27. Norton, B., Bomze, H., and Sharman, S. (1975): Correlation between gait speed and spasticity in the knee. *Phys. Ther.*, 155:355–359.
28. Perry, J. (1969): *The mechanics of walking in hemiplegia. Clin. Ortho.*, 63:23–31.
29. Richards, C., and Bodgardh, E. (1974): Gait analysis and relearning of gait control in hemiplegic patients. In: *Proceedings of the Conference on Physical Therapy*, pp. 443–453. Fed. Physio., Oslo.
30. Rood, M. S. (1954): Neurophysiological reactions as a basis for physical therapy. *Phys. Ther. Rev.*, 34:444.
31. Report of the Geriatric Working Group on Strokes (1974): Royal College of Physicians, London.
32. Weddell (1980): Applications of a stroke register in planning. In: *Proc. Conf. Neuroepidemiology*, edited by F. C. Rose, pp. 112–130. Pitman Medical, London.

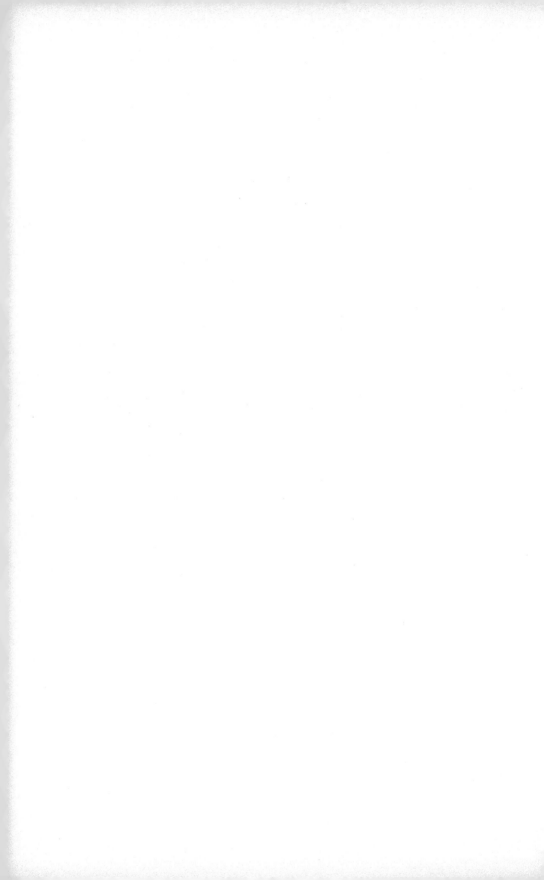

Advances in Stroke Therapy, edited by
F. C. Rose. Raven Press, New York © 1982.

Gait Assessment After Stroke:
The Polarised Light Goniometer

T. J. Steiner, Rudy Capildeo, and F. Clifford Rose

Department of Neurology, Charing Cross Hospital, London, W6 8RF, England

Recovery of leg function can be recognised as of the greatest significance in rehabilitating the hemiplegic stroke patient, that is, regaining the ability to walk with the least possible aid. On this alone may depend the patient's hopes for discharge from hospital and his subsequent level of independence. This is shown by the direct correlation between the time course of recovery of walking ability and duration of stay in hospital. Fortunately for the patient and the therapists involved in his treatment, the natural history of the disease is commonly on their side, and independent mobility can frequently be expected and eventually achieved.

ASSESSMENT

What purpose can be served in these circumstances by objective gait assessments? Complex machinery and paper charts are not necessary to tell whether or not a patient is walking. Nor may they be necessary to record whether a patient is walking better than at the last time he was seen, since often the patient can answer that for himself even if it is not readily apparent to an observer. Furthermore, where there is uncomplicated recovery, any amount of detailed assessment, however sophisticated, may not affect outcome.

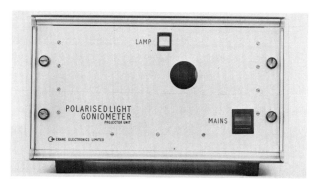

FIG. 1. Polarised light source (Crane Electronics, Ltd.).

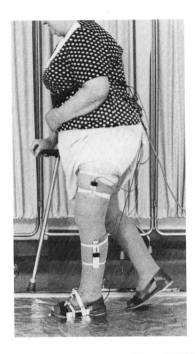

FIG. 2. Optical sensors securely attached to thigh, calf, and foot respond to the incident polarised light beam, each emitting an electrical signal proportional to its rotation from vertical during the walking action.

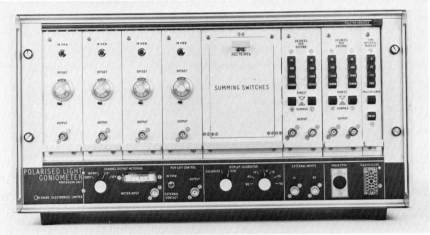

FIG. 3. Signal processing unit (Crane Electronics, Ltd.).

Three main purposes for objective assessment are envisaged for which the keeping of accurate records may be required beyond a simple statement of ability (e.g., "walks 10 yards in 20 sec") together with a neurological examination of the affected limb:

1. To aid in the recognition of specific problems where gait is abnormal but the nature of the difficulty is not clear from observation: this may help to direct physical therapy towards appropriate aims.

2. To record small changes in ability, which may be of particular importance in a condition where recovery is often very slow and the patient (and therapists) become disillusioned by long periods without apparent progress.

3. Where strict objective comparisons are necessary, e.g., in trials to assess the effects of particular treatments.

POLARISED LIGHT GONIOMETRY

Goniometry, the science of measuring angles, achieves particular value clinically when applied to an activity such as walking where the main components of the action consist of cyclical angular movements at three joints (hip, knee, and ankle), all essentially in one and the same plane. Various techniques have been described, but we find the polarised light goniometer to be the most effective (1,2).

A beam of polarised light shines on the patient from a special source (Fig. 1) as he traverses a walkway. The patient (Fig. 2) wears optical sensors that face the light source, one on the thigh, one on the calf and one on the foot. These have to be attached securely, but gain considerable advantage from the fact that no piece of apparatus has to cross any of the joints, as with other goniometric systems that use such devices to relate directly the angulations of the parts of the limb on each side of the joint. Indeed, no moving-part machinery has to be attached to the patient at all. With only a little care, it is possible to apply the sensors quite adequately

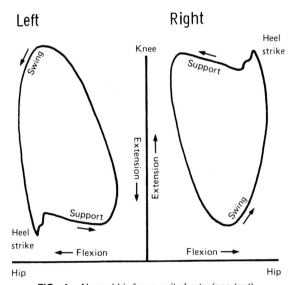

FIG. 4. Normal hip/knee gait charts *(see text)*.

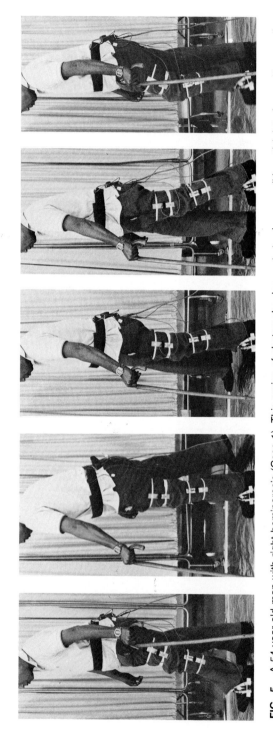

FIG. 5. A 54-year-old man with right hemiparesis (Case 1). This series of photographs demonstrates how a walking stick interferes with recording by obstructing the view of the sensors (*see text* for clinical details).

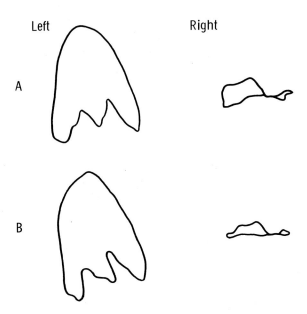

FIG. 6. Gait charts of patient in Fig. 5 *(see text)*.

over a patient's trousers (see Fig. 5), which greatly increases simplicity of use and acceptability to the patient. The one practical disadvantage of the system is that nothing may be interposed between the light source and the sensors during the recording, which prevents the use, e.g., of a walking stick such as the patient carries in Fig. 5. In a hemiplegic patient, this is not usually a problem when the affected side is recorded. Each sensor is masked by a polarising filter, so that the light it receives from the polarised source is directly related to its angular rotation away from a vertical reference. The outputs from the three sensors are fed to a system of summing amplifiers (Fig. 3) that can drive a recording device with the unadulterated signals or can be made to relate mathematically, e.g., thigh movement from vertical to that of the calf, to give a direct measurement of the angle formed at the knee. On an XY recorder, a chart can be plotted of thigh movement against calf movement or, alternatively, of angle at hip against angle at knee, recorded continuously in either case throughout the walking cycle. An immediate permanent record is obtained that is studied by the assessor (and often the patient).

NORMAL GAIT PATTERN

Figure 4 shows normal hip/knee charts. Thigh movement, equivalent to the angle at the hip if the trunk is assumed to remain vertical, is represented on the horizontal axis, and the angle at the knee is on the vertical axis. As the patient's leg moves through one gait cycle, the loop-shaped graph is traced in the direction of the arrows. The moment of heel ground-strike, if this occurs, always imposes a sharp reversal upon the tracing: This is very easy to understand for, all at that instant,

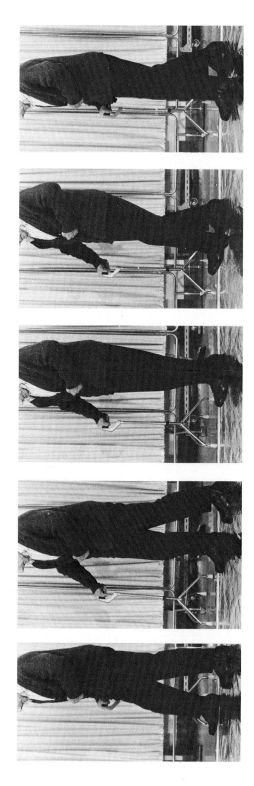

FIG. 7. A 66-year-old man with left hemiparesis (Case 2) (*see text* for clinical details).

Left   Right

A

B

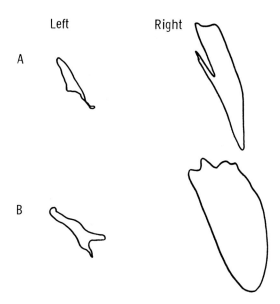

FIG. 8. Gait charts of patient in Fig. 7 *(see text)*.

the dorsiflexing foot begins to plantarflex, the extending knee begins to flex, and the flexing hip begins to extend. From the moment of heel-down, the tracing can be followed through the support phase (heel raised, then toe raised), into swing and back to heel-down. The left leg record drawn on the same axes as the right is reversed and inverted because the patient walks in the opposite direction through the light beam. Information provided by the tracing is both qualitative and quantitative. The width and height of the curve for each leg indicate the angular range of movement at hip and knee respectively, and asymmetry between the two legs can be readily seen. If there is any pathology affecting the gait, both size and shape of the curve are altered; the former can be translated using the calibrations of the machine into a precise anatomical description of the walking action, but clinical goniometry does not usually demand such sophistication.

ILLUSTRATIVE PATTERNS AFTER STROKE

Case 1

A 54-year-old male was referred for assessment 15 months after he had sustained a left cerebral infarction with severe right hemiparesis. He had been receiving little in the way of formal therapy. On examination, he had marked residual hemiparesis, especially of hip flexion, with only mild spasticity. His walking action is illustrated in Fig. 5. The gait charts (Fig. 6A) show a grossly abnormal pattern for the right leg: a back and forth swinging at the hip with very little angulation at the knee. On the left side, there is some approximation to the shape of a normal chart with

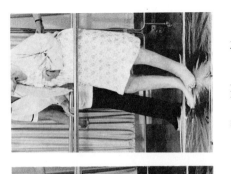
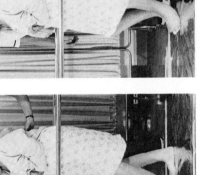
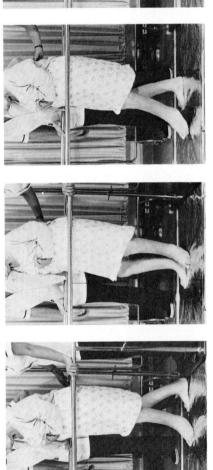

FIG. 9. A 77-year-old woman with left hemiparesis. Although she needed assistance to walk without a caliper, goniometry still could be used to define the active components of her walking (*see text* for further clinical details).

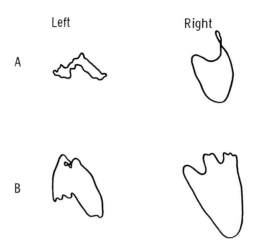

FIG. 10. Gait charts of patient in Fig. 9 *(see text)*.

wide angulation at both hip and knee. The most obvious abnormality is the marked oscillation at hip and knee during hip extension in the early support phase, an action induced by the patient's efforts to impart a swing to the paretic right leg by pelvic thrust. A second set of charts made 6 weeks later (Fig. 6B), with no treatment given to the patient in the intervening period, is essentially similar in all respects. As expected, there had been no change in the patient noticeable clinically, and the goniometric technique was able to confirm this.

Case 2

A 66-year-old man was referred with a severely spastic left hemiparesis following a right intracapsular haemorrhage 17 months earlier. Unlike the previous patient, this man had relatively good power on the affected side and with the marked spasticity was able to use the leg as a supporting strut whilst walking (Fig. 7). The effect of this, seen in the gait charts (Fig. 8A), was an obvious severe limitation of angulation on the affected side but, in addition, it restricted the normal swing on the other side. His spasticity was subsequently treated with baclofen for 12 weeks with some reduction assessed clinically. Improvement in the range of movements was recognisable in both legs when the charts were afterwards repeated (Fig. 8B), but especially on the unaffected right side with much closer approximation to a normal pattern than earlier.

Case 3

A woman of 77 had a severe left spastic hemiparesis following right cerebral infarction nearly 2 years earlier. Her walking was seriously impeded by spastic inversion of the affected foot (Fig. 9), and she used a caliper to correct this which also had a toe-lifting brace. Gait charts were made to show how this affected her walking pattern (Fig. 10). The initial records without the caliper (Fig. 10A) were grotesquely abnormal, but comparison with those obtained while the caliper was worn (Fig. 10B) shows improved movement. This woman's charts also show oscillation during the early support phase of the unaffected leg as she tries to swing the other leg forward.

SUMMARY

Polarised light goniometry is a sensitive method for objectively assessing gait and demonstrating changing ability of clinical significance in patients recovering from stroke. Three case reports have illustrated how it can be used:

1. to identify the nature of a gait abnormality

2. to provide feed back to therapist and patient of a change in walking action as an aid to its improvement

3. as a tool to assess the benefit from methods of physical therapy or to evaluate specific drug treatment.

REFERENCES

1. Capildeo, R., Mitchelson, D., and Rose, F. C. (1978): Assessment of hemiplegic gait. *Chest Heart Stroke J.*, 3:13–17.
2. Mitchelson, D. L. (1975): Recording of movements without photography. In: *Techniques for the Analysis of Human Movement*, edited by D. W. Grieve, D. I. Miller, D. L. Mitchelson, J. P. Paul, and A. J. Smith, pp. 33–69. Lepus Books, London.

Advances in Stroke Therapy, edited by
F. C. Rose. Raven Press, New York © 1982.

Trials of Speech Therapy

*G. P. Mulley, *N. B. Lincoln, †E. McGuirk, and
††J. R. A. Mitchell

*Department of Health Care of the Elderly, Sherwood Hospital; Nottingham NG5 1PD,
England; †Department of Speech Therapy; and ††Department of Medicine, University
Hospital, Nottingham, NG5 1PD, England*

The limits of my language are the limits of my world

—Wittgenstein

Loss of language is one of the most devastating effects of stroke. What can be done to help the aphasic patient? The obvious answer is speech therapy but, in the absence of evidence proving its efficacy, many clinicians remain sceptical about its value. Speech therapists are often unevenly distributed throughout a country, and in some areas therapy is not available. Consequently many stroke victims with language disorders do not see a speech therapist. If we are to provide optimum treatment for stroke patients and deploy therapists where their impact is greatest, we must determine whether speech therapy affects recovery and, if so, what the best way is of stimulating recovery of language.

Before scrutinising the studies of speech therapy, let us review its historical development and see what speech therapists actually do.

HISTORICAL BACKGROUND

Although it has been known for centuries that loss of speech occurs in association with apoplexy, and an impressive amount was known about aphasia by the year 1800 (4), it was only in the nineteenth century that our understanding of speech disorders really began to develop. In 1836, Dax observed that loss of speech occurred in association with right-sided hemiplegia. On the basis of autopsies, Broca placed the speech centre in the third left frontal convolution of the brain. Shortly afterwards, sensory aphasia was described and Wernicke associated it with a lesion of the first temporal convolution of the left hemisphere.

The first documented account of speech therapy was by Hun in 1851. A 35-year-old blacksmith with valvular heart disease sustained a stroke that rendered him stuporous for several days. Initially, he could only speak a few words although his understanding appeared to be good. Professor Hun described him as an amnesiac, and in an attempt to restore the "forgotten" words, he embarked on a course of language instruction: Hun wrote down words and had the patient try to pronounce them. The blacksmith did much of the therapy himself and by the end of 6 months, he could make himself understood although he did tend to use circumlocutions.

By the turn of the nineteenth century, language therapy had developed into systematic retraining. Mills (1904) developed a programme of education involving the repetition of letters and words. Subsequently more complex schooling took place with a phonetic approach and emphasis on grammar. In the early 1900s, specific forms of language training were used for individual speech disorders: For pure motor aphasia, reading and writing and the use of the phonetic alphabet were deemed to be of the greatest value. For sensorimotor aphasia (which proved very hard to treat), writing with the left hand, playing with picture cards, and drawing geometrical pictures "proved to be of greatest benefit," whereas constant repetition of letters, words, and sentences was recommended for those with a pure sensory aphasia (Weisenburg, 1904). The early workers enunciated prognostic factors in the recovery of aphasia: Those with traumatic aphasia did better than stroke patients; there was a correlation between the extent of the lesion and the extent of recovery and the intelligence of the patient was of key importance.

Although the efficacy of these classroom techniques was generally accepted, it was admitted that spontaneous recovery occurred and that it was hard to say how much improvement was due to education and how much to the natural course of events. The mechanism of recovery was a source of speculation: Did therapy educate the right side of the brain to take over the functions of the left, or was progressive shrinkage of the cerebral lesion the important factor?

After these pioneering days, interest in speech therapy was stimulated by the large numbers of soldiers who returned from the Great War with aphasia caused by traumatic brain damage. Aphasia centres were established and techniques of therapy were devised. At this time speech therapy was largely the province of physicians. After the Second World War, speech therapists came into their own and were subsequently influenced by the new sciences of speech pathology, behavioural psychology, and linguistics. The traditional method of teaching patients by classroom techniques was gradually replaced by new approaches.

An interesting development in recent years has been the recruitment of volunteers in helping aphasic patients. The use of volunteers has been championed by Valerie Eaton Griffith (11) who reported that 21 of 31 aphasic subjects improved in speech and understanding after regular contact with a volunteer. This study made no attempt to be scientific: the author acknowledged that spontaneous recovery may have occurred, that standard assessments were not used, and that some patients also received speech therapy. The report did however raise an important question: Was the *content* of speech therapy important as had previously been assumed, or was *contact* with someone, trained or untrained, the major factor in influencing language recovery?

WHAT IS SPEECH THERAPY?

Taylor (25) has described the varieties of language therapy and classified speech rehabilitation techniques under three main headings: nonspecific stimulation, specific stimulation, and the linguistic approach.

Nonspecific Stimulation

Nonspecific stimulation is a generalised approach whereby the patient is encouraged to speak by such techniques as playing games, taking part in group therapy, and being stimulated to talk about hobbies and interests. This form of therapy is widely used by untrained volunteers who are now deployed increasingly in the management of aphasic stroke patients (12).

Specific Stimulation

Specific stimulation is an attempt to encourage language production by using specific stimuli according to the nature of the language disorder. For example, if comprehension is the major problem, the therapist will use auditory stimulation to try to effect improvement. One recent development is Melodic Intonation Therapy (MIT) (1) which is used in aphasic patients with severe expression problems but relatively good comprehension. It has been known for decades that aphasic patients can sing and that, although they cannot speak, they can pronounce sung words without difficulty. The right hemisphere is dominant for music; by MIT, the therapist rhythmically accentuates words in an attempt to stimulate the patient to produce what he still knows about language and to stimulate the right hemisphere to take over language function.

The Linguistic Approach

The linguistic approach also involves detailed assessment of the patient. Drawing on principles from linguistic analysis, the therapist treats the patient by taking him stepwise through a hierarchy of skills starting with allegedly easy tasks (such as getting the patient to imitate body movements) before moving progressively up the scale to spoken language (17).

In this country, therapists tend to tailor the type of treatment to the individual, and there is not strict adherence to rigid schemes of management. This is one factor that makes the evaluation of language therapy difficult, since we cannot test language stimulation in the same way that we can evaluate a drug where the clinical indication and dose schedules are generally agreed upon and response can be more easily quantified. Language stimulation is but one of several components of speech therapy: The therapist also assesses the type and degree of language impairment; educates the patient, family and health professionals; often provides moral and social support and, particularly in dysarthric patients, provides appropriate communication aids. However, much time is spent in language stimulation, and it is important to determine whether this does improve language. While speech therapy has become

increasingly complex, physicians (who have little formal training in language disorders and speech therapy) have in recent decades paid little attention to the management of aphasia. Geschwind (10) has commented on the dearth of articles on
aphasia in the medical and neurological literature. He suggests that doctors consider
speech therapy to be exotic, not susceptible to expert analysis, and of little practical
value. The belief that the only benefit of speech therapy is psychological appears
to be widespread.

In a retrospective survey of 200 hospitalised stroke patients, Rose et al. (21)
found that only 31 of 73 patients who had a language problem were referred for
speech therapy. Perhaps doctors simply forget to involve the speech therapist.
Perhaps the paucity of referrals reflects the general nihilism about stroke. Whatever
the reason, it is unlikely that the management of aphasia will improve until we
have significant data on the natural history and on the effectiveness of speech
therapy.

IS SPEECH THERAPY EFFECTIVE?

It is only in the past 20 years or so that therapists or doctors with an interest in
aphasia have started to ask fundamental questions about speech therapy. Vignolo
(28) was one of the first to voice the basic question: Does speech therapy have a
decisive influence on the course and outcome of aphasia? Before reviewing the
clinical trials of speech therapy, we must be aware of the difficulties of its evaluation.

PROBLEMS IN ASSESSMENT

There are three major difficulties in designing studies to assess the value of
speech therapy (28): 1. the phenomenon of spontaneous recovery, 2. the large
number of variables which will influence improvement, and 3. the problems of
objective evaluation.

Recovery of language may occur in aphasic patients who have had no speech
therapy. Butfield and Zangwill (6) reported that most dysphasics make some spontaneous recovery most of which occurs in the first 3 months. Culton (7) compared
11 patients who had become aphasic in the previous month with 10 who had been
aphasic for 11 to 48 months. He confirmed that rapid recovery occurred in the first
month in the first group but found very little further recovery in the second group.

One classification of aphasia is based on verbal expression. Fluent or Wernicke's
aphasia is characterised by impaired auditory comprehension of fluently articulated
speech that may include neologisms and, in a severe form, may be meaningless
jargon. In nonfluent or Broca's aphasia, the articulation is awkward, the speech
slow, and the vocabulary limited. In global or total aphasia, the patient has severe
comprehensive and expressive difficulties. The slope of the recovery curve is different with the various types of aphasia: Whereas patients with fluent and nonfluent
aphasia show the greatest gain in communication skills in the first 6 months post-
stroke, those with global dysphasia show greatest improvement in the latter part of
the first year (14,23). However, global aphasics remain considerably more impaired

than other groups. This means that considerable improvement will occur independently of any effect of speech therapy and therefore it becomes more difficult to detect response to treatment.

In assessing recovery from aphasia, we must take into account the numerous factors that may influence improvement (8,28). The aetiology of the aphasia, the site and size of the lesion, the type and severity of the language disorder, the general health of the patient, his educational status and previous language skills, his social milieu (whether he is isolated or whether he lives in a stimulating environment); whether the left or right hemisphere is dominant, the interval between the stroke and the onset of therapy, the nature, duration, intensity, and type of therapy—all of these variables may have to be considered. Attempts have been made to determine the importance of some of these variables, e.g., age. In a small sample of aphasic patients, Kirkpatrick (16) found that the patients over 65 fared no worse than younger aphasics. It may be that other factors are also unimportant but since this has not yet been established, all variables have to be considered.

The problem of the large number of variables is daunting: it prompted a *Lancet* editorial (2) to suggest that assessing the value of speech therapy is virtually impossible. There are two possible solutions to this problem:

1. To recruit a sufficiently large number of subjects to allow for the great variation in response to treatment and to be able to examine subgroups within the sample. Because of the difficulties inherent in conducting multicentre trials, this would best be done in one major centre.

2. To do many highly selective studies on homogeneous samples of patients that attempt to examine individual variables in relation to response to treatment.

To evaluate therapy accurately, we must have standardised tests in order to measure improvement. The tests should not be too long, as the patient may become exhausted. The Minnesota Test for the Differential Diagnosis of Aphasia (24) takes approximately 2½ hr; an abbreviated version that takes only 40 min is a more useful clinical tool (27).

Assessments should have scoring systems so that progress can be quantified. The Porch Index of Communicative Ability (PICA) is one of the few tests which has a numerical scale. The PICA is a behavioural scale of communicative ability and is sensitive to slight change; it is probably the best test available for quantifying aspects of language.

Although objective tests of language performance are mandatory to assess effectiveness of therapy, the ability to perform a language test may tell us a little about the patient's ability to communicate in more natural circumstances. Attempts have been made to measure everyday language function. The Functional Communication Profile (26), which examines 50 aspects of communication (such as handling money, greeting people, understanding television), each item being scored on an 8-point scale, is an attempt to measure how the patient overcomes his language impairment.

We must also consider the devastating psychological impact aphasia may have on the patient and the family. In one of the few surveys of psychological and social effects of loss of language, Kinsella and Duffy (15) reported an increased incidence of psychiatric disturbance in spouses of aphasics. Evaluation of the efficacy of speech therapy ideally should include assessments of mood and general health of both patient and relatives, in addition to tests of language abilities.

TRIALS OF SPEECH THERAPY

There have been very few clinical trials of speech therapy. Sarno et al. (22) were one of the first to use a control group in a study of the effect of programmed instruction and nonprogrammed therapy on patients with severe aphasia. There were 31 patients in the study, and the aphasia was of at least 3 months' duration. There was no difference in outcome between the treated and control groups, supporting the clinical impression that patients with severe aphasia do not benefit from regular sessions with a speech therapist. However, Sarno suggested that the therapist may have an important role in helping the patient to adjust to his disability and in educating the family. Kertesz and McCabe (14) found no difference between untreated and treated patients, but advised caution in interpreting this, as there was no control of the amount, duration, or quality of therapy. They stressed the need for a controlled study of the effect of therapy on language parameters, with a randomised allocation of patients to avoid selection bias.

Placebo groups are needed to control for the effects of attention. In the past decade, a few studies have compared formal speech therapy with therapy given by untrained volunteers. Lesser and Watt (18) examined the impact of untrained helpers on 16 aphasic patients. Assessment of the type of language disorder was made by the Boston test, and the Functional Communication Profile was used to measure language ability. The interval between onset of stroke and initiation of voluntary support ranged from 11 to 185 months. Although the majority of subjects showed some language improvement, the main effect of volunteers was found to be in increasing patients' social confidence. Volunteers were considered not to be an alternative to formally trained speech therapists.

Meikle et al. (19) compared speech therapy with treatment by volunteers. The volunteers were given a short introductory course that included explanations about the nature of stroke and aphasia. Of the 87 patients recruited in the study, 56 were excluded, 17 were too ill to attend hospital regularly for therapy, 15 declined on hearing about the nature of the trial, and the others were excluded for a variety of medical, social, and language factors. The remaining 31 patients were randomly allocated to the two treatment groups and assessed on the PICA and a simple test composed of comprehension, verbal expression, writing, and spelling. Again there was variability between onset of stroke and entry to the trial ranging from 1 to 67 months. Because of the small numbers in the study, the authors were reluctant to draw any firm conclusions. However, they were unable to find any significant differences in outcome between patients allocated to volunteers and those to speech therapists.

David et al. (1979) are doing a well designed, multicentre study to compare speech therapy with untrained volunteers. In a report of the pilot study on 13 patients, they found that most recovery appeared to have taken place in the first month of treatment and that there were no apparent differences between the two groups in functional language. The results of the larger study are awaited with interest.

These studies must be interpreted with caution but do raise an important question: If speech therapy really is of no greater benefit than therapy by untrained volunteers, does it actually have any effect on language recovery? There has only been one large-scale study where aphasic patients were allocated treatment and no treatment groups. Basso et al. (3) studied 238 patients, 85% of whom had sustained a stroke. The patients were not randomly allocated to the two groups: Those with family and transport problems that prevented them attending for therapy three times a week for 5 months or more were allocated to the no-treatment group. Unfortunately, over 200 patients were withdrawn from the study, and the patients remaining were young—the mean age in the treatment group was only 48 years.

The conclusion of this study therefore cannot be accepted without reservations. Until further studies are done (and we in Nottingham are currently conducting a randomised, single-centre study to compare formal speech therapy with no therapy) it does appear that formal stimulation is more effective than no therapy in improving the language of aphasic patients.

CONCLUSIONS

Although it is 150 years since speech therapy began, we know little about its effectiveness. We are not certain that speech therapy has any impact on language recovery. We do not know if untrained volunteers are as effective (or as ineffective) as speech therapists in stimulating recovery in aphasics. If therapy is shown to be effective, we need to determine which type of treatment is efficacious, which groups of aphasics will respond, when to initiate and how long to continue therapy. If one-to-one speech therapy sessions are shown to be ineffective or no better than volunteer treatment, we must determine how best to utilise speech therapists in the assessment of patients, the education of relatives and staff, and in the support of the aphasic family.

At present, the only certainty is that speech therapists are courageously asking uncomfortable questions about their own effectiveness.

REFERENCES

1. Albert, M., Sparks, R. W., and Helm, N. A. (1973): Melodic intonation therapy for aphasia. *Arch. Neurol.*, 29:130–131.
2. Anonymous (1977): Prognosis in aphasia. *Lancet*, ii:24.
3. Basso, A., Capitani, E., and Vignolo, L. A. (1979): Influence of rehabilitation on language skills in aphasic patients. A controlled study. *Arch. Neurol.*, 36:190–196.
4. Benton, A. L. (1964): Contributions to aphasia before Broca. *Cortex*, 1:314–327.
5. Burr, C. W. (1904): Treatment of aphasia by training. *J.A.M.A.*, 158:1948.
6. Butfield, E., and Zangwill, O. L. (1946): Re-education in aphasia: a review of 70 cases. *J. Neurol. Neurosurg. Psychiatr.*, 9:75–79.

7. Culton, G. L. (1969): Spontaneous recovery from aphasia. *J. Sp. Hearing Res.*, 12:825–832.
8. Darley, F. L. (1972): The efficacy of language rehabilitation in aphasia. *J. Sp. Hearing Dis.*, 37:3–21.
9. David, R. M., Enderby, P., and Bainton, D. (1979): Progress report on an evaluation of speech therapy for aphasia. *Br. J. Dis. Comm.*, 14:85–88.
10. Geschwind, N. (1970): Aphasia. *N. Engl. J. Med.*, 284:654–656.
11. Griffith, V. E. (1975): Volunteer scheme for dysphasia and allied problems in stroke patients. *Br. Med. J.*, 3:633–635.
12. Griffith, V. E., and Miller, C. L. (1980): Volunteer stroke scheme for dysphasic patients with stroke. *Br. Med. J.*, 281:1605–1607.
13. Hun, T. (1851): A case of amnesia. *Am. J. Insanity*, 7:358–363.
14. Kertesz, A., and McCabe, P. (1977): Recovery patterns and prognosis in aphasia. *Brain*, 100:1–18.
15. Kinsella, G. J., and Duffy, F. D. (1979): Psychological readjustment in the spouses of aphasic patients. *Scand. J. Rehab. Med.*, 11:129–132.
16. Kirkpatrick, E. I. (1974): Recovery from aphasia as a function of age. *Aust. J. Hum. Comm. Dis.*, 2:56–61.
17. Lesser, R. (1978): *Linguistic Investigations of Aphasia.* Arnold, London.
18. Lesser, R., and Watt, M. (1978): Untrained community help in the rehabilitation of stroke sufferers with language disorder. *Br. Med. J.*, 2:1045–1048.
19. Meikle, M., Wechsler, E., Tupper, A., Benenson, M., Butler, J., Mulhall, D., and Stern, G. (1979): Comparative trial of volunteer and professional treatments of dysphasia after stroke. *Br. Med. J.*, 2:87–89.
20. Mills, D. K. (1904): Treatment of aphasia by training. *J.A.M.A.*, 158:1940–1949.
21. Rose, F. C., Boby, V., and Capildeo, R. (1976): A retrospective survey of speech disorders following stroke, with particular reference to the value of speech therapy. In: *Recovery in Aphasics*, edited by Lebrun and Hoops, pp. 189–197. Swets and Zeitlinger, Amsterdam.
22. Sarno, M. T., Silverman, M., and Sands, E. (1970): Speech therapy and language recovery in severe aphasia. *J. Sp. Hearing Res.*, 13:607–623.
23. Sarno, M. T., and Levita, E. (1979): Recovery in treated aphasia in the first year post-stroke. *Stroke*, 10:663–670.
24. Schuell, H. (1965): *The Minnesota Test for the Differential Diagnosis of Aphasia.* University of Minnesota, Minneapolis.
25. Taylor, M. L. (1964): Language therapy. In: *The Aphasic Adult—Evaluation and Rehabilitation*, edited by H. G. Burr, pp. 139–160. Wayside Press, Charlottesville.
26. Taylor, M. L. (1965): A measurement of functional communication in aphasia. *Arch. Phys. Med. Rehab.*, 46:101–107.
27. Thompson, J., and Enderby, P. (1979): Is all your Schuell really necessary? *Br. J. Dis. Comm.*, 14:195–202.
28. Vignolo, L. A. (1964): Evaluation of aphasia and language rehabilitation: A retrospective exploratory study. *Cortex*, 1:344–367.
29. Weisenburg, T. H. (1904): Treatment of aphasia by training. *J.A.M.A.*, 158:1947–1948.

Advances in Stroke Therapy, edited by
F. C. Rose. Raven Press, New York © 1982.

Controlled Trials in Remedial Therapy

T. W. Meade

*MRC Epidemiology and Medical Care Unit, Northwick Park Hospital,
Harrow, Middlesex, HA1 3UJ, England*

The randomized, controlled trial is the best way of assessing the effectiveness of treatment, whether by drugs or by nonpharmacological methods. Particular reasons for emphasizing the need for randomized treatment allocation in stroke rehabilitation studies have been discussed elsewhere (8).

This chapter reviews trials of remedial therapy (other than speech therapy) after recovery from acute stroke.

PREVIOUS TRIALS

Feldman et al. (3) randomly allocated 82 stroke patients admitted to hospital within 2 months of a hemiparesis to either a "formal rehabilitation program" or to "functionally oriented medical care" (the control group). Follow-up was for at least 1 year. The general conclusion was that formal rehabilitation did not confer any obvious advantages. Gordon and Kohn (6) randomly allocated 91 patients to either a general hospital under the management of a nurse trained in rehabilitation procedures, or to a rehabilitation centre (control group). Approximately one-third of the patients were recruited more than 6 months from the onset of disability. Again, there were no obvious differences in outcome between the two groups. The authors suggested that, if anything, the control group did better in terms of locomotion.

The trial described by Peacock et al. (9) was based on only 52 patients. Intensive rehabilitation was compared with standard care. Outcome was measured by success or failure in reaching a projected goal set at the time of entry to the trial. The average duration of observation was approximately 7 months. A larger proportion of the intensive rehabilitation group (79%) reached or surpassed personal care goals than the control group (61%) but the difference was not significant at a conventional level. At final evaluation, it was estimated that further improvement was still possible for a significantly larger proportion of the control group than the intensively rehabilitated experimental group. The authors concluded, however, that "despite these encouraging results... the long-range relative effectiveness of lengthy and expensive rehabilitation as applied to the type of population studied in this project had not been proven to be of value."

Several points should be borne in mind in interpreting these trials. First, the numbers of patients were small and none of the trials is likely to have had adequate statistical power. Second, there were long intervals between the onset of stroke and trial entry in a large proportion of the patients in at least one of the trials. If rehabilitation is only of value when started early, the inclusion of many patients with long intervals between disease onset and trial entry will make it difficult to detect beneficial effects. Finally, and perhaps most important, the measures of outcome used were diffuse and not easy to define precisely. Their repeatability is uncertain. These difficulties have both statistical and clinical implications. The three trials thus leave the matter unresolved. They do not suggest any obvious benefits attributable to rehabilitation nor do they establish that rehabilitation is ineffective.

NORTHWICK PARK TRIAL

The Northwick Park stroke rehabilitation trial, full details of which are given elsewhere (10), compared the effectiveness of three intensities of out-patient rehabilitation. Allocation of the patients to the three groups was made at random. The "intensive" regime (group 1; 46 patients) aimed at attendance in the rehabilitation department 4 whole days a week for both group and individual physiotherapy and for occupational therapy. The "conventional" regime (group 2; 43 patients) called for attendance three half days a week. Treatment in groups 1 and 2 lasted for up to 6 months. The third regime (group 3; 44 patients) involved no routine out-patient rehabilitation. Patients in this group were regularly visited at home by a health visitor and were encouraged to continue with exercises taught while in hospital. The main criterion for eligibility was that the patient should be able to manage the most intensive of the regimes—travelling, treatment sessions, etc.— even if he or she were eventually allocated to one of the other two regimes. Of the 1,094 patients with a recent confirmed stroke and considered for the trial, 30% were excluded by this criterion. Most of the patients in question were female and either too old or frail for intensive rehabilitation or suffering from other serious diseases besides stroke. One-third of the patients died while in hospital and 20% made a full, early recovery. Eventually, only 11% of all the patients considered for the trial were entered. This point has been discussed in more detail elsewhere (10,11) and is referred to again later.

The main measure of progress, or outcome, was an Activities of Daily Living (ADL) index. This is based (12) on 17 items of mobility, self-care, and simple household tasks. It is highly repeatable, subject to little within-person variability over short periods, and gives scores in hospital that correlate with those obtained at home (12). The index also correlates with other measures of disability or impairment (1,2,7). The ADL index was measured at entry to the trial and at 3 and 12 months after entry by therapists not involved in treatment. The maximum score on the index, 51, indicates almost total disability. The minimum score, 17, indicates none. The mean score on entry to the trial was about 21.5.

The mean interval between onset and entry to the trial was just under 6 weeks. Patients in group 1 received about twice as much physiotherapy and occupational therapy as those in group 2.

Table 1 shows the decrease in ADL scores (i.e., improvement) between entry and the 3 and 12 month follow-up examinations. At 3 months, the greatest improvement had occurred in patients in group 1, the improvement in group 2 being the next in magnitude, and least in group 3. Results at 1 year were similar. Because the mean level of disability at entry was not high (about 21.5 on the ADL scale, compared with a minimum of 17) the scope for improvement was limited. Each patient who deteriorated was therefore identified, deterioration being defined as any increase in ADL score between entry and the relevant follow-up visit. The results are shown in Table 2. The number of patients who deteriorated rose with decreasing intensity of rehabilitation. Among those who deteriorated, the extent of deterioration was greater in group 3 (especially at 1 year) than in groups 1 and 2. (Some patients who had deteriorated between entry and 3 months had improved at 12 months.

TABLE 1. *Decrease in total ADL scores*

	Group 1	Group 2	Group 3
Between entry and 3-month review			
Men	2.96 (27)[a]	2.80 (30)	1.88 (26)
Women	4.64 (14)	3.10 (10)	0.88 (16)
Total	3.54 (41)	2.87 (40)	1.50 (42)
Between entry and 12-month review			
Men	2.68 (25)	2.42 (26)	0.36 (22)
Women	5.36 (11)	4.10 (10)	1.00 (13)
Total	3.50 (36)	2.89 (36)	0.60 (35)

[a]Figures in parentheses are numbers of patients with ADL assessments at entry and at follow-up interval specified.

For all patients (both sexes): At three months: 1 vs 3, $p < 0.01$; 1 and 2 vs 3, $p < 0.01$. At 12 months: 1 vs 3, $p < 0.05$.

TABLE 2. *Numbers of patients who deteriorated*

	Group 1	Group 2	Group 3
Between entry and 3-month review			
Deteriorated	1 (1)[a]	4 (1)	10 (1.9)
Total	41	40	42
Test for trend, $p < 0.001$			
Between entry and 12-month review			
Deteriorated	2 (2.5)	4 (2.5)	8 (7.6)
Total	36	36	35
Test for trend, $p < 0.05$.			

[a]Figures in parentheses are mean increases in ADL scores for those who deteriorated.

Deaths during the trial and a few withdrawals account for the smaller numbers in Tables 1 and 2 than the original totals.)

Attention already has been drawn to the small proportion of the patients considered for the trial who were actually entered into it. This feature was almost certainly not the result of selection criteria which differ markedly from those used in day-to-day practice (11). It seems probable that only about 10% of district hospital stroke patients are in fact suitable for out-patient rehabilitation after account has been taken of those who die early on, those who recover quickly and those who are too old or frail to attend hospital regularly. The need for out-patient rehabilitation may therefore have been overstated in the past.

The trial strongly suggests that intensive rehabilitation is effective, not only in assisting improvement but also in preventing deterioration. The trial was chiefly one of different intensities of treatment and not of qualitatively different treatments. It is not, therefore, possible to say which parts of the overall regime—physiotherapy, occupational therapy or nonspecific care and attention—were responsible for the benefits. This is a subject for further trials.

The trial provides guidelines for day-to-day practice. First, some out-patient rehabilitation (groups 1 and 2) is undoubtedly better than none (group 3). Second, very intensive rehabilitation (group 1) is probably more effective than a conventional level (group 2). Availability of resources will determine what intensity actually can be provided. Third, improvement seems to occur within the first 3 months, though it is sustained for 1 year. The latter finding contrasts with the less sustained improvement described by Garraway et al. (4,5) in their comparison of a special stroke unit with medical ward management. Fourth, those who are suitable for out-patient rehabilitation will tend to be younger than stroke patients as a whole, and there will be more men than women (10,11).

A final point concerns the large proportion of mainly elderly female patients who are not suitable for out-patient rehabilitation. Although the question was not formally tested in a separate trial, it seems likely from the Northwick Park results that domiciliary physiotherapy will be effective in this group, at least to some extent. A domiciliary service for these patients has in fact been provided by Northwick Park for the past 5 or 6 years.

REFERENCES

1. Bebbington, A. C. (1977): Scaling indices of disablement. *Br. J. Prev. Soc. Med.*, 3:122–126.
2. Donaldson, S. W., Wagner, C. C., and Gresham, G. E. (1973): A unified ADL evaluation form. *Arch. Phys. Med. Rehab.*, 54:175–179.
3. Feldman, D. J., Lee, P. R., Unterecker, J., Lloyd, K., Rusk, H. A., and Toole, A. (1962): A comparison of functionally orientated medical care and formal rehabilitation in the management of patients with hemiplegia due to cerebrovascular disease. *J. Chron. Dis.*, 15:297–310.
4. Garraway, W. M., Akhtar, A. J., Hockey, L., and Prescott, R. J. (1980): Management of acute stroke in the elderly: follow-up of a controlled trial. *Br. Med. J.*, 281:827–829.
5. Garraway, W. M., Akhtar, A. J., Prescott, R. J., and Hockey, L. (1980): Management of acute stroke in the elderly: preliminary results of a controlled trial. *Br. Med. J.*, 280:1040–1043.
6. Gordon, E. E., Kohn, K. H. (1966): Evaluation of rehabilitation methods in the hemiplegic patient. *J. Chron. Dis.*, 19:3–16.

7. Grynderup, V. (1969): A comparison of some rating systems in multiple sclerosis. *Acta Neurol. Scand.*, 45:611–622.

8. Meade, T. W., and Smith, D. S. (1980): Assessing the effectiveness of rehabilitation following stroke. In: *Clinical Neuroepidemiology*, edited by F. C. Rose, pp. 163–167. Pitman Medical, Tunbridge Wells, Kent.

9. Peacock, P. B., Riley, C. P., Lampton, T. D., Raffael, S. S., and Walker, J. S. (1972): The Birmingham stroke epidemiology and rehabilitation study. In: *Trends in Epidemiology: Application to Health Services Research and Training*, edited by C. T. Stewart, pp. 231–345. Charles C. Thomas, Springfield, Illinois.

10. Smith, D. S., Goldenberg, E., Ashburn, A., et al. (1981): Remedial therapy after stroke: a randomised controlled trial. *Br. Med. J.*, 282:517–520.

11. Sheikh, K., Meade, T. W., Brennan, P. J., Goldenberg, E., and Smith, D. S. (1981): Intensive rehabilitation after stroke: service implications. *Comm. Med.*, 3:210–216.

12. Sheikh, K., Smith, D. S., Meade, T. W., Goldenberg, E., Brennan, P. J., and Kinsella, G. (1979): Repeatability and validity of a modified Activities of Daily Living (ADL) index in studies of chronic disability. *Internat. Rehab. Med.*, 1:51–58.

Advances in Stroke Therapy, edited by
F. C. Rose. Raven Press, New York © 1982.

Stroke Unit or Medical Units in the Management of Acute Stroke: Lessons from a Controlled Trial

W. M. Garraway

*Department of Medical Statistics and Epidemiology, Mayo Clinic,
Rochester, Minnesota 55905*

The rationale of initially admitting stroke patients to medical units is to confirm the diagnosis in circumstances where all the necessary investigative techniques, skills, and equipment are available. But thereafter, is the general physician the best person to provide optimal care for the stroke patient? It can be postulated that medical units, with their emphasis on the diagnostic investigation and "cure" of disease, may not be equipped in terms of staff or facilities to handle the "care" problems inherent in the detailed planning required for the management of stroke. This was recognised by a Report from the Geriatrics Committee of the Royal College of Physicians which recommended setting up a few stroke units based on existing departments of neurology, rehabilitation, or geriatric medicine (38). This report emphasized that any scheme designed to establish stroke units must include a method of assessing their value. Several studies already have attempted to assess the effectiveness of stroke units (1,8,22,26,27,35) but a recent review of the literature concluded that the relative effectiveness of a stroke unit compared with a general medical unit in the management of stroke remains controversial (13). Accordingly, a study was set up in Edinburgh in 1974 to evaluate the effectiveness of a stroke unit compared with medical units in the management of acute stroke as an essential first step to establishing the most effective method of organising stroke rehabilitation. This chapter describes the methods used, outlines the results obtained, and summarizes the conclusions that can be drawn from the study.

METHODS

The Hypothesis

The study was designed as a randomised controlled trial to test the hypothesis that the proportion of patients who could be returned to independence after admission to a stroke unit would be higher than the proportion of patients who were admitted to medical units.

The Allocations

The traditional way of managing acute stroke in Edinburgh is by emergency hospital admission to a medical unit shortly after onset for investigation, diagnosis, and treatment. Admissions are accomplished through an Emergency Bed Bureau run by the Lothian Health Board which facilitates admission on behalf of referring general practitioners. Each medical unit has access to a full range of diagnostic facilities for investigating stroke as well as access to rehabilitation staff and facilities, either within its parent institution or in an affiliated hospital.

A stroke unit was created by changing the function of a ward of 15 beds within the Geriatric Unit at the Royal Victoria Hospital, Edinburgh. A rehabilitation team was established from existing staff already working in the hospital, under the direction of A. J. Akhtar who took no part in the assessment of outcome. No new staff were appointed specifically to the stroke unit, and particular emphasis was placed on not attempting to achieve unrealistic levels of staffing that could not be attained elsewhere. The stroke unit had been in operation for 1 year before the study commenced and had evolved an operational policy that initially was based on the work of Isaacs (21). See Akhtar et al. (2) for a full description of the clinical organization of the stroke unit.

Patients

Patients were eligible for the study from a defined population of 470,000. All general practitioners were contacted, mostly through personal visits by one of the investigators, but also by explanatory tours of the stroke unit and other stroke related meetings. Of the 277 practising doctors serving the catchment population at the beginning of the study, 275 agreed to notify appropriate patients using the definition of stroke as the onset of a focal neurological deficit of presumed vascular origin present for at least 6 hr but not longer than 3 days. There was no upper age limit, but a lower age limit of 60 was employed because the stroke unit was operating under the auspices of a geriatric unit. Practitioners were encouraged to notify all patients who appeared to be suitable. Medical staff from the study were on call 24 hr a day to undertake home visits to confirm the practitioner's diagnosis and establish clinical eligibility to participate. Only first strokes were considered for the study.

Selection Criteria

Stroke presentations seen on home visits were divided into a triage of three bands: "upper," "middle," and "lower" using selection criteria derived from previous studies of the natural history of stroke (11,23,25,37). Patients placed in the middle band of strokes using the criteria illustrated in Table 1 were eligible for the study. The upper band contained patients who were likely to do poorly whether they were rehabilitated or not. The lower band contained patients who were likely to recover spontaneously and who would not require a sustained period of rehabilitation. Concentrating on the middle band of strokes allowed a more realistic comparison

TABLE 1. *Triage used to select strokes for the stroke unit vs medical units study*

	Stroke presentation	Prognosis	Eligibility
Upper band	Unconscious at onset Already dependent in daily living activities	Bad for survival Likely to remain dependent	Excluded
Middle band	Conscious at onset Established or developing hemiplegia present	Good for survival Spontaneous recovery of independence unlikely	Included
Lower band	Conscious at onset Able to walk without human assistance	Good for survival Spontaneous recovery of independence likely	Excluded

Reproduced with permission of the *Journal of Epidemiology and Community Health.*

to be made of the relative effectiveness of a stroke unit and medical units in rehabilitating those patients whose prognosis in terms of years of life was good, but who were likely to have residual disability that would require ongoing support. Five hundred and eighty-four patients received domiciliary visits of whom 311 were placed in the middle band. All agreed to participate in the study. The mean duration of stroke in these patients from onset to the time of admission to the study was 26 hr.

Randomization

The options were allocated in a series of sealed envelopes at the beginning of the study using a system of restricted randomization and were unknown to the investigators until a patient was accepted into the trial. This was accomplished by opening the envelopes in numerical sequence during the domiciliary visit after patients' eligibility to participate had been established. Patients were then either admitted directly to the stroke unit or referred immediately to the Emergency Bed Bureau for placement in a medical unit. The management of patients during the acute phase of rehabilitation was determined by the staff of the appropriate unit; no attempt was made to restrict the clinical freedom of any medical, nursing, or therapy staff.

Outcome

The outcome of the acute phase of rehabilitation was assessed when discharge was imminent, or at a cut-off point of 16 weeks after admission. The assessment was made using a purpose-built Activities of Daily Living (ADL) unit designed to reproduce the home or other circumstances to which the patients were being discharged. The aids or adaptations that had been prescribed for patients were included in the replication of the circumstances at discharge. Patients were assessed on their ability to perform the seven basic activities of getting in and out of bed, dressing, indoor mobility, toileting and personal hygiene, cooking a simple hot meal, feeding, and control of environment. Patients were classified as independent if they could perform all seven activities without human assistance, and dependent if they required human assistance to complete at least one activity or if they failed to carry out the activity altogether. A description of the planning and use of the ADL unit has been reported elsewhere (30).

Follow-Up

The follow-up started once patients had been discharged from hospital or at a cut-off point 16 weeks after admission and lasted for 1 year. During this period, all patients were visited at monthly intervals and an index of nursing dependency administered. This index was designed to establish the degree of assistance that patients received when performing activities of daily living during the 24 hr preceding each visit. The design, composition, and use of the index are described elsewhere (34). The functional outcome at the end of the follow-up was assessed by the same criteria and methods that were applied at hospital discharge (30). A log book was kept by all patients (or their caring friend or relative) living at home during any part of the follow-up in which all personal contacts that occurred between patients and any member of the community health or social services were recorded. Details in the log books were checked for completeness and collated on each monthly visit when the nursing dependency index was administered.

RESULTS

Outcome of the Acute Phase of Rehabilitation

One hundred and fifty-five patients were admitted to the stroke unit and 156 patients to medical units from October, 1975 to April, 1978. There were four postrandomization drop-outs, all from medical units. The mean age of the remaining 307 patients was 73 years, with an age range of 60 to 91 years. There were no differences between patients in the two allocations in age, sex, social class, marital status, home or family situation, prestroke activities, or duration of stroke present on admission to the study. The degree of hemiplegia present was remarkably similar in the two allocations on entry to the study. A difference in mean duration of hospital stay of 55 days in the stroke unit and 75 days in medical units occurred as a result of medical units having a higher residue of patients with an extended stay beyond the 16 week cut-off point. Thirty-two patients admitted to medical units were transferred during the acute phase of rehabilitation to rehabilitation or geriatric assessment units, all of which contained a varied case mix. No deaths occurred in this group. Transfers occurred at a mean interval of 33 days after admission and involved a further stay in the transfer unit of 75 days. The mean duration of stay of the 72 survivors who remained in admitting medical units throughout was 96 days.

Table 2 summarizes the outcome of the acute phase of rehabilitation. Seventy-eight (50%) of patients admitted to the stroke unit were assessed as independent compared with 49 (32%) patients admitted to medical units ($p < 0.01$. χ^2 10.49 on 2 df). When only survivors of the acute phase of rehabilitation were considered, the proportions of independent patients rose to 62% for the stroke units and 45% for medical units ($p < 0.05$. χ^2 6.46 on 1 df). The outcome of patients from medical units who were transferred for further rehabilitation and survivors who remained in their admitting medical units was the same, 47% being assessed as independent and 53% as dependent.

Investigation, Diagnosis and Drug Therapy

Similar proportions of patients in each allocation had investigations performed, supplementary diagnoses made, or drug therapy prescribed. The only medical input that revealed any statistical difference was the mean number of stroke-related investigations performed. This happened because staff in the stroke unit carried out more chest and skull X-rays and screened more patients for neurosyphilis. A very low proportion of patients received lumbar puncture, electroencephalography, brain scanning, or computer assisted tomography in either allocation.

Nursing Dependency

Nursing dependency was measured using a modified version of the Dundee chart, patients being classified into low, medium, and high levels of nursing dependency (10). All patients in the stroke unit were concentrated in the middle range of dependency whereas medical units that had a heterogeneous case mix had patients spread over all three bands of nursing dependency. Nursing activity times for tasks such as washing and toileting patients in the stroke unit were higher than times for similar activities that had been collected in a previous nursing study of medical and surgical units in Edinburgh hospitals (19).

TABLE 2. *Outcome at end of acute phase of rehabilitation [figures are numbers (%) of patients]*

	Stroke unit	Medical units
	(N = 155)	(N = 152)
Independent	78 (50)	49 (32)
Dependent	47 (31)	60 (40)
Dead	30 (19)	43 (28)

Significance of difference: $p < 0.01$ (χ^2 = 10.49, df = 2).
Reproduced with permission of the *British Medical Journal*.

Social Work

A much higher proportion of stroke unit patients required social work, but more time was spent on medical unit patients who were referred. The nature of the contacts that social workers had with patients, relatives, other members of the hospital staff, community services etc. was similar in both allocations as was the distribution of time used in these contacts.

Physiotherapy

High levels of referral for physiotherapy were achieved in both the stroke unit and medical units. As Table 3 demonstrates, there were significant differences in favour of the stroke unit in the proportion of patients receiving any physiotherapy and in having the shorter delay between admission and physiotherapy commencing. Medical unit patients using physiotherapy had a longer period of therapy and consumed a significantly greater number of hours of treatment. These latter differences were due to the longer mean duration of stay of medical unit patients, 57% of all physiotherapy consumed being used by patients who had an extended hospital stay. When these patients are excluded, the differences in therapy duration and time consumption disappear.

Important differences in the use of physiotherapy occurred among patients transferred from medical units when they were compared with those who remained in the initial admitting hospital, the mean consumption of physiotherapy among these transfer patients being more than double that of stroke unit survivors. Seventy-three percent of physiotherapy consumed by this group took place after transfer from the medical unit.

Occupational Therapy

Major differences in the use of occupational therapy between allocations occurred and are summarized in Table 4. The differences between the proportion of patients receiving any occupational therapy and particularly, the mean intervals between hospital admission and the commencement of occupational therapy were striking. Put another way, 66% of all patients had begun occupational therapy within 1 week

TABLE 3. *Use of physiotherapy[a]*

	Stroke unit	Medical units	Significance of differences
	(N = 155)	(N = 152)	
No. (%) of patients receiving any physiotherapy	149 (96)	134 (88)	$p < 0.05$
Delay in starting treatment (days)	3.0 ± 0.3	3.8 ± 0.2	$p < 0.05$
Duration of treatment (days)	49.3 ± 3.3	70.5 ± 7.8	$p < 0.05$
No. of hrs of treatment	21.0 ± 1.5	36.4 ± 4.0	$p < 0.001$

[a]Figures are means ± S.E.
Reproduced with permission of the *British Medical Journal*.

TABLE 4. *Use of occupational therapy (Mean results expressed ± S.E.)*

	Stroke unit (N = 155)	Medical units (N = 152)	Significance of differences
No. (%) of patients receiving any occupational therapy	136 (88)	71 (47)	$p < 0.001$
Mean delay in starting treatment (days)	6.4 ± 0.5	21.1 ± 3.8	$p < 0.001$
Mean duration of treatment (days)	46.9 ± 3.2	68.6 ± 10.3	$p < 0.05$
Mean no. of hrs of treatment	33.3 ± 2.4	48.2 ± 6.1	$p < 0.05$

Reproduced with permission of the *British Medical Journal.*

of admission to the stroke unit compared with only 18% of all admissions to medical units in the same time period. The pattern of medical unit patients who were referred as having a longer duration and a higher overall consumption of therapy seen in physiotherapy was repeated.

The proportion of transfer patients from medical units who received occupational therapy approached the level of that obtained by survivors in the stroke unit. Transfer patients had more than double the consumption of occupational therapy compared with stroke unit patients, but no less than 89% of this occupational therapy was provided after the transfer from medical units had occurred.

Speech Therapy

There were no dramatic differences in the use of speech therapy between allocations to match those seen in the use of occupational therapy. Only 13% of stroke unit and 18% of medical unit patients received any speech therapy. The mean delay to commencement, mean duration and mean amount of time used was 9 days, 61 days, and 17 hr respectively for patients in the stroke unit, and 6 days, 65 days, and 11 hr respectively for patients in medical units.

Aids and Adaptations

Prescribing aids to daily living and providing adaptations to patients' home environment may have an important bearing on the outcome of stroke rehabilitation. Table 5 summarizes the provision of aids and adaptations to the survivors of the acute phase of rehabilitation and highlights the significant differences between the stroke unit and medical units in this respect. Patients may derive no benefit from special aids and adaptation if their "accessory" aids such as spectacles, hearing aids, and dentures are not in working order. There was a striking difference in the proportions of patients in the two allocations who had their accessory aids modified or replaced during the acute phase of rehabilitation.

Communication

Family members of stroke patients are an important resource that should be used by hospital staff. To make full use of this resource requires the active involvement

TABLE 5. *Use of aids and adaptations*

	Stroke unit		Medical units		Significance of differences
	No.	%	No.	%	
Aid(s) and/or adaptation(s) prescribed during hospital stay	103	82	61	56	$p < 0.001$
Accessory "aids" modified or replaced by hospital staff[a]	68	54	12	11	$p < 0.001$

[a]Spectacles, hearing aids, and dentures.

of all members of the hospital rehabilitation team in reassuring, discussing the prognosis, and describing the plan of treatment to key family members. There were significant differences between the allocations in the proportion of caring persons who reported that they had contact with members of the hospital staff, particularly medical consultants and therapists. These differences were much less pronounced when the contacts were separated into those initiated by the caring person themselves and those in which the hospital staff made the initial approach.

Completing the Triage of Stroke Rehabilitation

All study patients placed in the upper and lower bands were followed up and their outcome noted at the time of hospital discharge. It was also necessary to look for all cases of stroke that were not referred to or accepted by the study in order to complete the triage. It was particularly important to identify middle band strokes who were admitted to hospital directly by their G.P.s or through an accident and emergency department. The identification of all cases of stroke was limited to those admitted to hospital during the years 1976 to 1977, although the intake period of the trial extended from October 5, 1975 to April 30, 1978. All stroke admissions among patients age 60 and over from the defined population during 1976 to 1977 were identified from case listings of Scottish Hospital Inpatient Statistics. A one-in-three random sample was drawn and the medical records of these patients examined to determine where they would have been placed in the triage and to ascertain their outcome on hospital discharge. This was undertaken using the Rankin Disability Scale, a more subjective assessment of stroke dependency that has been widely used in other studies based on reviews of medical records, but which was compatible with the Activities of Daily Living classification used in the trial (29). Seventeen medical records could not be traced. It was not possible to establish the position in the triage of stroke patients from the defined population who were retained at home throughout by general practitioners.

INCIDENCE OF STROKE

The total number of strokes among persons age 60 and over in the defined population who were admitted to hospital in 1976 to 1977 was 1,429. Upper band strokes accounted for 43% of all strokes, middle band strokes 24%, and lower band strokes 33%. Seventy-one percent of all middle band strokes were referred to the study compared with 18% of upper and 23% of lower band strokes.

The average annual age- and sex-specific incidence rate for hospital admission of stroke was 7.3 per 1,000 persons age 60 and over. This rate comprised 3.1, 1.8, and 2.4 per 1,000 person-years for upper, middle, and lower band strokes respectively.

THE SIZE OF A STROKE UNIT

Basing the study on hospital admissions from a defined population and completing the triage of stroke rehabilitation for all such admission enabled an estimate to be made of the number of beds that would be required for a stroke unit per unit of population. The steps taken in estimating the size of a stroke unit required to admit acute strokes in the middle band is presented in Table 6. This estimate is made assuming the same criteria for placement in the middle band of stroke, that all middle band strokes occurring in the defined population are referred to hospital, the same case fatality ratio is present, the same mean duration of stay that applied to the stroke unit in the study occurs, and the bed occupancy rate is that which applied to medical units in Scotland during 1976 to 1977 (20). If these assumptions are applied, the number of beds required for a stroke unit in a standard population would be four beds for every 10,000 persons age 60 and over, or 15 beds for a stroke unit located in a district general hospital serving a population of 250,000, 18% of whom were age 60 or over.

OUTCOME OF THE CONTINUING PHASE OF REHABILITATION

Eighteen patients from the stroke unit and 12 from medical units died during the follow-up period of 1 year. Six patients in each group were lost to follow-up, leaving 101 patients from the stroke unit and 91 patients from medical units whose outcome was reassessed 1 year later. The initial improvement in outcome brought

TABLE 6. *Size of a stroke unit*

Average annual incidence rate of middle band stroke in persons ages $\geqslant$60 = 1.8 per 1,000 person-years[a]

Assuming the mean hospital stay in the stroke unit = 55 days

Assuming the bed occupancy ratio = 0.85[b]

Number of beds required for a stroke unit to serve a population of 10,000 persons aged $\geqslant$ 60

$$= \frac{55 \times 1.8 \times 10}{7 \times 52 \times 0.85} = 4 \text{ beds}[c]$$

[a]Age and sex adjusted to the Scottish population ages 60 and over at the 1971 census.
[b]Based on bed occupancy of medical units in Scotland, 1976.
[c]Rounded to the nearest whole number.
Reproduced with permission of the *Journal of Epidemiology and Community Health*.

about by the stroke unit as shown by the increased proportion of patients assessed as independent at discharge had disappeared by 1 year, with 56 patients (55%) from the stroke unit being reassessed as independent compared with 52 (57%) of the patients discharged from medical units. Thirteen of 67 previously independent patients from the stroke unit (19%) became dependent. On the other hand, 11 of 45 previously dependent patients from medical units (24%) were classified as independent.

We identified two factors that may have contributed to these changes. Over 80% of all surviving patients lived in their own homes at any point during the follow-up, the overwhelming majority living with relatives or friends. We compared the activities of daily living these patients were actually performing with those they were capable of performing. Human assistance was provided for all patients living at home who were dependent when discharged from hospital. There were appreciable differences, however, between the proportions of independent patients who had been treated in the stroke unit and those treated in medical units who received help when performing activities of daily living. At the beginning of the follow-up, 58 (58%) of the patients discharged from the stroke unit and 34 (37%) of those discharged from medical units received assistance for at least one activity in which they had been assessed as independent at hospital discharge. When dependent patients were examined, a higher proportion from medical units were carrying out activities unaided as the follow-up progressed compared with patients from the stroke unit. Thus, independent patients from the stroke unit were allowed to do less during the follow-up than independent patients from medical units, and dependent patients from medical units were allowed to do more than similar patients from the stroke unit.

The second factor was the early discharge of patients from medical units. Mean duration of hospital stay was 47 days for patients judged at discharge from medical units to be dependent who were reassessed as independent at the end of follow-up compared with 91 days for patients from medical units whose outcome did not change. Hence the patients from medical units whose functional outcome changed to independent during the follow-up received less physiotherapy (a mean of 26 hr over 34 days) than the other patients discharged from these units (a mean of 42 hr over 89 days). A similar trend occurred in the use of occupational therapy (a mean of 40 hr over 31 days compared with 51 hr over 78 days). These trends did not apply to patients treated in the stroke unit.

USE OF COMMUNITY SERVICES DURING THE CONTINUING PHASE OF REHABILITATION

The use of community-based health and social services by patients located at home during any part of the follow-up is summarized in Table 7. The proportions of patients who used services were similar in both allocations with the exception of health visitor involvement, where there was a significant difference in favour of the stroke unit. The general practitioner was seen by the highest proportion of

TABLE 7. *Continuing phase of rehabilitation: The use of community services*

Service	Stroke unit ($N = 112$)			Medical units ($N = 93$)			Significance of differences
	No.	%	Number of contacts mean ± S.E.	No.	%	Number of contacts mean ± S.E.	
General practitioner	99	88	9.4 ± 0.7	81	87	9.2 ± 0.7	NS
Health visitor	85	76	4.0 ± 0.4	32	34	3.1 ± 0.7	$p < 0.001$
Community nurse	61	54	20.7 ± 2.6	37	40	23.1 ± 3.8	NS
Social worker	11	10	2.3 ± 0.5	13	14	2.5 ± 0.8	NS
Home help	41	37	111.1 ± 9.9	29	31	98.3 ± 12.7	NS
Chiropodist	46	41	3.8 ± 0.3	30	32	2.8 ± 0.3	NS
Meals on wheels	2	2	59.0 ± 9.0	6	7	61.2 ± 13.2	NS
Voluntary agencies	9	8	33.7 ± 11.4	14	15	20.5 ± 11.9	NS

Significance of differences is between percentages of patients receiving each service: NS = not significant ($p > 0.05$).
The mean (± S.E.) number of contacts refers only to those patients who received any contact with the relevant community service.
Reproduced with permission of *Age and Ageing*.

TABLE 8. *Continuing phase of rehabilitation: The use of hospital services*

Service	Stroke unit ($N = 112$)			Medical units ($N = 93$)			Significance of differences
	No.	%	Number of contacts mean ± S.E.	No.	%	Number of contacts mean ± S.E.	
Hospital out-patient clinic attendance	75	67	9.0 ± 2.6	49	53	13.6 ± 4.1	NS
Day hospital attendance	27	24	38.2 ± 6.4	9	10	36.9 ± 13.9	$p < 0.05$
Physiotherapist	85	76	34.4 ± 3.1	45	48	34.2 ± 6.7	$p < 0.001$
Occupational therapist	59	53	20.7 ± 3.8	40	43	14.6 ± 3.2	NS
Speech therapist	14	13	32.1 ± 5.9	13	14	20.3 ± 6.5	NS

Significance of differences is between percentages of patients receiving each service: NS = not significant ($p > 0.05$).
The mean (± S.E.) number of contacts refers only to those patients who received any contact with the relevant hospital service.
Reproduced with permission of *Age and Ageing*.

patients in both allocations, but did not have the highest frequency of contact. This was provided by the home help service, which averaged two contacts per week among one-third of patients from each allocation.

USE OF HOSPITAL SERVICES DURING THE CONTINUING PHASE OF REHABILITATION

Significant differences occurred in the proportions of stroke unit and medical unit patients who received any out-patient physiotherapy or attended a day hospital (Table 8). Further differences in the proportion of patients who attended hospital out-patient clinics and received out-patient occupational therapy occurred, but the differences did not reach conventional levels of statistical significance. The proportion of patients receiving out-patient speech therapy was similar to the proportion who received it as hospital in-patients during the acute phase of rehabilitation. During follow-up, there was no repetition of the imbalance that had occurred between the allocations in the mean amount of physiotherapy and occupational therapy used during the acute phase of rehabilitation by the group of patients with an extended hospital stay.

Functional Outcome and Services Used

The use of services was examined in relation to the functional performance of patients at the time of hospital discharge. The level of use of community-based services was not related to outcome expressed as independence or dependence in performing activities of daily living. There were three statistically significant differences in the proportion of independent versus dependent patients who received services, but none when the mean number of contacts for different community services was considered. Community nursing was the only service where both the coverage and frequency of contacts were higher in dependent patients. Surprisingly, this did not apply to the home help service. A higher proportion of independent rather than dependent patients received contact with the general practitioner and health visitor. There was evidence that the use of hospital services was related to patients' functional performance. With one exception (attendance at medical out-patient clinics), a higher proportion of dependent patients received hospital services than independent patients. This trend also applied to the mean number of contacts which stroke unit patients received, dependent patients having more contacts than independent patients for all hospital services.

DISCUSSION

Establishing a special unit improved the natural history of stroke by increasing the proportion of patients who were returned to functional independence. The difference in outcome is statistically significant, and may be clinically important in the context of the future organisation of services for the care and rehabilitation of acute stroke.

Utilization of Therapy

Differences in the utilization of therapy were found that could have contributed to the improved outcome of patients admitted to the stroke unit. It is not possible to say whether the optimum level or mix of therapy was used to achieve the improvement in functional prognosis. This information can only come from a series of trials that examine the impact of different levels of each component of stroke rehabilitation in turn while maintaining the input of all other components constant.

Admission to the stroke unit did not result in the intensive use of therapy that might have been implied by the creation of such a unit. What was achieved in the stroke unit was almost universal coverage of physiotherapy and occupational therapy and shorter delays before commencing treatment. The mean use of 21 hr of physiotherapy and 33 hr of occupational therapy for each referred patient in the stroke unit is quite modest. It was also significantly less than the mean consumption of occupational therapy and particularly physiotherapy among referred patients in medical units. The low level of speech therapy involvement is not surprising, being similar to the level reported to be used in stroke rehabilitation by other workers and in line with the prevalence of dysphasia found in stroke (5,7). The policy of transferring a selected group of patients from medical units after a number of weeks have passed and then subjecting them to intensive therapy must be seriously questioned. The failure to improve the functional outcome of this group of transfer patients compared with survivors who remained in admitting medical units throughout is further evidence that wider coverage of stroke patients with rehabilitation potential accompanied by earlier intervention might be a more effective answer to the problem than a late, concentrated effort (16). Other important questions that need to be answered are which patients will benefit from continued therapy over a long period of time? Is the present policy of treating most patients for the total zlength of their hospital stay making the best use of scarce resources, or should attention be focused on early referral of selected patients for more coordinated treatment by therapists and nursing staff? In some cases, consideration might usefully be given to greater involvement of relatives in maintenance therapy, provided that therapists are readily available to give advice and check progress.

Triage System Criteria

A group of patients were identified as those likely to derive the most benefit from intervention in the provision of rehabilitation services after acute stroke. The development of a system of triage that defined a middle band of stroke was probably an important factor in being able to accept the hypothesis that a stroke unit could return a higher proportion of patients to independence after onset of acute stroke than could medical units. Comparing the outcome of middle band strokes with upper and lower band strokes at the time of hospital discharge indicated that the criteria used in the triage were broadly correct. Further development of the triage is required in order to reduce or eliminate the inconsistencies that resulted in the outcome of 5% of upper band strokes being independent and 15% of lower band strokes not surviving or remaining dependent. This might be achieved by refining the selection criteria used, and there is an urgent need to develop ways of predicting functional outcome following stroke that would be clinically useful in selecting those patients who are most likely to benefit from management in a stroke unit (17). An attempt to develop a standard neurological examination that could be useful in this context was made in this study and has been reported elsewhere (28). The experience of this group of investigators in attempting to reduce the considerable observer variation present in using this standard neurological examination has also been described (15).

Alternatively, the efficiency of the triage might be improved by altering the timing at which it has applied. The triage was applied in the study at a mean period of 26 hr after stroke onset in order to satisfy the requirements of general practitioners and hospital staff who participated in the study. A delay of 3 or 4 days would probably have eliminated or greatly reduced the inefficiency of the triage process because more strokes would have stabilised and certain patients proved their ability to survive. This also would be a better time to select patients for admission to a stroke unit because it is unlikely that a domiciliary service similar to that used to admit patients to the study could be contemplated in routine clinical practice. It also would enable the present desirable policy of admitting acute strokes to medical units in order to confirm the diagnosis and initiate relevant treatment for concomitant conditions to continue. Completing the triage of stroke rehabilitation for all hospital admissions from the defined population enabled an estimate to be made of the number of beds required for a stroke unit to serve a standard population. What is striking is the comparatively low incidence of middle band strokes in this population which, if confirmed by studies conducted on other defined populations, would suggest that only one-fourth of strokes, at least among persons ages 60 years and over, might be suitable for admission to a stroke unit. Thus, it may be possible to consider stroke units as a realistic policy in the National Health Service in the same way that it has been suggested recently that intensive out-patient rehabilitation may be feasible for the small proportion of stroke patients who would benefit from it (32).

Follow-Up Results

The results of the follow-up are both surprising and disappointing. They emphasize the importance of follow-up of patients over a sufficiently long period to be certain that improvements in the natural history of a disease produced by interventions in the working of health services do not disappear when the intervention is withdrawn. Thus, while intervention in the management of stroke at an early stage after onset through the establishment of a stroke unit created a temporary improvement in the natural history of the disease, it did not provide a sustained or long-term advantage over more conventional management in medical units. The data do not provide conclusive reasons why this should have occurred. A larger number of patients assessed as independent at discharge from the stroke unit subsequently regressed to functional dependence compared with patients discharged from medical units. This may have occurred as a result of the greater protection given by the caring relatives and friends who provided more assistance than necessary and thereby did not permit patients from the stroke unit to carry out activities of daily living of which they were capable. Relatives and friends of patients who had been in the stroke unit may have had a heightened awareness of the patients' disabilities as a result of the better communication that existed with members of the staff of the stroke unit. Thus the opportunity was available to give adequate orientation and instruction to the families of patients in the stroke unit about the need to maintain gains made during the acute phase of rehabilitation. But the extent to which this opportunity was taken and the reasons why families might have adopted a more protective role to the detriment of the long-term functional outcome of these patients are not known.

The other factor that contributed to the final outcome was the larger number of patients from medical units who were dependent at hospital discharge but who gained their independence during the follow-up. This group stayed in hospital for a much shorter period than other patients in the medical units. Consequently they received less physiotherapy and occupational therapy and their full rehabilitation potential may not have been realized when they were discharged from hospital. Pressure on medical-unit beds created predominantly by patients with strokes has been recognised as a problem (33) but the extent to which this was responsible for early discharge from the medical units of patients whose rehabilitation potential might not have been fully realized is not known. The results of the follow-up confirm that management of stroke continues well beyond the acute phase in hospital and further suggest that if the input of only one factor in the chain of stroke rehabilitation is inappropriate, incomplete, or missing, the contribution of all other factors may not lead to the successful long-term maintenance of patients with stroke returned to independence in the community.

Use of Health and Social Services

No clear conclusions can be drawn about the use of health and social services in the long-term management of stroke patients. A higher proportion of stroke unit patients living at home compared with medical unit patients at home used services during the follow-up. This applied to virtually every individual hospital and community service, although many differences were not statistically significant. There is no information available to explain why the consistent pattern of higher use of services by stroke unit patients occurred, although better levels of communication with general practitioner and community services, combined with the higher level of hospital follow-up arranged prior to hospital discharge must have been contributory factors (14). Yet, it was a higher number of patients from medical units whose functional performance improved following hospital discharge while more stroke unit patients regressed to become dependent in daily living activities. The overall levels of contact with virtually all services were low and confirm the findings of previous reports that the involvement of health and social services in the long-term management of stroke patients is not very extensive (4,36). By far the most frequent contribution was made by the home help service, and particular attention should be paid in the future to assessing the role of home help in the long-term management of stroke.

Interpreting the Results

The planning, conduct, and interpretation of the results of this study are subject to some of the limitations that apply to controlled trials in health care (18). Even though the study was undertaken in a defined population, it cannot be assumed that the findings of the study would be useful in other areas. Different geographical areas may have different local priorities that could render the clinical importance of being able to accept the hypothesis that was tested less relevant to a local situation. For example, the fact that the short term improvement in functional outcome among stroke unit patients was achieved by using more occupational therapy may rule out the possibility of establishing a stroke unit if there were no occupational therapists available in the area concerned.

The inferences that can be drawn from the study and applied to patients in other locations are also restricted because many other factors relating to the management of acute stroke that were involved in this study must be taken into consideration. The pattern of hospital care for stroke in the defined population was similar to Scotland as a whole except that a higher proportion of admissions were placed in medical units. This does not exclude the possibility that hospital admission and discharge policies for stroke patients that could influence outcome might be different in other centers. Longer delays between onset and hospital admission might occur, or patients could be discharged early before their full rehabilitation potential had been realised. The policy of who, where, when, and how to provide treatment for acute stroke in hospital might also differ in other locations. Additional factors other than hospital admission, treatment, and discharge policies might affect the outcome of stroke rehabilitation. For example, knowledge, opinions, and attitudes towards stroke among members of hospital staff and patients' families may not be similar in other centers. Thus, just because the study has demonstrated that a stroke unit can return a higher proportion of patients to functional independence at the end of the acute phase of rehabilitation does not mean that this would occur wherever stroke units are set up. This study can only point the way to the need for further evaluation at other centres, and if similar findings are made elsewhere, wider inferences may be justified.

Double blind procedures when neither patient nor doctor know which treatment is being given are widely used in therapeutic trials in order to avoid the possibility of bias. Blindness could not be introduced into the design of this study because it involved the use of different facilities as the alternative forms of health care being compared. One major source of bias that might have arisen in the study (as a result of being unable to implement blindness) could have been a change in the performance of medical units as a result of heightened awareness of participating in the study over time. A careful search of the data was made for supporting evidence that this might have occurred, but none was found. The fact that several medical units were involved and that each contained other stroke patients who were not participating in the study might have helped to avoid the potentially serious bias that could have arisen as the study progressed. Lack of blindness also limited the methods of data collection that could be employed; in particular, direct observation of events that occurred during the acute phase of rehabilitation could not be considered, as this would have been accompanied by the risk of influencing treatment through a heightened awareness of the study. A consequence of being unable to make direct observations because of the lack of blindness was the absence of information on four important aspects of the acute phase of stroke rehabilitation.

1. *Methods of rehabilitation employed in the stroke and medical units.* While the study has provided information on the timing, duration, and amount of therapy used by patients in the stroke and medical units, it was not possible to obtain any information about the actual methods of rehabilitation used. In particular, no data is available to indicate whether active or remedial therapy was employed, to what extent an individual or group approach to therapy was used, or which of the techniques of Brunnstrom (6), Bobath (3), or Knott (24) formed the basis for physiotherapy treatment in either allocation.

2. *The stroke unit as a therapeutic community.* An important contribution to the difference in outcome between the stroke and medical units might have been the psychological and therapeutic effect that the stroke unit had on patients. The stroke unit can be envisaged as a community where the close relationship between the hospital staff and patients played an important part in achieving a higher level of functional independence in its patients than occurred in medical units which offered a more conventional institutional approach. The study has provided no insight into this important aspect of stroke rehabilitation.

3. *Input of different members of the rehabilitation team.* A major advantage that has been put forward for setting up stroke units is the opportunity to develop a collaborative policy for stroke rehabilitation (21). This should form the basis for constant and active teamwork between the different members of the rehabilitation team (12). While the study was able to obtain information on the use of several of the components that are advocated for the rehabilitation of acute stroke such as diagnostic investigations, drug therapy, social work involvement, nursing dependency, aids and adaptations prescribed, as well as the use of physiotherapy, occupational therapy and speech therapy, no data could be obtained on the relationship between the contribution of these various components. For example, to what extent were the longer nursing activity times in the stroke unit due to nursing staff providing additional physiotherapy, or occupational therapy to patients when the trained therapy staff had gone off duty? Answering questions of this nature would have required the kind of direct observations that could not be considered in this study.

4. *Difference in mortality between the stroke and medical units.* The difference in mortality between the stroke unit (19%) and medical units (28%) cannot be explained satisfactorily. Confirmation of previous reports (9) that this difference might have occurred as a result of the stroke unit reducing the number of secondary complications due to stroke would again have required the kind of direct observation likely to encourage treatment bias in the absence of blindness.

CONCLUSION

The hypothesis that a stroke unit could discharge a higher proportion of patients following acute stroke who were independent in daily living activities compared with the proportion of such patients who were discharged from medical units can be accepted. Differences in the use of some of the components of rehabilitation including almost universal coverage of physiotherapy and occupational therapy and shorter delays before commencing treatment could have contributed to the improved outcome of patients admitted to the stroke unit. However, the improvement in outcome amongst stroke unit patients at the time of hospital discharge had disappeared by the end of 1 year. Factors that may have contributed to this final result are overprotection by the families of patients who were not permitted to carry out activities of daily living in which they were independent, and the early discharge from medical units of patients whose full rehabilitation potential had not been realised. Thus, while intervention in the management of stroke at an early stage after onset through the establishment of a stroke unit created a temporary improvement in the natural history of the disease, it did not provide a sustained or long-term advantage over more conventional management.

Stroke rehabilitation is a continuing process and prolonging the benefits of short term gains made in functional outcome through the intervention of a stroke unit requires that all the links in the chain of rehabilitation are maintained including the proper orientation of patients' families before home discharge is arranged. Appropriate levels of support from community health and social services based on criteria of need are required to support families who are carrying the burden of stroke dependency in the community. Completing the triage of stroke rehabilitation has enabled the size of a stroke unit per unit of population to be calculated, and this should form a useful baseline for establishing stroke units once all the links in the chain of stroke rehabilitation have been completed. Because of the limitations inherent in carrying out controlled trials in health care, the inferences that have been drawn from this study must be widened by attempting to replicate the findings in other centers before any policy to establish stroke units for the management of acute stroke can be adopted universally.

ACKNOWLEDGMENTS

This study was carried out in collaboration with Dr. A. J. Akhtar, Dr. R. J. Prescott, and Dr. L. Hockey. We are grateful to the following people for advice and help without which this study could not have been undertaken: the members of the Division of Medicine, North Lothian District, who agreed to the establishment of the stroke unit and subsequently participated in the study, and their colleagues in the Division of Medicine, South Lothian District; the staff of the geriatric assessment unit, Royal Victoria Hospital; the staff of the Emergency Bed Bureau, Lothian Health Board; general practitioners; hospital medical records staff, nursing staff, social workers, and therapists; staff in the Information Services Division, Common Services Agency, for numerous ad hoc tabulations of Scottish hospital in-patient statistics; the Scottish Health Education Unit; Mr. C. J. A. Andrews, Department of Ergonomics, Napier College of Commerce and Technology, for designing the activities of daily living assessment unit; the Department of Medicine, Western General Hospital, for providing office accommodation; and the research staff who worked on the project between 1974 and 1979.

We acknowledge the financial support given to the study by the Scottish Home and Health Department and Lothian Regional Council.

REFERENCES

1. Adams, G. F. (1974): Prognosis and prospects of strokes. In: *Cerebrovascular Disability and the Ageing Brain.* Churchill Livingstone, Edinburgh and London.
2. Akhtar, A. J. (1982): Clinical organisation of a stroke unit. *(this volume).*
3. Bobath, B. (1970): *Adult Hemiplegia: Evaluation and Treatment.* Heinemann Medical, London.
4. Brocklehurst, J. C., Andrews, K., Morris, P. E., Richards, B., and Laycock, P. J. (1978): *Medical, Social and Psychological Aspects of Stroke: Final Report.* Department of Geriatric Medicine, University of Manchester.
5. Brocklehurst, J. C., Andrews, K., Richards, B., et al. (1978): How much physical therapy for patients with stroke? *Br. Med. J.,* i:1307–1310.
6. Brunnstrom, S. (1964): *Movement Therapy in Hemiplegia, a Neurophysiological Approach.* Harper and Row, New York.
7. Brust, J. C. M., Shafer, S. Q., Richter, R. W., et al. (1976): Aphasia in acute stroke. *Stroke,* 7: 167–174.
8. Dow, R. S., Dick, H. L., and Crowell, F. A. (1974): Failures and successes in a stroke program. *Stroke,* 5:40–47.
9. Drake, W. E., Hamilton, M. J., Carlsson, M., et al. (1973): Acute stroke management and patient outcome: the value of neurovascular care units (NCU). *Stroke,* 4:933–945.
10. Eastern Regional Hospital Board (1973): Instruction Manual. *Patient Dependency: Extracted from a Routine Nursing Report.* Dundee.
11. Eisenberg, H., Morrison, J. T., Sullivan, P., and Foote, F. M. (1964): Incidence and survival rates in a defined population, Middlesex County, Connecticut. *JAMA,* 189:107–112.
12. Feigenson, J. S., and McCarthy, M. L. (1977): II: Guidelines for establishing a stroke rehabilitation unit. *N.Y. State J. Med.,* 34:1430–1434.
13. Garraway, W. M. (1981): Management of cerebrovascular disease: a community perspective. In: *Cerebral Arterial Disease* (2nd Ed.), edited by R. W. Ross Russell, Churchill Livingstone, London *(in press).*
14. Garraway, W. M. (1980): *M.D. Thesis.* University of Edinburgh.
15. Garraway, W. M., Akhtar, A. J., Gore, S. M., and Prescott, R. J. (1976): Observer variation in the clinical examination of stroke. *Age Ageing,* 5:223–240.
16. Garraway, W. M., Akhtar, A. J., Prescott, R. J., and Hockey, L. (1980): Management of acute stroke in the elderly: preliminary results of a controlled trial. *Br. Med. J.,* 280:1040–1043.
17. Garraway, W. M., Akhtar, A. J., Smith, D. L., and Smith, M. E. (1981): The triage of stroke rehabilitation. *J. Epidemiol. Comm. Health,* 35:39–44.
18. Garraway, W. M., and Prescott, R. J. (1977): Limitations of the controlled trial in health care. *Health Bull. (Edinb.),* 35:131–134.
19. Grant, N. K. (1979): *Time to Care: a Method of Calculating Nursing Workload Based on Individual Patient Care.* Royal College of Nursing, London.
20. Information Services Division, Common Services Agency for the Scottish Health Service (1978): *Scottish Health Statistics, 1977.* H.M.S.O., Edinburgh.
21. Isaacs, B. (1977): Five years' experience of a stroke unit. *Health Bull. (Edinb.),* 35:93–98.
22. Isaacs, B., and Marks, R. (1973): Determinants of outcome of stroke rehabilitation. *Age Ageing,* 2:139–149.
23. Katz, S., Ford, A. B., Chinn, A. B., and Newill, V. A. (1966): Prognosis after strokes. Part II: Long-term course of 159 patients. *Medicine,* 45:236–246.
24. Knott, M. (1967): Introduction to and philosophy of neuromuscular facilitation. *Physiotherapy,* 53:2–12.
25. Marquardsen, J. (1969): *The Natural History of Acute Cerebrovascular Disease.* Munksgaard, Copenhagen.
26. McCann, C., and Culbertson, R. A. (1976): Comparison of two systems for stroke rehabilitation in a general hospital. *J. Am. Geriatrics Soc.,* 24:211–216.
27. Peacock, P. B., Riley, C. P., Lamptom, T. D., Raffel, S. S., and Walker, J. S. (1972): The Birmingham stroke epidemiology and rehabilitation study. In: *Trends in Epidemiology. Application*

to *Health Service Research and Training*, edited by G. T. Stewart. Charles C Thomas, Springfield, Illinois.

28. Prescott, R. J., Garraway, W. M., Akhtar, A. J., and Smith, D. L. (1981): Predicting functional outcome following stroke. *Stroke (in press)*.
29. Rankin, J. (1957): Cerebral vascular accidents in patients over the age of 60. II: Prognosis. *Br. Med. J.*, 200–215.
30. Smith, M. E., Garraway, W. M., Akhtar, A. J., et al. (1977): An assessment unit for measuring the outcome of stroke rehabilitation. *Br. J. Occ. Ther.*, 40:51–53.
31. Smith, M. E., Garraway, W. M., Smith, D. L., and Akhtar, A. J. (1982): The impact of therapy on functional outcome in a controlled trial of stroke rehabilitation. *Arch. Phys. Med. Rehab.*, 63:21–24.
32. Smith, D. S., Goldenberg, E., Ashburn, A., et al. (1981): Remedial therapy after stroke: a randomised controlled trial. *Br. Med. J.*, 282:517–520.
33. Sutherland, A. (1972): A study of long-stay admissions to the acute medical wards of the Aberdeen hospitals. *Scottish Health Services Studies No. 22.* Scottish Home and Health Department, Edinburgh.
34. Walton, M. E., Hockey, L., and Garraway, W. M. (1978): How dependent are stroke patients? *Nurs. Mirror*, 147:56–58.
35. Waylonis, G. W., Keith, M. W., and Aseff, J. N. (1973): Stroke rehabilitation in a midwestern county. *Arch. Phys. Med. Rehab.*, 54:151–155.
36. Weddell, J. M., and Beresford, S. A. A. (1979): *Planning for Stroke Patients: A Four-year Descriptive Study of Home and Hospital Care.* H.M.S.O., London.
37. Whisnant, J. P., Matsumoto, N., and Elveback, E. 1973): Transient cerebral ischaemic attacks in a community—Rochester, Minnesota, 1955 through 1969. *Mayo Clin. Proc.*, 48:194–198.
38. *Working Group on Strokes, Geriatrics Committee.* (1974): Report. Royal College of Physicians, London.

Advances in Stroke Therapy, edited by
F. C. Rose. Raven Press, New York © 1982.

The Dover Stroke Rehabilitation Unit: A Randomised Controlled Trial of Stroke Management

R. S. Stevens and N. R. Ambler

The Royal Victoria Hospital, Dover, Kent, England

It was decided in 1974 to convert an unused ward, situated above a geriatric day hospital in Dover, into a 20-bed stroke rehabilitation unit, which was opened in November, 1977.

Stroke illness involves a vast diversity of symptoms and effects, uses a wide range of resources, and presents clinicians, nurses, therapists, social workers and, above all, patients with a complexity of problems. It may on the face of it be more effective and efficient to coordinate a multidisciplinary team to treat patients in a single department with appropriate facilities than to look after these patients in the hectic environment of a medical ward. Such a focus of attention may prove more advantageous for both patients and staff and for the optimum use of resources. This is the crux of the arguments adduced in favour of special stroke rehabilitation centres, as first developed in Britain by Adams (1), in Belfast by Isaacs (5), in Glasgow, and by several physicians in the United States (2,6,7).

Coincidentally with the planning in Dover, the Royal College of Physicians published (10) a report by a Working Group on Strokes in which one suggestion was that research should be undertaken to investigate the value of specialised units. At that time, there were no reports of appropriately controlled trials of the performance of such stroke centres. However, a randomised controlled trial was begun in Edinburgh in 1975 (3).

With the agreement of physicians and management in South East Kent, it was decided that the new unit should be used for a research project with the object of comparing the progress of patients rehabilitated there with that of patients treated along conventional lines in general or geriatric wards. Furthermore in a 1971 WHO report on cerebrovascular diseases (12), it was stated that "the registration of strokes might serve as a basis for comparative studies of various types of management." This suggestion was adopted since a register of all strokes occurring in the health district would provide more complete detail about the total problem of stroke and the resulting use of health services in a defined population.

THE DOVER STROKE REHABILITATION CENTRE

The unit is not an expensive creation with elaborate facilities and expanses of space; despite alterations and some rebuilding, the facilities remain modest and restricted.

The nursing establishment is similar to that for a general medical ward. Senior posts are held in physiotherapy, occupational and speech therapy, and medical social work. Rehabilitation elsewhere in the District was supplemented rather than devalued by this innovation.

METHOD

The programme was developed in two sections: the register of strokes and a longitudinal study of patients referred for rehabilitation.

The Register

The stroke register has been constructed from notifications by general practitioners, consultant physicians, house officers, ward sisters, statistics of hospital activity analysis, and mortality returns. Coroners allowed access to their reports from pathologists. The information in every case was checked in detail to ensure that we registered only those cases defined as "a focal neurological deficit of cerebrovascular origin with resultant limb weakness lasting at least 24 hr." We omitted those hemiplegias dead in less than 24 hr and certain undoubted cerebrovascular catastrophes which we added to a supplementary register.

Management

The physicians agreed to refer to the research team all stroke patients whom they deemed "fit for rehabilitation." Only patients over the age of 90 or those who were moribund would be excluded, and it was accepted that patients making very rapid and complete recovery might not need to be transferred. Referred patients were randomly assigned to either: the stroke centre, or to the control group whose course of treatment would be continued in one of the five other appropriate hospitals in the district.

The medical research fellow examined all patients soon after referral, noting clinical and demographic data. He visited them at 4-month intervals, recording progress to 1 year, or earlier death. The research associate studied the patients' adjustment to the event, resettlement after discharge, and the formal and informal support given in the community. Treatment sessions were recorded by the therapists whether in the stroke centre or the control series.

RESULTS

The Register

During 1978 and 1979, 1,812 notifications of possible strokes were scrutinised, and from a population of 248,000 persons (18% over 65 years of age), 839 cases of acute onset of (mono-) or hemiplegia were registered, indicating an annual incidence of 16.9 per 10,000 local population.

The preponderance of elderly victims is confirmed in that exactly three-fourths were 70 years of age or more. The average age was 75 years. The male to female ratio of 2:3 reflects the proportions of the sexes in that segment of the population most at risk.

The study of a group of patients undergoing rehabilitation for stroke is necessarily practised in a diminishing population. After 2 weeks, one-third of the registered patients had died, and after 52 weeks, two-thirds had died.

Referral for Rehabilitation

Referral ranged from the day of onset to day 59, the average being on day 12. The average age was 72 and the sex ratio was the same as that recorded on the register, i.e., 2:3. Two hundred and twenty-eight referrals were accepted into the study and randomised; 112 were assigned to the stroke centre, and 116 became controls. Seven other referrals were excluded because their symptoms did not meet the definition. A patient who refused transfer to the stroke unit was also excluded. The two groups were well matched for age, sex, severity of stroke, and side affected. Because the majority of the patients were elderly, many of them suffered preexisting conditions, some of which were aggravated by the stroke. Four examples of the concomitant diseases noted are shown in Table 1.

Examples of clinical conditions that also balanced well between the two groups are homonymous hemianopia (25% overall) and dysphasia (more than 40% overall). The range of severity of these cases can be summarized by reference to the Rankin scale (9), Table 2.

TABLE 1. *Examples of concomitant diseases*

	No. patients	
	Stroke centre	Control
Diabetes mellitus	13	11
Heart disease	36	34
Hypertension	39	42
Previous completed stroke	26	29

TABLE 2. *Rankin scale[a]*

	I	II	III	IV	V	Total
Stroke centre	2(2)	0(0)	8(7)	54(48)	48(43)	112
Control	1(1)	4(3)	16(14)	30(26)	65(56)	116

[a]Numbers in parentheses represent percent of total.

While the distribution of patients along the scale is not identical in the two groups, the average is the same. This assessment was made soon after assignment, and may have been modified by the early effects of the different regimes of management in the two groups.

Length of Stay in Hospital

Table 3 indicates the difference in total length of hospital stay in each group from admission until 365 days after onset or earlier departure. On average, the stroke centre patients spent 13 more days in hospital during this first year after onset.

A third group of the registered cases were those who were not referred for rehabilitation. While the central theme of this research has been to examine the performance of the stroke unit, early results necessarily will be confined to its use, since many aspects must be considered in combination to provide a useful and balanced assessment. These issues, including follow-up by the research team, will be the subject of future reports.

DISCUSSION

This was not an empirical study of stroke illness but a practical recording of its incidence and management in a mixed urban and rural health district spread over 433 square miles.

The crude incidence of strokes as defined can be compared with that reported from other European studies (4,8,11) if related to structure of population and definition.

Twenty-seven percent of registered patients were subsequently referred for rehabilitation, a proportion that would be considerably higher if those who did not survive the acute phase of the illness were excluded.

The average length of hospital stay was different in the two groups. Patients in the stroke centre spent nearly 2 weeks longer in hospital than controls, but this

TABLE 3. *Total hospital stay*

Weeks in hospital	Stroke centre N (%)	Control N (%)
0–3	15(13)	33(29)
4–7	22(20)	31(27)
8–12	26(23)	11(10)
13–25	24(21)	14(12)
26+	25(22)	25(22)
Total and (means)	112(118)	114[a](105)

[a]Two cases excluded from original 116: 1 never admitted, 1 transferred to stroke centre group after referral for further stroke.

difference may be offset over an extended period by the larger number of control patients transferred to continued nursing care.

No advance assumptions were made about the relative benefit that might be gained by patients grouped according to the severity of their symptoms. Despite such selection as the physicians may have exercised, there was a wide range of severity and concomitant illness amongst referrals.

There was a high mortality during the period of study but, in the absence of clear and reliable prognostic indicators, this should not be allowed to detract from full commitment to treatment of all stroke victims for the sake of those who will survive.

ACKNOWLEDGMENTS

With great pleasure we acknowledge the research grants from South East Thames Regional Health Authority, the cooperation of the physicians and District Management Team of South East Kent, and especially, we record our gratitude to Professor M. D. Warren, director of the Health Services Research Unit at the University of Kent at Canterbury, for his encouragement and advice, and for introducing us to computing and other facilities at the the University.

REFERENCES

1. Adams, G. F. (1971): Clinical outlook for stroke patients. *Gerontol. Clin.*, 13:181–188.
2. Feigenson, J. S., McDowell, F. H., Meese, P., McCarthy, M. L., and Greenberg, S. D. (1977): Factors influencing outcome and length of stay in a stroke rehabilitation unit. *Stroke*, 8:651–662.
3. Garraway, W. A., Akhtar, A. J., Prescott, R. J., and Hockey, L. (1980): Management of acute stroke in the elderly. *Br. Med. J.*, 280:1040–1043.
4. Herman, B., Schulte, B. P. M., van Luyk, J. H., Leyton, A. C. M., and Frenken, C. W. G. M. (1980): *Stroke*, 11:162–165.
5. Isaacs, B., and Marks, R. (1973): Determinants of outcome of stroke rehabilitation. *Age Ageing*, 2:139–149.
6. Jarrett, S. R. (1981): Stroke patient: home or hospital? *Lancet*, i:45.
7. McCann, B. C., and Culbertson, R. A. (1976): Comparison of two systems for stroke rehabilitation in a general hospital. *J. Am. Geriatric Soc.*, 24:211–216.
8. Marquardsen, J. (1976): An epidemiologic study of stroke in a Danish urban community. In: *Stroke*, edited by F. J. Gillingham, C. Mawdsley, and A. E. William, pp. 62–71. Churchill Livingstone, Edinburgh.
9. Rankin, J. (1957): Cerebral vascular accidents in patients over the age of 60: prognosis. *Scot. Med. J.*, 2:200–215.
10. Royal College of Physicians of London (1974): *Report of the Geriatrics Committee Working Group on Strokes*.
11. Weddell, J. M., and Beresford, S. A. A. (1979): Planning for stroke patients. London HMSO.
12. World Health Organization (1971): Cerebrovascular Diseases. Technical Report Series, No. 469. Geneva.

Advances in Stroke Therapy, edited by
F. C. Rose. Raven Press, New York © 1982.

Establishment of a Stroke Rehabilitation Unit

*A. J. Akhtar, †Margaret Height, ‡Shelagh Dunbar, and
*†Linda Mitchell

*Department of Geriatric Medicine, Royal Victoria Hospital and University of Edinburgh;
†Stroke Unit; ‡Physiotherapy; and Occupational Therapy; Royal Victoria Hospital,
Edinburgh, Scotland*

As a consequence of the Edinburgh Stroke Rehabilitation Study (1), a Research Rehabilitation Unit was established in the Royal Victoria Hospital, Edinburgh. This is a Geriatric Assessment Hospital in which the use of 15 beds was changed from the assessment of geriatric patients to the admission and management of acute hemiplegia in patients 60 years of age and over, with the approval of the Division of Medicine of the North Lothian district. The purpose of this chapter is to describe the way in which this unit was organized. The creation of this unit did not involve the recruitment of extra staff, and any difference in performance was to be due to its organisation rather than to increased staffing. In a 31 month period commencing October 1975, 155 patients with acute stroke were admitted.

The patients were admitted from the community shortly after having had the stroke. The mean interval between the onset of the stroke and admission was 25.8 hr. A doctor visited the patient at home before admission so that contact between the unit and caring relatives was established early. A system of triage was used in the selection of patients into the study and only "middle band" strokes were admitted (2). The admission of patients directly from the community had the considerable advantage of not inheriting patients and relatives in whom expectations of poor recovery and long-term care had been established elsewhere.

THE TEAM

The management of stroke may be looked upon as a model for diseases that give rise to a mixture of medical, social, functional, and psychiatric disorders requiring the team approach to achieve the best results possible. The personality attributes of the individual members of the team probably influence the performance of the unit in a disorder such as stroke more than in illness requiring specific medical and nursing expertise, with little or no longer term functional impairment.

Three consultant physicians in geriatric medicine were in charge of the patients, although one was in administrative charge of the stroke unit for the duration of the study. Apart from his purely medical contribution, the doctor was closely involved in all decision-making by other members of the team, thus playing an important part in the overall coordination of the unit.

One senior full-time nurse, the ward sister, was in charge of the stroke unit. This appointment was held by the same nurse for the duration of this exercise. The contribution of the nurse extended much beyond her nursing expertise. She was not only responsible for creating an atmosphere of optimism among the patients and relatives, but the performance of the members of the rehabilitation disciplines in the ward depended much on how she saw their role. The personal attributes of the nurse in charge of the ward are probably of greater importance than those of any other member of the team. She must be hospitable and outward-looking and not excessively preoccupied by questions of professional boundaries. She had to bridge the gulf between the purely medical and nursing management of the patient and the management of functional impairment and social circumstances. The ward sister had working under her one staff nurse, one senior enrolled nurse, and one or two auxiliaries at any given time.

There was one part-time physiotherapist who was in post for the duration of the project. Treatment was given in the ward and in the physiotherapy department. Two occupational therapists were attached to the unit and, as with physiotherapy, treatment was given in the ward and in the occupational therapy department. The occupational therapists, unlike the physiotherapist, did not function exclusively in the stroke unit. The ward sister, the physiotherapist, and the occupational therapist worked closely together in planning rehabilitation and also in the functional assessment of the patient at the time of discharge from hospital. The rehabilitation policy of the unit initially was to achieve a universal coverage of the patients rather than to give a small number more intensive treatment.

One part-time speech therapist was available to the unit, but because of the size of her commitment, her expertise was sought in patients unequivocally in need of speech therapy because of significant impairment of language. One medical social worker was attached to the unit, but, like the speech therapist, this constituted a part of her commitment only which included other ward and out-patients.

ADMISSION PROCEDURE

The patient was examined by the admitting doctor in the usual way, and the relatives were interviewed by the doctor and the nurse. The physiotherapist and occupational therapist assessed the patient as quickly as possible after admission, but it was not usually considered necessary for them to see the patient outside normal working hours. The relatives were asked to bring the patient's outdoor clothes and shoes as soon as possible. They were asked about the height and type of bed at home and its position and also the type of house and the number of occupants. After questioning the relatives, the doctor answered questions about stroke and explained to them in simple terms the nature of the illness. They were not to be over-burdened by information at this stage.

The relatives were given tea while the patient was settled. Positioning of limbs was done in conjunction with the physiotherapist. A bed cradle was used on the paralysed side to keep the bedclothes off the affected foot. The ward was equipped with King's Fund beds and all patients were given ripple mattresses or full length sheepskins to prevent pressure sores. The relatives were then invited to unpack the patient's belongings and were given a brief and simple account of the rehabilitation programme within the patient's hearing. Quite often, this had to be repeated several times during subsequent visits because of the age of the relatives.

THE PATIENT'S DAY

One of the important aims of the stroke unit was to make every activity involving the patient of rehabilitational value. Dressing in the morning was supervised by the occupational therapist, and the patients were made to dress themselves whenever possible, even if it was expedient to do it for them in order to save time. Ward routine was adjusted to suit the rehabilitation requirements of the patient rather than the opposite. Every patient not acutely ill was walked to the lavatory if at all possible. The physiotherapist was able to impart her expertise to the nursing staff in this, and in time, was able to delegate the performance of very basic physiotherapy to the nurses in the ward. In the early stages of the illness when the patient could not be walked to the lavatory, the use of bed pans was avoided. The patient was either taken to the lavatory by wheelchair or a bedside commode was used. One of the advantages of a stroke rehabilitation unit lies in the relative uniformity of the nursing and rehabilitation requirements of the patients. The consequent repetition of the way in which patients are managed results in greatest efficiency.

A policy of open visiting was adopted and relatives were invited to care for patients in the ward where appropriate. Ex-patients were encouraged to visit the ward and talk of their recovery to in-patients in the hope that this would prove motivating and reassuring.

MEETINGS AND WARD ROUNDS

In order to maintain a high level of enthusiasm and motivation among the members of the team, regular and frequent meetings were considered necessary. By this means, the functioning of the unit was monitored. During these meetings, opinions were expressed freely, and each team member was able to educate the rest by imparting specialised knowledge and expertise. This was especially true during sessions in which the patient was also present. Because most of the members of the stroke team were in post for the duration of the stroke study, the educational benefits of these meetings were cumulative and by the end of this exercise each member got to know a great deal about other disciplines.

The grand round took place once a week. Each patient was fully discussed by the team and was examined medically if appropriate and put through his paces by the physiotherapist and occupational therapist.

Two patients were selected each week for full discussion by the entire team, when the patients were invited to attend and ask questions of individual members. During these meetings, the doctor examined the patient neurologically and the patient's function was demonstrated by the physiotherapist and occupational therapist. The team found these sessions of educational value and almost all the patients seen approved of them. After the patients had finished asking questions, the relatives were invited to join the team, and the patient was escorted back to the ward. The permission of the patient was always sought before the relatives were asked to come. These sessions had several advantages. The team was able to prepare the relatives for the patient's discharge and the relatives were able to air their anxieties about the patient's future. They were able to ask each member of the team relevant questions and often came prepared with a list. Where appropriate, planning for discharge was given emphasis and if the relatives seemed apprehensive at the prospect of having the patient home, readmission was guaranteed. This underwriting of the patient's care and support in the event of deterioration or a further stroke gave the relatives confidence.

DISCHARGE

Planning for discharge began early in the course of the patient's admission. Whenever possible the relatives were firmly and repeatedly given to understand that the patient would be returning to the community unless something unforeseen occurred. The caring relatives were encouraged to participate in the patient's rehabilitation and to get the feel of the patient's disability. They were shown how to handle the patient correctly so that by the time of discharge, the caring relatives and the patient felt confident. The caring relatives and the patient were invited to a predischarge meeting, when they were given the opportunity to air opinions and anxieties, and to ask relevant questions of the team members. Where appropriate the district nurse, who was to help look after the patient at home, was invited to discuss the patient's nursing needs with the ward sister. All patients were tested in an Activities of Daily Living Unit before discharge (3).

In almost every case, the patient was taken on at least one home visit by the occupational therapist and physiotherapist to observe his performance before final discharge, when the need for aids and adaptations was determined. The patient and the caring relatives found this to be reassuring. In a few instances, the patient was discharged on a trial basis and readmitted if this proved to be unsuccessful. This course of action was necessary in precarious discharges only and a substantial number of these were successful. The arrangements for domiciliary support were undertaken by the social worker.

After discharge, patients were seen in the Out-Patients Department by the consultant and were followed up at home by a hospital health visitor, who reported progress to the consultant. Precarious discharges continued to receive out-patient physiotherapy for a finite period, which varied between 4 and 12 weeks. A stroke club was established for patients and their relatives which was well attended.

EDUCATION OF THE CARING RELATIVES

Elderly, caring relatives take time to assimilate the traumatic and totally alien circumstances surrounding a stroke. Relevant questions come to them slowly and it is for this reason that frequent contact with staff is important. The multidisciplinary meetings with the caring relatives present were of considerable educational value. Individual contributions by team members to the relatives' understanding of the illness and its management occurred during the participation of the relatives in the patient's day. In patients where prospects of discharge appeared to be good, the relatives were invited to listen to a tape recording that described the pathogenesis of stroke in simple language followed by the verbatim statements of patients who had made a good recovery describing their experiences during the illness. The words were spoken by an actor. They could listen to the tape at their leisure and it often suggested questions.

ACKNOWLEDGMENTS

We are grateful to the members of the Division of Medicine, North Lothian District, who agreed to the establishment of the stroke unit, and we would like to thank Dr. David Player of the Scottish Health Education Unit for providing the tape recording for the education of relatives. It is a pleasure to acknowledge the financial support given to the study by the Scottish Home and Health Department and Lothian Regional Council.

REFERENCES

1. Garraway, W. M., Akhtar, A. J., Hockey, L., and Prescott, R. J. (1980): Management of acute stroke in the elderly: follow-up of a controlled trial. *Br. Med. J.*, 280:1040–1043.
2. Garraway, W. M., Akhtar, A. J., Smith, D. L., and Smith, M. E. (1981): The triage of stroke rehabilitation. *Epidemiol. Commu. Health*, 35:39–44.
3. Smith, M. E., Garraway, W. M., Akhtar, A. J., and Andrews, C. J. A. (1977): An assessment unit for measuring the outcome of stroke rehabilitation. *Br. J. Occ. Ther.*, 40:51–53.

Advances in Stroke Therapy, edited by
F. C. Rose. Raven Press, New York © 1982.

The Stroke Units at Greenwich: Why, Which, and How

Peter Blower

Department of Rheumatology, Greenwich District Hospital, Greenwich, London

WHY

I start with the assumption that stroke care can be arbitrarily divided into two phases—an acute medical/neurological phase, usually (though not in all cases) followed by a rehabilitation phase. The distinction here is not absolute in that rehabilitation can begin while neurological investigation is still underway, and similarly, some patients will need continuing medical treatment during their rehabilitation phase (e.g., hypotensives, anticoagulants, and antiarrhythmic agents). In any hospital, the care in either or both phases may be less than ideal, but in the United Kingdom, the greater deficit is likely to be in the rehabilitation phase. A relative indifference to this field of medical care may be partly responsible for this state of affairs, but of at least equal importance is the sheer difficulty of providing optimum care for some stroke victims. Their residual neurological deficit may be complex; there may be associated or independent medical disorders requiring active management; the patients are often elderly and may have lost their life partners and live alone with all the problems that this presents to a disabled person.

Effective help for a disabled stroke survivor, in whom hemiplegia/hemiparesis is the commonest major residual deficit, may involve the skills of a number of disciplines. In hospital, doctors, nurses, physiotherapists, occupational therapists, speech therapists, social workers and orthotists may all be involved, and outside hospital, the general practitioner, the local nursing service, and various community services may all be needed. Such a multiplicity of agents inevitably provides scope for confusion, lack of coordination, and the flowering of interprofessional rivalries. The result may be suboptimal rehabilitation of the stroke patient. This is unfortunate because strokes are a major medical problem and the commonest cause of severe permanent disability in the United Kingdom (4).

The controlled trial at Edinburgh (3) has shown that a stroke unit produced better rehabilitation results than when management of patients was diffused throughout a number of medical units. From the data presented, it is not absolutely clear why this result occurred, but common sense would suggest that the creation of a spe-

269

cialised stroke unit allows the many members of a rehabilitation team the opportunity to develop their individual expertise in this demanding field and, more pertinently, the chance to apply those skills more effectively. But need such a unit be sited in a hospital? Spinal cord injuries are dealt with very effectively in supraregional units—why not strokes?

London and the Home Counties have a population of approximately thirteen and two-thirds million people and in 1980, the four major residential rehabilitation centres serving this area treated a total of 453 hemiplegic patients (Farnham Park 55, Garston Manor 104, Passmore Edwards, Clacton 159, and the Wolfson, Wimbledon 135).

Table 1 shows that in this large population, using an incidence for hemiplegia of 150/100,000/year that a total of 20,000 new cases would be expected annually. The arithmetic in the rest of the table is less certain but it seems likely that a minimum of 6,000 to 8,000 new disabled stroke victims occur annually. Four hundred and fifty-three of these, less than 10%, went to a residential rehabilitation centre in 1980. The corollary is that more than 90% did not go and, as no major expansion of such centres is planned, this pattern will continue in the future. But even if such centres were to be expanded dramatically, the service they provide might still fall short of the ideal. Stroke rehabilitation is predominantly concerned with elderly people and for those admitted to hospital, the commonest major goal is return home. Often this entails one or more home visits by rehabilitation staff to assess the local situation and at least one trial at home for one or two nights by the patient so that any major problems may be recognised before final discharge is attempted. These measures are difficult to achieve from a residential rehabilitation centre situated some miles from the patient's home.

The message is clear. The vast majority of stroke rehabilitation must be done and is probably best done, locally. This being so, the evidence from Edinburgh (3) and common sense suggest that it would be done more effectively if every major general hospital had its own specialised stroke unit.

WHICH

At Greenwich, we have had three different systems of stroke care (Table 2) and these exemplify the main choices open to any general hospital. Greenwich District Hospital is a new hospital of approximately 700 beds and its separate phases were completed between 1969 and 1976.

TABLE 1. *London and home counties—13,660,000 population: expectations for hemiplegia*

Hemiplegia 150/100,000/yr:	20,000
Deaths (20–40%):	4,000–8,000
Survivors:	12,000–16,000
Residual disability:	6,000–8,000

Hemiplegics in rehabilitation centres = 453.

TABLE 2. *Stroke care at Greenwich*

All physicians (pre 1972):	Total care
Stroke rehabilitation unit (1972–1977):	Rehabilitation only
Comprehensive stroke unit (1977–):	Acute care
	Rehabilitation
	Placement of reha-bilitation failures

TABLE 3. *Pros and cons: stroke rehabilitation unit and comprehensive stroke unit*

For	Against
Stroke rehabilitation unit, 1972–1977	
Rehabilitation only	Small unit
No acute care	Severe cases
No placement problems	Slow turnover
Comprehensive stroke unit, 1977– ?	
Separate ward	Acute care
Early rehabilitation	Deaths
Mild and severe cases	Placement of failures

Before 1972, as in most general hospitals, nearly all strokes were admitted under the care of general physicians. Although management in the acute phase was generally adequate, in the rehabilitation phase, the interest and commitment of the medical staff were often low. In 1972 when the second phase of the new hospital opened, we were able to create a small six-bedded Stroke Rehabilitation Unit on a 33-bedded acute medical ward. Strokes continued to be admitted under the general physicians who were responsible for their acute medical care and neurological screening. Once the acute phase had passed, patients who still had a significant neurological deficit were assessed with a view to transfer to the Stroke Rehabilitation Unit. Patients were accepted only on a trial basis and if return home was impossible, they were returned to the referring physicians to await long-term placement. In 1977 following the opening of the last phase of the new hospital, the Stroke Rehabilitation Unit was replaced by a Comprehensive Stroke Unit situated in a new ward of only 20 beds (in addition to three six-bedded bays and two single rooms, there were also a large day room, a small conference room, and the usual ward facilities). This unit accepted strokes directly from the community and was thus responsible for acute medical care and neurological screening, any necessary rehabilitation, and for the placement of those who failed to become sufficiently independent to return home. Shaukat Ali, the Consultant Geriatrician, and I were the consultants in charge.

Both units had pros and cons (Table 3). Our first unit, the Stroke Rehabilitation Unit, could concentrate solely on rehabilitation because the acute phase management had been completed elsewhere and it had no responsibilities for long-term placement of its failures. The disadvantages were that it was only a small part of the work of a busy medical ward and we dealt only with moderate or severe cases because mild ones had been sent home directly by the physicians who had admitted them. As such, turnover was sometimes slow. We were very lucky in that the ward sister was extremely interested in this work and what she could have dismissed as being a mere fringe activity became instead one of major importance to her; this was probably the single biggest factor in our success.

The Comprehensive Stroke Unit opened in 1977. We were now able to admit stroke patients directly and thus to be sure that they started on an adequate rehabilitation programme at the earliest possible moment. Some mild cases were admitted and discharged quickly. As seeing patients go home is one of the things that creates good morale in both staff and patients, this was a considerable benefit. We did have new responsibilities as we now undertook all acute medical care and neurological screening; inevitably a number of our patients died shortly after their admission and we were now responsible for the disposition of survivors.

I thus have no complete or easy answer to the question, "What type of stroke unit should a hospital have?" We like to think that both our units have been successful but that the Comprehensive Stroke Unit is better than the Stroke Rehabilitation Unit. Some information about the working of these units has been described elsewhere (1,2).

HOW

Three things are necessary for any effective rehabilitation unit: a doctor or doctors, other rehabilitation personnel, and physical facilities. The doctor is at the top of the list, not because he does most of the work (we all know he doesn't), but because the creation of any unit within a hospital influences the use of resources, including beds, within that hospital. However keen the rehabilitation personnel or however good the physical facilities, without the support of an interested doctor, nothing can happen.

In this country, the most likely candidates to run a stroke unit would probably come from neurology, general medicine, geriatric medicine, or rheumatology and rehabilitation. The most important quality is enthusiasm for the work, but one or two points are worth making. There are only 150 full-time equivalent neurologists in England and Wales, which constitutes one neurologist for every one-third million people, and the opportunities for many neurologists to become involved in rehabilitation are limited. However, if you create a comprehensive stroke unit, then the support of an interested neurologist is invaluable because although the major deficit in stroke care is in the field of rehabilitation, it would be less than honest to say that the neurological/diagnostic side is always well performed. If a comprehensive unit is going to run at a high level with respect to both medicine and rehabilitation, then a neurologist is a key figure.

Similarly, the physician in geriatric medicine may also have a unique contribution to make. Of hospital stroke survivors, 20 to 25% remain heavily dependent, and some of these will be unable to return home. If a stroke unit is responsible for the long-term placement of all admissions, then without the cooperation of the local geriatrician it will quickly silt up with heavily disabled rehabilitation failures.

The next key appointment is the ward sister. Many disciplines are involved in stroke care but in hospital, no unit will work effectively without the right ward sister. She must be interested not only in nursing patients but in rehabilitating them and have the ability to work closely and amicably with other professional groups.

CONCLUSION

Stroke victims often present complex neurological, medical, and social problems and are best dealt with by a team interested and experienced in this field. Strokes are so common that they cannot be dealt with effectively by regional or supraregional units. The work must be done locally, and probably every major general hospital would provide a better service to stroke patients if it had its own specific stroke unit. Whether this is a simple stroke rehabilitation unit or a comprehensive stroke unit is a secondary issue dependent on local facilities and local personalities. The physician or physicians in charge could come from a number of medical disciplines but it is worth noting that if you create a comprehensive stroke unit, then the help of an interested neurologist is invaluable and the cooperation of the local geriatrician is essential.

REFERENCES

1. Blower, P. (1980): Stroke rehabilitation. *Hosp. Doctor*, 4:8.
2. Blower, P., and Ali, S. (1979): A stroke unit in a district general hospital: the Greenwich experience. *Br. Med. J.*, 2:644–646.
3. Garraway, W. M., Akhtar, A. J., Prescott, R. J., and Hockey, L. (1980): Management of acute stroke in the elderly: preliminary results of a controlled trial. *Br. Med. J.*, 280:1040–1043.
4. Office of Population Censuses and Surveys (1971): *Handicapped and Impaired in Great Britain, Part I*, London, HMSO.

Advances in Stroke Therapy, edited by
F. C. Rose. Raven Press, New York © 1982.

The Bristol Stroke Unit

R. Langton-Hewer

Frenchay Hospital, Bristol, England

In 1974, the Royal College of Physicians Working Group on Strokes produced its report (13). One of its main recommendations was that there should be a few experimental stroke units that might have the following objectives:

1. to act as a focal point for the development of facilities for disabled stroke patients
2. to act as an educational centre for doctors, social workers, and therapists
3. to initiate research.

The report coincided with a decision of the Department of Health and Social Security to establish an experimental stroke unit in Bristol. The main initial objective of the D.H.S.S. was to enable it to decide whether or not it was worthwhile having similar units elsewhere throughout the country.

The Bristol Unit (now called the Avon Stroke Unit) was built in 1974 and opened in 1975. It is a single storey building of about 6,500 square feet and incorporates various rehabilitation services (physiotherapy, occupational therapy, speech therapy, together with social work), and also offices, workshop, and laboratories. The Avon Stroke Unit (A.S.U.) is part of Frenchay Hospital, a District General Hospital, and also contains the sub-regional centre for neurology and neurosurgery. The A.S.U. is adjacent to the medical and neurological wards. No additional beds were provided for the A.S.U. and to some extent, this has determined the type of service that can be provided. However, the unit has been able to use the beds of the Neurology Department and also deals with patients who are in general medical beds. The unit has its own ambulance and crew.

Over 500 stroke patients have been treated in the stroke unit during the first 6 years of its existence. Most patients have been followed up for 2 years, and careful records have been kept of their progress.

When the A.S.U. opened, it was virtually the only stroke unit of its kind in the United Kingdom. A number of important developments have occurred during the last 6 years as part of a process of evolution. Some of these are as follows:

1. Computer and data handling facilities have been developed.
2. Strong links have been developed with various departments in the University of Bristol, notably electrical engineering, anatomy, and physiology. A number of postgraduate students have worked in the unit and three have obtained a Ph.D. or equivalent degree.

275

3. The Department of Medical Physics at Frenchay has taken on the running of the workshop and has provided much help with data handling and the maintenance of electronic equipment.

4. The Department of Neurology has recently moved into the A.S.U. building. The A.S.U. and the Department of Neurology have been effectively fused, thus giving substance to our view that neurological rehabilitation should develop within the speciality of clinical neurology.

5. A principal psychologist has been appointed with a 50% commitment to research, and this has proved to be a particularly valuable development. Besides providing the neuropsychological skills that are important to any unit dealing with brain damaged patients, the psychologist, together with members of the Department of Medical Physics, has provided the on-site capability to handle the statistical side of the unit's activities (e.g., construction of recovery curves, prediction of outcome, etc.).

6. A strong lay support group has been established under the auspices of the Bristol Council for Voluntary Service. This group has raised funds, recruited volunteers to help with stroke survivors (currently, over 100 volunteers are working with stroke patients), and has constructed a specially designed garden for disabled patients. Similar stroke support groups are now being set up in association with the other hospitals in Bristol. A Bristol stroke foundation, with the objectives of providing more funds for both research and support of stroke survivors, was launched in the autumn of 1981.

PRACTICAL MANAGEMENT

The objective of any rehabilitation programme is to produce the best possible outcome in terms of recovery and adaptation to residual disability, at the least possible cost to the patient and to the state. A rehabilitation service, whether it is based upon a hospital ward, the patient's home, a stroke unit, or a combination of these, probably should be based upon a number of principles, discussed below. It does not necessarily follow that such a programme as this will produce "better" results than some other ad hoc arrangement.

Home or Hospital

The patient should be looked after in the most appropriate place. A recent study (1) indicates that this does not always happen. A case can be made for admitting all patients with a severe acute stroke to hospital initially, so that a firm diagnosis can be made and the acute crises allowed to resolve. Many disabled patients can be managed at home if there is a competent domiciliary team, and there is little doubt that some patients become demoralised by being kept in hospital for many weeks, which is also very expensive.

Assessment

The first assessment involves making a diagnosis in terms of pathology, site of lesion, and functional implications. Other conditions such as subdural haematoma, tumour, and meningitis, must be excluded.

Most of the survivors of an acute stroke will have a hemiplegia. Other deficits such as dysphasia, agnosia, and spatial disorientation, are of equal, and possibly greater, importance. Medical assessment involves the identification of these problems. It is also necessary to take note of the patient's general health (for example, angina, heart failure, emphysema), the health of the spouse, the prestroke situation, and details of his housing.

Record Keeping

The proper keeping of records is essential if good communication is to exist between the various professional groups involved. Records should ideally be "problem-oriented," simple, and kept in one place (preferably the patient's notes).

Communication

Good communication should exist between all the various staff involved. It is particularly important that links should be developed between the hospital and the community, between the medical and paramedical staff and the patient and his family, and between community-based staff (for example, the general practitioner, social worker, and district nurse). There are virtually no published reports of community teams dealing with stroke patients.

Staff Deployment and Training

All staff should undergo a period of training in the management of stroke-induced disability. The staff should understand the significance of the various neurological deficits (for instance, hemianopia and spatial disorder), and must be capable of dealing with the various psychological problems faced by the patient and his relatives. Each also must be capable of working in a team.

A Programme of Rehabilitation

Active rehabilitation, particularly when given in hospital, should not consist simply of a few minutes of remedial therapy each day. A proper programme should be planned and written down. The patient himself should be given certain targets, and an "achievement chart" should be hung in a prominent place, for instance, over the patient's bed.

Support for the Family

The main burden of looking after a disabled stroke patient is likely to ultimately fall upon the spouse, or possibly the daughter. The spouse should be involved at every stage of rehabilitation. He/she should attend the remedial departments and should learn how to handle the patient, for instance, getting him/her from chair to bed and back again.

Complications

The avoidable complication rate should be low. Complications, when they do occur, must be recognised early and dealt with promptly. Examples include a stiff painful shoulder, contractures, limb fractures and severe depression.

Home Alterations and Services

Severely disabled patients will require considerable help at home. Aids (e.g., wheelchair, calipers), home alterations (e.g., an additional stair rail), and services such as Home Help and Meals on Wheels should be provided promptly.

Psychosocial Problems

Specific provision should be made for dealing with psychological problems. The social worker probably will be the person most involved, but every member of the rehabilitation team must be familiar with this aspect of care.

Long-Term Management

Some stroke patients survive for many years. Specific provision should be made for helping the patient to make the most of his residual capabilities. The patient should not be allowed to sit at home doing nothing—except in unusual circumstances.

The various points discussed above have been drawn up as a result of working in the stroke unit, and a "good" rehabilitation programme should include them. Most are common sense and are already operative in some geriatric departments.

RESEARCH

Research and "service" go hand in hand. It is impossible to conduct meaningful research in this field without having access to a large number of patients. The following is a summary of projects being undertaken in the A.S.U. Funding has been provided by a variety of bodies, including the Department of Health and Social Security, the Medical Research Council, the Science Research Council, and the Chest, Heart and Stroke Association. In addition, local industry and many others have generously contributed.

Course of Recovery

One hundred and sixty-two consecutive patients who were referred to the A.S.U. between 1977 and 1979 have been followed up for at least 2 years. Assessments have been undertaken at regular intervals following the stroke—an initial assessment, then at 1 month, 3 months, 6 months, 1 year, 2 years, and 3 years (not all patients have been seen at 3 years). The data is being used for a variety of purposes, and should provide valuable information about the duration and speed of recovery. A data bank is being built up using this and other material that should allow us to make predictions of outcome at an early stage following a stroke.

Upper Limb Project

Our interest in the hemiplegic upper limb stems from the fact that only 10 to 15% of hemiplegic patients with an initially paralysed arm will achieve anything like normal function in the relevant upper limb. The work in this field has involved extensive collaboration with members of the university (notably S. Miller, Department of Anatomy, now Professor of Anatomy at the University of Newcastle, G. A. L. Reed and P. A. Lynn of the Department of Electronic and Electrical Engineering, and K. W. Ranatunga, Department of Physiology).

A battery of assessment tests has been developed, and keeps track of what is known as the physiology of neural control of the upper limb. Most of the tests are summarised in two recent publications (4,5): a series of simple clinical tests (4,5); a pursuit tracking task (4); the ability to turn a cranked wheel (7); surface electromyography (9,10); and the recording of isometric tension of elbow flexor muscles (8).

The group has been investigating the natural history of recovery in the paralysed arm and is currently involved in a study of the development of spasticity (11,12). The assessment battery is being used to investigate the effect of therapeutic procedures including visual and auditory feedback, the elimination of gravity by suspending the paralysed limb, and the effect of passive movement.

Domiciliary Care

Hospitals are by far the most expensive resource involved in the management of stroke-induced disability. At present, there is no consistent national pattern relating to hospital admission (the admission rate varies between 40 and 75% in various series). Furthermore, hospital admission is often unrelated to the severity of the stroke (1). The role of domiciliary rehabilitation has received little attention, none of it in the United Kingdom.

We are embarking upon a project that is assessing the potential for domiciliary care. The project has three aims: 1. To observe the present pattern of management of acute stroke. 2. To set up a domiciliary Stroke Rehabilitation Team (S.R.T.) with the objectives of increasing the number of patients who can be managed at home. 3. To monitor the changes produced by 2.

The project has three hypotheses to be tested: 1. That the new service (i.e., that provided by the S.R.T.) will result in a net financial saving. 2. That the patient and his family will make the best possible psychological adjustment. 3. That the patients in the experimental group will make an equally good physical recovery.

The population to be studied is the 207,000 patients on the lists of 88 general practitioners whose practices lie within Frenchay health district. The district is subdivided so that half of the practices form the control group and the other half the trial group. The trial group will have access only to the domiciliary team, but both groups will be monitored.

The Value of Speech Therapy

There have been few published attempts to ascertain whether therapy has an important influence on the course of recovery of dysphasia following a stroke. A multicentre project involving fourteen centres has been organised jointly from the A.S.U. and the Department of Speech Therapy at Frenchay Hospital. The hypothesis tested in this study is that any improvement in communication in stroke-induced dysphasia results not from any specific skills related to speech therapy but from nonspecific support and encouragement. The study compares the level of performance in patients with dysphasia following a stroke who have been randomly allocated to either a speech therapist or a volunteer. Details of this study have been published (3,6), and results of the final study are in press (2).

FINAL COMMENTS

The process of setting up a stroke unit takes much time, and many lessons are learned in the early stages. The best chance of making significant advances lies in allowing a unit to evolve over a period of years. In some instances, elsewhere, similar units have been disbanded after the completion of a single project, a policy that is wasteful.

The management of post-stroke disability is important, both because of the large number of patients who survive with a disability, and because of the expense involved. The subject is still in its early stages, and advances are not dramatic. A stroke unit of the type described gives the opportunity to concentrate expertise in one place, to evaluate the different components of the rehabilitation service, and to undertake clinical research.

REFERENCES

1. Brocklehurst, J. C., Andrews, K., Morris, P. E., Richards, B., and Laycock, P. J. (1978): Medical, social and psychosocial aspects of stroke. *Final Report 1978.* University of Manchester.
2. David, R. M., Enderby, P., and Bainton, D. (1982): Treatment of acquired aphasia: speech therapists and volunteers compared. *J. Neurol. Neurosurg. Psychiatr.* (in press).
3. David, R. M., Enderby, P., and Bainton, D. (1979): Progress report on an evaluation of speech therapy for aphasia. *Br. J. Dis. Comm.,* 14:(2) 85–88.
4. De Souza, L. H., Langton-Hewer, R., Lynn, P. A., Miller, S., Reed, G. A. L. (1980): Assessment of recovery of arm control in hemiplegic stroke patients. 2. Comparison of arm function tests and pursuit tracking in relation to clinical recovery. *Int. Rehab. Med.,* 2:10–16.
5. De Souza, L. H., Langton-Hewer, R. and Miller, S. (1980): Assessment of recovery of arm control in hemiplegic stroke patients. 1. Arm function tests. *Int. Rehab. Med.,* 2:3–9.
6. Enderby, P., and David, R. M. (1976): Proposed evaluation of speech therapy for acquired aphasia. *Br. J. Dis. Comm.,* 11:(2)144–148.

7. Gandy, M., Johnson, S. W., Lynn, P. A., Miller, S., and Reed, G. A. L. (1979): The use of a stirring wheel in the study of patterns of arm and trunk movements in normal subjects and hemiplegic patients. *J. Physiol.*, 269:18–19P.
8. Ismail, H. M., and Ranatunga, K. W. (1981): Isometric contractions of normal and spastic human skeletal muscle. *Muscle Nerve*, 4:214–218.
9. Johnson, S. W., Lynn, P. A., Miller, S., and Reed, G. A. L. (1979): Reflex electromyographic response to random limb displacement. *J. Physiol.*, 292:2–3P.
10. Johnson, S. W., Lynn, P. A., Miller, S., and Reed, G. A. L. (1977): A skin mounted preamplifier for recording the surface electromyogram. *J. Physiol.*, 269:16–18.
11. Langton-Hewer, R. (1979): How does arm movement recover? *Practitioner*, 223:800–803.
12. Lynn, P. A., Miller, S., Reed, G. A. L., and Langton-Hewer, R. (1978): Research in rehabilitation of stroke patients: a team approach at Bristol University and the Avon Stroke Unit. *J. Chest Heart Stroke Assoc.*, 3:25–31.
13. Lynn, P. A., Reed, G. A. L., Parker, W. R., and Langton-Hewer, R. (1977): Some applications of human operator research to the assessment of disability in stroke. *Med. Biol. Eng. Comput.*, 15:184–188.
14. Royal College of Physicians (1974): *Report of Working Group on Strokes*.

Advances in Stroke Therapy, edited by
F. C. Rose. Raven Press, New York © 1982.

A Stroke Unit in Bordeaux: L'Unité de Pathologie Vasculaire Cérébrale

J. M. Orgogozo, J. P. Castel, J. F. Dartigues, J. J. Péré,
L. de Coninck, P. Y. Henry, F. Cohadon, and P. Loiseau

*Unité de Pathologie Vasculaire Cérébrale, Department of Neurology and Neurosurgery,
Hôpital Pellegrin, Université de Bordeaux II, Bordeaux, France*

Intensive care units for stroke patients are particularly difficult to evaluate, since early mortality and functional outcome—the important end-points—vary more with patient selection than with particular therapeutic procedures. For example, Norris and Hachinski (6) reported a figure of 7% early deaths in their first annual report on the McLachlan stroke unit in Toronto, which compared favorably with other reports of 47% (8) to 49% (9), but the following year, their early death rate was 24% (plus 12% after discharge), which simply reflected the trend towards admission of patients more critically ill (Hachinski and Norris, *personal communication*, 1978).

We shall not make another attempt to demonstrate the clinical usefulness of the acute stroke units from our data, but describe the general organization of such a medical–surgical setting, the data collected in the first year from a comprehensive number of patients, the possibilities offered by the unit in terms of improvement of medical and surgical care, and the scientific evaluation of treatment.

GENERAL ORGANIZATION

The aim of this unit was to take care of a significant proportion of the *treatable* cases of strokes occurring in the Bordeaux area. By "treatable" we mean cases in which reasonable benefit can be expected from a relatively aggressive (and expensive) use of diagnostic and therapeutic procedures not easily and rapidly available in more conventional medical and neurological wards. This includes early access to CT scan and round-the-clock use of angiography, intensive care facilities, and vascular and neurological surgery. This concept of treatable strokes does not exclude very old, or otherwise critically ill patients (i.e., with dementia, severe heart disease, or cancer), but it obviously limits their admission in order to avoid occupying beds with patients not likely to be discharged home or to a rehabilitation center after the acute phase. In no case was a patient referred to the unit refused if a bed was available, but doctors who wanted to have their stroke patients sent there soon understood that in order to keep the unit capable of accepting treatable patients, they had to avoid excessive referral of the more numerous "hopeless" cases.

In France, medical care in the public hospitals is organized in wards of 30 to 60 beds on average, each being under the medical and administrative responsibility of one head. In university hospitals like ours, this head is also a faculty member who usually teaches the specialty corresponding to his clinical work so that no medical–surgical ward can be run without a consensus among different heads and the hospital administration. This stroke unit was founded by Prof. Pierre Loiseau, Chairman of Neurology, Prof. agr. Patrick Henry, Head of Neurology, and Prof. François Cohadon, Head of Neurosurgery and Chairman of Experimental Medicine.

The Stroke Unit

The stroke unit includes 29 beds in a single ward dedicated to cerebrovascular disorders. Six of these beds are located in an intensive care room where comatose patients, acute completed strokes, and postoperative patients are kept. Two rooms of two beds are devoted to the monitoring of patients not critically ill but whose condition is likely to deteriorate rapidly: among these are patients just recovering from transient ischemic attack (TIA), or having several TIAs, patients with uncomplicated recent subarachnoid hemorrhage, and patients with heart problems. These two rooms can be changed to one with four beds by removing a mobile wall, and these four beds can be electronically monitored in the same way as the intensive care beds. The last 19 beds are for patients recovering from a stroke, or investigated after a TIA or a small stroke. Six rooms have two beds, and seven have one bed.

Staff

The medical responsibility of the unit is shared by a neurologist (J.M.O.) and a neurosurgeon (J.P.C.), both being full-time in the hospital, and faculty members. They are helped by a neurologist (J. F. D.) who also works at the University Department of Statistics, Epidemiology, and Computer Science. Another neurologist (J.J.P.) works part-time as stroke data coordinator, and is responsible for most of the clinical trials. The 24-hr duty in the intensive care section rests on a team of three specialists (L. de C. being the senior) working part-time for the unit. This medical staff is completed by two interns in training, two specialists in rehabilitation, one cardiologist making one round a week, and one Doppler specialist making the controls after surgery and at the time of follow-up.

The nonmedical staff consists of one head nurse, 18 nurses who work alternately in the I.C. section and in the ward, and 17 nurse-helpers. Also two full-time physiotherapists, one part-time speech therapist, and one part-time Doppler technician work for the unit.

Equipment

Most of the special equipment is located in the intensive care section, and in the adjacent intensive monitoring section. This includes eight individual electronic monitors (EKG, two pressure inputs, respiration, temperature) connected to a central processing computerized monitor (Kontron Roche) that manages the alarms and edits periodically the trend curves for each parameter; two automatized mechanical respirators (SF 4); four automatic cuff arterial pressure monitors with two recorders (Dinamap); and two capnographs (Datascope). The rest of the equipment comprises the Doppler lab (with a Delalande DUD 400 and a Mira Dop 8000), an intracranial pressure lab, a cerebral blood flow lab using intracarotid and intravenous xenon techniques, a rehabilitation room with the usual apparatus and one tilting bed (Stricker), and a microcomputer used for research purposes.

Associated Facilities

A stroke unit of this kind cannot function in isolation because of the need for other specialists to deal with specific aspects of the problem. The Department of Neuroradiology accepted to carry out CT examinations within 48 hr of admission for almost all patients who need it. Cervical and cerebral arteriography can be performed at any time as in other places, but are decided according to an explicit strategy (1). The CBF lab is located in this department. Two rehabilitation wards collaborate with the unit which enables us to refer patients to them as early as 2 to 3 weeks after onset, even when some investigations, like follow-up Holter monitoring or CT scan, still need to be performed. The heads of these rehabilitation centers both come weekly in order to control early rehabilitation techniques and to decide when a patient can be admitted to their centers. As previously mentioned, we collaborate with the Department of Statistics, Epidemiology, and Computer Science, through J.F.D., who also runs the dedicated microcomputer. Last, we collaborate with the hospital laboratory of pharmacology for the pharmacokinetic studies of drugs on trial.

Teaching

Medical students and junior medical staff attend the three teaching rounds in the unit; one of the rounds is jointly held with neuroradiologists and neuroanesthesiologists and open to residents and interns not working in the unit for discussion of stroke problems managed elsewhere.

RESULTS

With the help of the University of Bordeaux Computer Center, a significant amount of data has been analyzed concerning patients managed in the unit during the first year, from March 4, 1980 to April 30, 1981.

These data indicate that 668 patients have been admitted during this first year, 412 of them being stroke patients. This figure reflects the fact that at this time, we have been obliged to admit a number of nonstroke patients (most of them being head injuries) because of the previous organization of the neurosurgery ward. These patients are now only exceptionally admitted to the unit.

As in many other series, we found more males than females comprising stroke patients [260 (63%) vs 152 (37%)]. The mean age of these patients was 59.3 years, which is considerably less than expected from population studies. The vast majority of patients were between 50 and 80 years, and 43.5% were below 60, which reflects a strong tendency towards referral of the younger—presumably more treatable—patients.

The mean duration of stay was only 14.3 days, due mainly to the easy access to rehabilitation centers and nursing homes for the more severe cases. This is to be compared with the mean lengths of stay of 37.7 days in general hospitals and 42.1 days in the university hospitals (3). Delay between onset and admission was less than 24 hr in 40% of cases, between 1 and 5 days in 32%, and more than 5 days in 28%, these last cases being mostly secondary referrals for further investigation or surgery.

Considering how these patients were admitted, only 7% came via the hospital emergency ward, while 37% were referred directly by their family practitioners, and 42.5% were sent by another ward where they first had been admitted. Only 10% were admitted through the outpatient clinic, mainly for nonacute problems such as previous TIAs.

The final diagnoses are presented in Table 1. Following our formal strategy, a Doppler examination, an EKG, and routine laboratory tests were performed in all patients, whereas CT scan was performed in 250, angiography in 209, Holter monitoring and echocardiography in 88, and angiocardiography in 11. It is interesting to note that even with these investigations, the cause of brain infarction could not be elicited in 52 of 211 cases (25%). Artery-to-artery embolism and hemody-

TABLE 1. *Stroke unit diagnoses*[a]

Infarction		211 (55%)
Atheroma:	72	
Cardiac emboli:	46	
Lacunes:	28	
A–A emboli	2	
Hemodynamic:	2	
Unknown origin:	52	
Rare causes:	9	
TIAs		34 (9%)
A–A emboli:	11	
Cardiac emboli:	3	
Hemodynamic:	2	
Various and unknown:	14	
Vert.–Bas. TIA:	4	
I.C. hematomas		60 (16%)
Spontaneous:	41	
A.V. malformation:	8	
Other causes:	11	
Angiomas		10 (2.5%)
S.A.H.		35 (9%)
Vascular malformation:	25	
No malformation:	11	
Unclassified		28 (7.5%)

[a]$N = 412$.

namic problems were documented in only vary rare instances. In many cases classified as "atheroma" (34%), they may have played a role but without direct proof, such as seeing an occluded intracranial artery distal to an ulcerated plaque, or the occurrence of a stroke during an hypotensive episode with a known occlusion or tight stenosis of an appropriate extra- or intracranial artery.

The surgery performed in the unit is described in Table 2. Discrepancies between the number of aneurysms and angiomas in Tables 1 and 2 arise from the fact that some of these malformations are not revealed by cerebrovascular accidents but by other symptoms such as epilepsy and headache. The small number of operations on carotid arteries reflects our tendency to operate on only tight stenoses giving hemodynamic consequences. The rare occurrence of subclavian stenosis or occlusion as a cause of C.V.A. is obvious in this series (no case amenable to surgery).

The outcome of the stroke patients was as follows: 39% returned home, which means without significant disability; 21.5% were referred to one of the two rehabilitation centers; 20% died in the ward; 12.5% were referred to other wards, either for some medical problems or as a first chance before going to a nursing home; 5% were sent directly to a chronic care facility. The 20% deaths in the ward represent 82 cases. Of these, 57% died during the first 5 days after admission, and the mean delay between admission and death was 8.5 days. The proportions of the four main causes of death are shown in Table 3.

When comparing the outcome between cerebral infarction and hemorrhage we confirmed (Table 4) that the early prognosis is definitely worse in intracerebral bleeding if one considers early deaths (4) or good recovery.

CONCLUSIONS

In accordance with Millikan (5), we think that it is difficult to prove that mortality and morbidity of acute stroke may be improved significantly in stroke intensive care units when compared with nonspecialized wards or other intensive care units. In the past, different authors came to completely opposite opinions concerning the usefulness of such units: Drake et al. (2) reported a 50% reduction of secondary complications after strokes in neurovascular care units while Pitner and Mance (7)

TABLE 2. *Stroke unit, surgery[a]*

Aneurysms	31
EC/IC By-pass	29
Intracerebral hematomas	18
Internal carotid (neck)	17
Angiomas	15
Vertebral artery (neck)	1
Subclavian artery	0
Total	111

[a]$N = 412$.

TABLE 3. *Proportions of the four main types of stroke causing death*

Brain infarction:	29.5%
Intracerebral hemorrhage:	25%
Unknown types of strokes:	26%[a]
Subarachnoid hemorrhage:	17%[b]

[a]Mostly patients whose condition is so severe at admission that they die before they can have a CT scan. Due to French law it is not always possible to obtain an autopsy for patients dying in the hospital.
[b]3 out of 5 deaths due to early rebleeding.

TABLE 4. *Stroke unit—outcome*

	Recovery	Rehabilition	Nursing home	Dead	Total
Infarction	85 (40.5%)	55 (26%)	47 (22%)	24 (11.5%)	211
Hemorrhage	8 (13.3%)	24 (40%)	8 (13.3%)	20 (33.3%)	60

$Chi^2 = 28.3$; $p < 0.001$.

found no difference in mortality between stroke patients treated in a specialized unit and those treated elsewhere.

The collection of stroke patients in a special hospital area stimulates interest of medical and nonmedical personnel in this category of patients and provides excellent opportunities for teaching because of the variety of demonstrable focal neurological deficits and the variety of diseases that can be associated with strokes. In such a setting, the junior medical staff rapidly understands that "stroke" is not a diagnosis, but rather a complication of several different conditions that may be difficult to recognize. Last, the data collected from our patients are necessary for further research in stroke therapy. As efficient therapy for completed stroke is still almost entirely lacking, much effort has been given to prevention, but completed strokes will continue to occur. As discussed by Capildeo et al. *(this volume)*, only proper methodology can help solve the problem of clinical therapeutic trials. This means a precise and early classification of stroke patients according to their nature, extent, localization, vascular territory, mechanism, causes, and time course. To achieve this, some kind of training and expertise is mandatory. Aided by the appropriate diagnostic and laboratory facilities, we think that stroke units like the one described may contribute significantly.

REFERENCES

1. Caillé, J. M., and Orgogozo, J. M. (1981): Exploration des accidents vasculaires cérébraux. *Proceeding of the 6° Congrès Annuel de la Société Française de Neuroradiologie*, Tours, May, 1981.
2. Drake, W. E. (1973): Acute stroke management and patient outcome: the value of neurovascular care units. *Stroke*, 4:933–945.

3. Feigenson, J. S., Feigenson, W. D., Gitlow, H. S., et al. (1978): Outcome and cost for stroke patients in academic and community hospitals. *J.A.M.A.*, 240:1878–1880.
4. Kennedy, F. B., Pozen, T. J., Gabelman, E. H., et al. (1970): Stroke intensive care—an appraisal. *Am. Heart J.*, 80:188–196.
5. Millikan, C. H. (1979): Stroke intensive care units: objectives and results. In: *Cerebrovascular Disease and Stroke, Advances in Neurology, Volume 25*, edited by M. Goldstein, pp. 361–366. Raven Press, New York.
6. Norris, J. W. and Hachinski, V. C. (1976): Intensive care management of stroke patients. *Stroke*, 7:573–577.
7. Pitner, S. E., and Mance, C. J. (1973): An evaluation of stroke intensive care: results in a municipal hospital. *Stroke*, 4:737–741.
8. Stallones, R. A., Dyken, M. L., Fang, H. C., et al. (1972): Epidemiology for stroke facilities planning. *Stroke*, 3:360–371.
9. Taylor, R. R. (1970): Acute stroke demonstration project in a community hospital. *J. S.C. Med. Assoc.*, 66:225–227.

Advances in Stroke Therapy, edited by
F. C. Rose. Raven Press, New York © 1982.

Subarachnoid Hemorrhage in a Community

Jack P. Whisnant

Department of Neurology, Mayo Clinic and Medical School, Rochester, Minnesota 55905

The published information concerning subarachnoid hemorrhage (SAH) from intracranial aneurysms has come primarily from medical referral centers. Each center has its own sampling bias based on the condition of the patient when seen by his own physician, by the distance the patient has to travel, perceived interests and skills of the surgeons in the center to which the patient is sent, and a number of other variables, all of which significantly affect the mortality of the whole sample of patients referred to, or received at, a particular center. Alvord has emphasized this point very well (1).

Recently, some investigators have begun to discuss and report the total mortality of all patients admitted to their centers (2). This is a positive step in that it recognizes the bias in the selection of relatively favorable patients for surgery, but it does not allow for satisfactory comparisons of total experience between two different centers.

In 1967, Pakarinen (8) first reported a population study of SAH from aneurysms for Helsinki. Since few patients had surgery during the first two months, that study does reflect natural history for that period of time (Fig. 1).

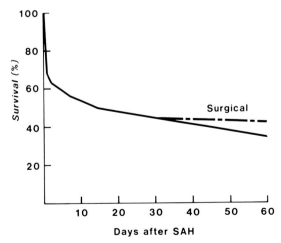

FIG. 1. Probability of survival among 589 patients with subarachnoid hemorrhage from the population of Helsinki, 1954–1961. (From ref. 10.)

Some of the statements in this chapter come from a study of SAH from aneurysms in the population of Rochester, Minnesota over a 30-year period in collaboration with my colleagues, Lawrence Phillips, Michael O'Fallon, and Thoralf Sundt (10). We are able to identify cases for the whole population of Rochester because of the large percentage of persons in the community cared for by Mayo physicians, the high level of neurological expertise in the community for many years, a record linkage system with all other medical care units in the city, and the fact that over half of the patients who die have an autopsy. All autopsies in the city are done by Mayo pathologists including coroner's cases such as sudden deaths.

During the 30 years, there were 129 patients who had their first SAH while a resident of Rochester. Five of those had an arteriovenous malformation and five had a disorder of hemostasis, so our concern will be with the remaining 119 who had rupture or presumed rupture of an intracranial aneurysm. This is a small proportion of all patients with aneurysms seen at Mayo, where now there are about 100 per year who have surgery by either of two neurosurgeons.

The average annual incidence rate for new cases was about 11/100,000 population per year and in contrast to other types of stroke in the same community which have shown a declining incidence, the incidence for SAH was almost exactly the same for each of the three decades from 1945 through 1974. The incidence rate in women was about 50% higher than the rate for men, as 12 compared to 8/100,000 persons per year. Another important observation was that the incidence rate increased with age, being about 40/100,000 per year in those over the age of 75 (Fig. 2). Pakarinen (8) indicated that he suspected that this circumstance might be the case, as he thought the diagnosis might often have been missed in older patients in Helsinki.

It is no surprise that patients in better condition had better survival. By using the Hunt and Hess (6) five grades of alive classification, those patients who were grade 1 or 2 on admission had a 60-day survival of about 70%, grade 3 had about a 45% 60-day survival, and grades 4 and 5 patients barely more than 15%. These were precisely the same at 30 days (Fig. 3).

The other primary factor that affects survival is time. Figure 4 is a graph of this community's patients with SAH from the onset and shows: 1. all the patients from onset (40%), a number close to the Pakarinen data, 2. those who survived 24 hr after SAH (55–60%), 3. those who survived to 48 hr (70%), and so forth, until we get to those who survived 2 weeks, at which time there is a very good long-term survival, regardless of what is done to the patients.

These data were used to develop a model from which the results of surgical treatment could be judged, but it was necessary to know the hours after SAH to make a satisfactory judgment: 8% died prior to being seen for medical attention. Among those who survived 6 hr, 12% didn't survive 24 hr, with a similar survival slope up to 48 hr. When patients are dying at this rate, the problems of judging treatment effect are considerable.

Starting not long prior to 1970, one neurosurgeon did essentially all the aneurysm surgery at Mayo, and did so until 1976, which covers the period of this study. He is recognized as an expert in the field by his colleagues at Mayo, and by his peers in neurosurgery. For the 5 years after 1970, 43% of the patients in the Rochester

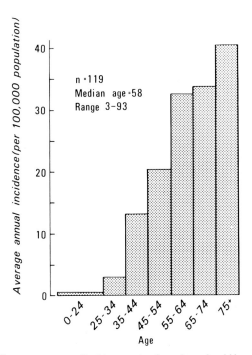

FIG. 2. Age-specific average annual incidence rates for subarachnoid hemorrhage from aneurysm or presumed aneurysm, Rochester, Minnesota, 1945–1974. (From ref. 6).

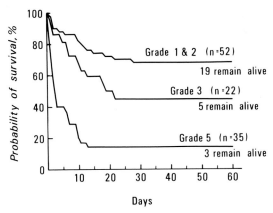

FIG. 3. Probability of survival after subarachnoid hemorrhage from aneurysm or presumed aneurysm by clinical grade at the time of first medical attention (Rochester, Minnesota, 1945–1974). Grade 1 is least severe and grade 5 most severe clinical symptoms. (From ref. 6.)

population had surgery, as compared to only 16% in the 25 years before that time [Drake (3) estimates that currently 30% are operated on in Ontario and only 13% in Japan]. Although there was an observed, modest increase in overall survival for those 5 years (1970–1974), it was not a significant difference (Fig. 5). Looking back over the earlier 25 years, there was another 5-year period in which the survival

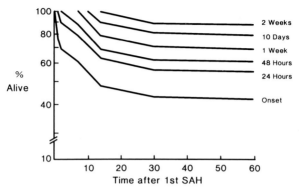

FIG. 4. Probability of survival after subarachnoid hemorrhage from aneurysm or presumed aneurysm and probability of survival among those who survived for 24 hr, 48 hr, 1 week, 10 days, and 2 weeks, Rochester, Minnesota, 1945–1974.

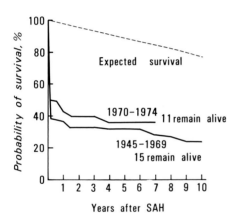

FIG. 5. Probability of survival after subarachnoid hemorrhage from aneurysm or presumed aneurysm, comparing those patients whose SAH occurred during the period 1945–1969 with those from 1970–1974, Rochester, Minnesota. (From ref. 6).

was very similar to that in 1970 to 1974 so the difference noted certainly could be a random one.

One might ask then what has been happening to mortality from SAH overall. Mortality from SAH as judged from death certificate data has been shown to be the most accurate among all the categories of stroke, so I think that the trends in this regard are probably reliable. Mortality rates from SAH in Rochester have held steady and without a change in incidence rates. There was no significant difference in mortality in men and women when comparing three 10-year periods from 1945–1974 (Fig. 6). This is not true for the United States white population, in which there may be underreporting if compared with the Rochester rates. The mortality rate in the United States has almost doubled since 1950 for men and women (13). Prior to 1950, one could not distinguish SAH as a distinct entity. Perhaps there has been a levelling off of the mortality rate since about 1970, or even a downturn for women. The trend in mortality is similar to that noted for England and Wales in 1978 by Roy Acheson (1).

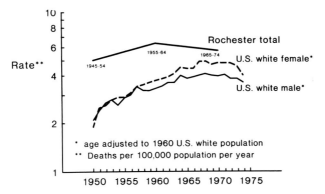

FIG. 6. Mortality rates for subarachnoid hemorrhage for United States white males and females compared with mortality rates for subarachnoid hemorrhage in Rochester, Minnesota. All rates are age adjusted (United States) or age and sex adjusted (Rochester) to the 1960 United States white population.

If we assume that the incidence rate has remained steady over the years in the United States as it has in Rochester, the increasing mortality implies increasingly ineffective overall management by all of us who deal with this problem. That may not be the case for those patients managed by a few experienced and capable neurosurgeons, but it seems to be the case overall.

It is clear that this disorder is not congenital, since it is manifested at the highest incidence rates in the oldest age groups. It is by no means clear what the factors are that influence its development. In our experience, prior hypertension is present to about the same extent as in a comparable age–sex matched sample in the population as a whole. Cigarette smoking has recently been implicated as a significant risk factor both by Pettitti and Wingard (9), and by Bell and Symon (2). It would be difficult to think of this as the major consideration in view of the incidence rate being 50% higher in women than in men. Oral contraceptives (9) also have been suggested as a contributor, but again, it is hard to think of this as a major contributor in view of a nonchanging incidence rate since 1945. Recently, it has been suggested that there is an association between SAH and influenza A infection (7). Eighty percent of those with confirmed SAH showed elevated antibody titers to influenza A compared with 12% of an age–sex matched control sample and 17% of a group of patients with other neurological disorders. It is apparent that not enough attention has been paid to the factors that may contribute to aneurysms and subsequent SAH, perhaps because of the ingrained assumption of a congenital origin.

The high early mortality is difficult to cope with. In most medical centers, surgery is done at 10 to 14 days. In Rochester, death after documented rebleeding accounted for less than one-half of deaths in the first 10 days. Rebleeding is difficult to document in clinical grades 4 and 5 patients. When documented rebleeding (for 10 years in terms of cumulative rebleeding) among survivors among grades 1, 2, or 3 patients is examined, all the action is in the first 30 days (Fig. 7). For the first 10 days, the slope of survivors who have not rebled shows a drop of nearly 2½%

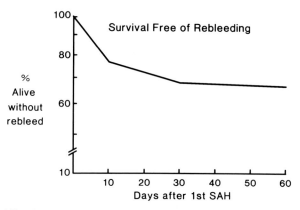

FIG. 7. Probability of survival free of rebleeding after the first subarachnoid hemorrhage among patients who were clinical grades 1, 2, or 3 at first medical attention, Rochester, Minnesota, 1945–1974.

per day. After 30 days, and all the way to 10 years, the slope is at a rate of about 2% per year. From 10 days to 30 days, the slope is a little less than ½% per day.

The mileage for salvage is in those first 10 days during which time, most surgeons are waiting for a more favorable surgical risk and after which time, there must be a very low surgical mortality to affect the overall mortality of the group.

In the last few years, increasing attention has been given to surgery within 1 or 2 days after SAH, as popularized by Suzuki (7) and Sano (11) and others in Japan. Some highly regarded, experienced neurosurgeons have suggested that this approach simply may rediscover the very high risk of operating too early. Looking at our overall clinical experience without regard to the population study, the risk certainly seems acceptable in grades 1 and 2 patients, but it is less clear in higher grade patients. Fisher et al. (5) and Eisentrout (4) and others now have pointed out good prognostic consideration that can be determined from CT evaluation that should help select those who are acceptable, early surgical risks. Unless we get a better idea of causative factors that we can influence, attention to this early period would appear to give the best chance of altering overall mortality and morbidity from aneurysmal SAH.

REFERENCES

1. Acheson, R. M., and Williams, D. R. R. (1980): Epidemiology of cerebrovascular disease: Some unanswered questions. In: *Clinical Neuroepidemiology*, edited by F. C. Rose. Pitman Medical, London.

1a. Alvord, E. C., Jr., Loeser, J. D., Bailey, W. L., and Copass, M. K. (1972): Subarachnoid hemorrhage due to ruptured aneurysm. A simple method of estimating prognosis. *Arch. Neurol.*, 27:273–284.

2. Bell, B. A., and Symon, L. (1979): Smoking and subarachnoid hemorrhage. *Br. Med. J.*, 1:577–578.

3. Drake, C. G. (1980): Perspectives on cerebral aneurysms with historical, current and future elements. Presented at the *5th J. Int. Conf. on Stroke and Cerebral Circulation*, Lake Buena Vista, Florida.

4. Eisentrout, C., Tomsick, T. A., and Tew, J. M. (1980): Computed tomography findings as a prognostic factor for ruptured cerebral aneurysms. *Stroke (abstr.)*, 11:124.
5. Fisher, C. M., Kistler, J. P., and Davis, J. M. (1980): The relation of cerebral vasospasm to subarachnoid blood by computerized tomography. *Stroke (abstr.)*, 11:124.
6. Hunt, W. E., and Hess, R. M. (1968): Surgical risk as related to time of intervention in the repair of intracranial aneurysms. *J. Neurosurg.*, 28:14–19.
7. Jones, D. B. (1979): An association between subarachnoid hemorrhage and influenza A infection. *Postgrad. Med.*, 55:853–855.
8. Pakarinen, S. (1967): Incidence, etiology, and prognosis of primary subarachnoid hemorrhage. *Acta Neurol. Scand. (Suppl.)*, 43:29.
9. Pettitti, D. B., and Wingard, J. (1978): Use of oral contraceptives, cigarette smoking, and risk of subarachnoid hemorrhage. *Lancet* ii:234–236.
10. Phillips, L. H., Whisnant, J. P., O'Fallon, W. M., and Sundt, T. M. Jr. (1940): The unchanging pattern of subarachnoid hemorrhage in a community. *Neurology*, 30:1034–1040.
11. Sano, K., and Saito, I. (1978): Timing and indication of surgery for ruptured intracranial aneurysms with regard to cerebral vasospasm. *Acta Neurochir.*, 41:49–60.
12. Suzuki, J., Yoshimoto, T., and Onuma, T. (1978): Early operations for ruptured intracranial aneurysms—study of 31 cases operated on within four days after ruptured aneurysm. *Neurol. Med. Chir. (Tokyo)*, 18:82–89.
13. United States Vital Statistics. United States Department of Health, Education and Welfare. 1950–1974.

Advances in Stroke Therapy, edited by
F. C. Rose. Raven Press, New York © 1982.

Role of Domiciliary Care Services for Acute Stroke Patients

Derick T. Wade and R. Langton-Hewer

Department of Neurology, Frenchay Hospital, Bristol, England

Stroke-induced illness is expensive and hospitals are by far the most expensive single resource involved. As most patients have their strokes at home, and most survivors will return home with their residual disability, it is perhaps surprising that there have been no controlled trials designed to assess the value of domiciliary care for patients who have suffered an acute stroke. This chapter outlines the background to the subject, and briefly outlines the first United Kingdom trial to be attempted.

ROLE OF THE HOSPITAL

Hospital admission is recommended by the W.H.O. and is considered essential by some neurologists in the United States (6). Indeed, in the United States, it is thought that only 5% of stroke patients remain at home (23). The reasons given for this policy include the following:

a. Hospitalization allows a full and accurate diagnosis to be made. Not only would the general diagnosis of a "cerebrovascular accident" be confirmed, but its type would be distinguished (e.g., haemorrhage, lacunar infarct), and its aetiology established, with particular regard to treatable factors.

b. Drug treatments, both general and specific, and expert nursing care can be given more easily in hospital.

c. Expert rehabilitation then can occur, maximising the patient's potential for recovery.

Similar reasons were once given for the policy of hospitalising patients with an acute myocardial infarction, yet since the Bristol study by Mather et al. (17), there has been considerable debate about the need for admitting such patients to hospital. We think that there is a need for a similar debate about stroke patients.

Returning to the reasons for hospitalisation given above:

a. It is uncertain how many remediable lesions can be identified by intensive investigation. In a personal series of 220 referrals to our stroke unit over two years, only two patients were found to have an alternative diagnosis—both having subdural haematomas.

A recent report (25) stated that only four tumours were present among 1,000 patients initially diagnosed as having a stroke. This represented a misdiagnosis rate of 0.4% in an elderly population, and this is likely to be more realistic than the rate of 2 to 3% suggested by Bull (5) or Groch (14).Another study has suggested a misdiagnosis rate of 8.1 (28). It is notable that in these last three studies, the populations were younger than the whole stroke population, and that all the misdiagnoses occurred in the younger patients.

Furthermore, there seems to be little evidence that knowing more detail about the type and extent of the stroke will materially alter management. However, this admittedly rather negative view about the value of investigating acute stroke patients requires to be examined further in the light of routine CT scanning on unselected patients from the general population who have suffered an acute stroke.

   b. At present, there are no drug treatments that benefit acute stroke patients (18).

   c. The process of formal rehabilitation yet has to be proved beneficial, although there is reasonable evidence to suggest that it is useful (16,24). However, there is no reason to suppose that this therapy has to be given in hospital.

Consideration of the reality of stroke care in the United Kingdom shows that patients are not usually admitted for the reasons suggested above. Very few stroke patients are cared for by specialist neurologists, and not many are admitted to hospitals with a CT scanner. Special stroke rehabilitation units are also uncommon.

Brocklehurst et al. (3) found that special investigations are notable for their rarity. They also found that general practitioners gave social reasons as the main reason for hospital admission in 89% of cases. Medical reasons were present in 50%. The recent debate about the role of hospital care (13,15,26,29) shows that these points are now being considered seriously.

We would suggest that the following circumstances dictate whether the patient be admitted to hospital: 1. when there is diagnostic doubt; 2. when there is the possibility of active therapy (e.g., the young patient with a good recovery and a unilateral carotid bruit); 3. when social circumstances dictate it. This would cover most patients living alone and those with a severe disability and an unfit spouse.

Patients who are unconscious or likely to die within a few hours often will not need to be admitted, and those patients with a mild completed stroke probably do not require immediate admission. It is clear that currently in the United Kingdom, it is usually home circumstances and not medical necessity that dictates hospital admission.

THE DISADVANTAGES OF HOSPITAL CARE

It has been suggested that moving a patient immediately after a stroke increases the risk of death if he has had an intracerebral haemorrhage (26,29), but there does not appear to be any evidence to support this. Obviously the patient is also at risk of iatrogenic disease associated with any special investigations or treatments given, and he may acquire unusual infections while in hospital.

Apart from these physical risks, there are psychological consequences associated with hospital care. A small study made in London (9) found that depression was extremely common after discharge from the hospital, and that many patients felt rejected by the medical profession. This may be due in part to inappropriate therapy being given in hospital without due regard to the home circumstances. Patients may appear to be able to achieve more in hospital surroundings than they actually do when they return home (2).

For the National Health Service (NHS), there are considerable costs associated with the process of hospitalising strokes. Stroke is the third single commonest cause for hospital admission (11) (after tonsillectomy and myocardial infarction), being responsible for 2.3% of the total number of admissions.

Strokes consume 4.6% of all NHS resources, being responsible for 6% of hospital running costs, occupying 6.4% of all bed days, 13% of general medical bed days, and 25% of geriatric bed days (7).

Figures from a district general hospital suggest that strokes account for 8 to 11% of all acute medical ward admissions (1). In the Frenchay Health District (207,000 people), our recent figures suggest that 280 strokes are hospitalised each year. Those discharged alive occupied 4,500 bed days each year, staying in hospital for an average (mean) of 6 weeks, with a median length of stay of about 4 weeks.

PRESENT ROLE OF DOMICILIARY CARE

Facts about the current nature and scale of domiciliary care for acute strokes are not readily available. It has been suggested that possibly only 40% of stroke patients in South Wales are admitted (8), but surveys in Surrey (27) and Manchester (3) suggest that as many as 75% of stroke patients are eventually admitted to hospital. A survey in Bristol 5 years ago suggested that only 40% of all stroke patients were admitted to hospital. The National Survey of General Practitioners (19) found that only 42% of all new episodes of cerebrovascular disease were referred to hospital for admission.

Strokes form 8 to 11% of a district nurse's workload (1,3), although not all of this work will be with acute strokes. In those areas with domiciliary physiotherapy services, stroke is probably responsible for 14 to 32% of the workload (10,12,22). It is second only to osteoarthritis. Again, these figures probably refer largely to nonacute stroke. Social services are also heavily involved with stroke patients (3), e.g., providing 40% of all stroke patients at home with Meals on Wheels.

FUTURE ROLE OF DOMICILIARY CARE FOR ACUTE STROKES

If it is accepted that hospitals in themselves have no special advantages to offer the patient, then it is important to consider how the necessary nursing care and later rehabilitation can be given most economically to the patients. This question has been asked several times recently (3,20,27,29), but has not yet been answered.

A retrospective case-controlled study on hospitalised patients in America (4) showed that the use of a domiciliary physiotherapy service reduced hospital stay by an average of 5 days and led to a better functional recovery. In addition, there was a net reduction in costs. No other studies looking at the role of domiciliary care for acute strokes have been published.

Domiciliary care for acute stroke patients may offer several advantages:

a. If the family can be helped to cope with the immediate problems, they will gain considerable confidence. They then will be in a good position to manage the more long-term problems that often arise. However, if the patient returns home from hospital with some problems extant, the family will often feel unable to cope and may reject the patient or force further hospital admission.

b. Any rehabilitative therapy given can be made relevant to the patient's home circumstances. Furthermore, the family can be involved more closely which should help some gain more satisfaction from their caring role, and may also mean that the patient receives more therapy.

c. Early involvement of a caring team with the whole family in their own home may diminish the psychological problems that inevitably arise.

d. There may be a considerable economic advantage. Costing of health care in the NHS is notoriously difficult. The difference in cost between an empty bed and a full bed, termed the marginal cost, is probably very small. But, as there is considerable pressure on hospital beds, the emptying of beds will free resources for other use and so it is reasonable to price the cost at the average cost of a hospital bed.

For the Frenchay Health District, we have estimated the cost of providing a domiciliary care service for acute strokes at between £25,000 to £30,000 per year. The cost of a general medical hospital bed is at present £60 per day. Therefore, the team needs to save 500 bed days per year to pay for itself. This represents 12% of all bed days devoted to stroke survivors and could be achieved either by preventing 34 (of 280) admissions, or by shortening the hospital stay by an average of 8 days.

One must realise that an increase in the number of patients kept at home has potential disadvantages:

a. Domiciliary services (e.g., district nursing or social services) may be used more, and this cost must always be considered.

b. Economic savings may be bought at the price of a reduced standard of patient care (21).

c. There may in fact be more stress, rather than less, upon the relatives.

THE FRENCHAY DOMICILIARY STROKE PROJECT

The Frenchay Domiciliary Stroke Project was set up at the end of 1980 and started in March 1981 and is due to run for 3 years. It has three aims:

1. To observe the present pattern of management of acute strokes with particular reference to the use of domiciliary and hospital resources.

2. To develop a new service to help in the management of acute stroke patients. This service is designed to increase the number of patients able to be kept at home, and also to facilitate early discharge from hospital. The service will be provided by a team, whose members will include a nurse, a physiotherapist, an occupational therapist, a speech therapist, and a social worker.

3. To monitor the change in the pattern of care that this service produces.

Three hypotheses are to be tested:

1. That the new service will cause a net saving in money.

2. That the team will help the patient to make the best possible psychological adjustment to the stroke.

3. That those patients receiving the services of this team will make an equally good functional recovery.

The population to be studied is the 207,000 people on the lists of the 96 general practitioners whose practices are within the Frenchay Health District. The district will be subdivided so that one-half of the practices form the control group, establishing a present pattern of management, and the other half, the trial group, who will have access to this team.

All strokes will be studied, regardless of age or severity. The diagnosis will be purely clinical and the study will accept all patients referred with strokes, withdrawing later those found to have another diagnosis. It should be stressed that this is not a trial of home against hospital care but an observational study that includes a trial of a more home orientated pattern of care. At no point does the study dictate the place of care, and clinical control remains entirely with the general practitioner and/or consultant.

All patients in both groups will have medical, functional, and psychological research assessments performed upon them: as soon as possible, at three weeks, and at six months. Costing data will be collected from all domiciliary and hospital services involved.

The team will start work in July 1981, and the study will end in December, 1983.

CONCLUSIONS

It can be said that the case for mandatory admission for all stroke patients is unproven, quite apart from being unrealistic. In practice, hospital admission primarily reflects home circumstances and, if the family can be helped at home, then probably more patients could be kept at home throughout, and those admitted to hospital could be discharged earlier. Though it remains to be proved, this policy could well benefit the patient, his family, and the N.H.S.

REFERENCES

1. Acheson, J., Acheson, H. W. K., and Talwright, J. M. (1968): The incidence and pattern of cerebrovascular disease in general practice. *J. R. Coll. Gen. Prac.*, 16:428–436.

2. Andrews, K., and Stewart, J. (1979): Stroke recovery: he can but does he? *Rheumatol. Rehab.*, 1843–1848.
3. Brocklehurst, J. C., Andrews, K., Morris, P. E., Richards, B., and Lacock, P. J. (1978): Medical, social and psychological aspects of stroke. Final report, University of Manchester.
4. Bryant, N. H., Candland, L., and Lowenstein, R. (1974): Comparison of care and cost outcomes for stroke patients with and without home care. *Stroke*, 5:54–59.
5. Bull, J. W. D., Marshall, J., Shaw, D. A. (1960): Cerebral angiography in the diagnosis of acute stroke. *Lancet*, i:562–565.
6. Buonanno, F., and Toole, J. F. (1981): Management of patients with established ("completed") cerebral infarction. *Stroke*, 12:7–16.
7. Carstairs, V. (1976): Stroke: resource consumption and cost to the community. In: *Stroke*, edited by F. J. Gillingham, C. Maudsley, and A. E. Williams. pp. 516–528. Churchill Livingstone, London.
8. Cochrane, A. L. (1970): Burden of cerebrovascular disease. *Br. Med. J.*, 3:165.
9. Court, C., Capildeo, R., and Rose, F. C. (1970): Medico-social aspects of stroke: a domiciliary follow-up study. In: *Progress in Stroke Research 1*, edited by R. M. Greenhalgh, and F. C. Rose, pp. 237–244. Pitman Medical, London.
10. Frazer, F. W. (1980): Domiciliary physiotherapy, cost and benefit. *Physiotherapy*, 66:2–7.
11. Garraway, W. M. (1976): The size of the problem of stroke in Scotland. In: *Stroke*, edited by F. J. Gillingham, C. Maudsley and A. E. Williams. pp. 72–82. Churchill Livingstone, London.
12. Glossop, E. S., and Smith, D. S. (1979): Domiciliary physiotherapy; a report to the DHSS. Northwick Park Clinical Research Centre.
13. Greenhouse, A. H. (1980): Patients with stroke: home or hospital? *Lancet*, ii:646.
14. Groch, S. N., Hurwitz, L. J., Wright, I. S., and McDowell, F. (1960): Intracranial lesions simulating cerebral thrombosis. *J.A.M.A.*, 172:1469–1472.
15. Jarrett, S. R. (1981): Stroke patient: home or hospital? *Lancet*, 146.
16. Lehmann, J. F., Delateur, B. J., Fowler, R. S., Warren, C. G., Arnold, R., Schertzer, G., Hurker, R., Whitmore, I. J., Masock, A. J., and Chambers, K. H. (1975): Stroke: does rehabilitation affect outcome? *Arch. Phys. Med. Rehab.*, 56:375–382.
17. Mather, H. G., Pearson, N. G., Read, K. L. Q., Shaw, D. B., Steed, G. R., Thorne, M. G., Jones, S., Guerrier, C. J., Eraut, C. D., McHugh, P. M., Chowdhury, N. R., Jafary, M. H., and Wallace T. J. (1971): Acute myocardial infarction: home and hospital treatment. *Br. Med. J.*, 3:334–338.
18. Matthews, W. B. (1978): The treatment of acute ischaemic stroke. In: *Recent Advances in Clinical Neurology 2*, edited by W. B. Matthews and G. H. Glaser, pp. 9–14. Churchill Livingstone, London.
19. Morbidity Statistics from General Practice—2nd National Study 1970–71. (1974): Studies on Medical and Population Subjects 26. *Office of Population Censuses and Surveys*, London HMSO.
20. Mulley, G., and Arie, T. (1978): Treating stroke; home or hospital? *Br. Med. J.*, 2:1321–1322.
21. Opit, L. J. (1977): Domiciliary care for the elderly sick—economy or neglect? *Br. Med. J.*, 1:30–33.
22. Partridge, C. J., and Warren, M. D. (1977): *Physiotherapy in the Community. A Descriptive Study of 14 Schemes*. Health Services Research Unit, University of Kent at Canterbury, Kent. Campfield Press, St. Albans.
23. Robins, M., and Weinfeld, F. D. (1981): Study design and methodology. In: *The National Survey of Stroke*, pp. 7–12. American Heart Association.
24. Smith, E. S., Goldenberg, E., Ashburn, A., Kinsella, G., Sheikh, K., Brennan, P. J., Mead, T. W., Zutski, D. W., Perry, J. B., and Riback, J. S. (1981): Remedial therapy after stroke: a randomised controlled trial. *Br. Med. J.*, 282:517–520.
25. Twomey, C. (1978): Investigating stroke. *Br. Med. J.*, 2:637–638.
26. Vetter, N. J. (1980): Home or hospital for the stroke patient. *Lancet*, ii:1254.
27. Weddell, J. M., and Berrisford, S. A. A. (1979): Planning for stroke patients. A four year descriptive study of home and hospital care. *Department of Health and Social Security*. HMSO.
28. Weisberg, L. A., and Nice, C. N. (1977): Intracranial lesions simulating the presentation of cerebrovascular syndromes. Early detection with cerebral computed tomography. *J.A.M.A.*, 63:517–524.
29. Wright, W. B., and Robson, P. (1980): Crisis procedure for stroke at home. *Lancet*, ii:249–250.

Advances in Stroke Therapy, edited by
F. C. Rose. Raven Press, New York © 1982.

The Continuing Needs of Stroke Patients

Bernard Isaacs

Department of Geriatric Medicine, University of Birmingham, Birmingham, England

HARD AND SOFT DATA

Clinical science demands objectivity. The material that medical scientists communicate to one another is called "hard data," and it is obtained by measurement, using methods that have been validated and checked for "interobserver" and "intraobserver" variation. The data is capable of being recorded on computer, presented as graphs and tables, and tested for significance by statistical methods. Hard data comprises the bulk of the material that is published in this volume, journals, and textbooks, and that is taught to medical students and required back from them in examinations. Hard data forms the basis of the treatment of disease and of the identification of service needs.

Clinical information that lacks the qualities of hard data is called "soft" or "anecdotal" data. It is looked upon as inferior and its dissemination is generally discouraged. Clinical observations based on "soft" data are largely debarred from publication. Soft data is suspect.

Most collections of hard data are about lots of people, e.g. the incidence of stroke illness in the United Kingdom, or about bits of people, e.g. the cerebral blood flow in patients with stroke. Soft data on the other hand is concerned with individuals, with whole people, such as the last patient you or I saw who had a stroke. Soft data is the stuff of clinical medicine, the patients we treat, those we show to our students and talk about over our coffee. Yet our permanent communications to the medical literature record only what we measure. The collection and analysis of hard data is the hard task we set ourselves and pride ourselves on.

A FAILURE OF COMMUNICATION

Ten years ago, my colleagues and I in Glasgow were struck by the paradox that our stroke patients who did very well in hospital did very badly at home. We obtained a research grant to undertake a 3-year follow-up study of the quality of life of 100 patients, but we were unable to recruit a qualified research worker to undertake the fieldwork. Instead we employed a housewife with no professional qualification. She visited the homes of our discharged patients, listened to them, and brought back reports of the intensity and diversity of their suffering that far transcended the boundaries of the little boxes into which the data was to have been compressed. She told stories of ruined lives, destroyed marriages, broken families, bizarre and altered behaviour, bewilderment, and perplexity. She brought back stories too of courage and resolve, of ingenuity and determination, of patience and gratitude. Her stories added a new dimension to my understanding of stroke illness. But when we came to prepare the material for publication in a medical journal we found that it was "soft," and in its soft form, unacceptable for publication. So we did a nice hardening job, turned it into scales and tables, and it duly took its humble place in the medical literature (1). But rereading that study, I am reminded of the words of Eliot's J. Alfred Prufrock

> That is not what I meant at all.
> That is not it, at all . . .

A SECOND TRY

I did not attempt a second survey, but instead I asked the Chest, Heart and Stroke Association to send me a selection of the enquiries they received from stroke victims, and asked a number of colleagues who worked closely with stroke patients to tell me their views on continuing needs. The material came from doctors, physiotherapists, occupational therapists, speech therapists, helpers in stroke clubs, stroke victims, and their relatives. I shall quote selectively from their comments, and shall begin with a summary of a case history supplied to me by a physiotherapist.

CASE HISTORY

In March 1979, a 70-year-old retired nursing sister suffered a stroke with loss of speech and use of right limbs. Within 7 days, her speech had returned to normal except for slight slurring when she was tired, and movement began to return to her arms and legs within 4 days. By June she was able to walk unassisted using a stick out of doors and in the garden. Her arm movements were good, but there was a little loss of power in the hands. Recovery of the trunk was poor, and she had some scoliosis and backache. Her initial recovery was thus better than in most patients of her age. But a year after onset, she fell in the garden and lost confidence. By November 1980 after a fall in the house when alone, she lost her ability to walk independently without holding on to the furniture.

What did this mean to the patient and to the friend with whom she shared a bungalow and who was still working as a physiotherapist?

The patient's problems are identified as:

Housebound
Frustration

> She can no longer fulfill her role in the household, i.e., shopping, gardening and housework.
> She can no longer follow her hobbies of gardening and hill walking.
> The poor quality of her writing, knitting, and sewing are not acceptable.

Boredom	She lacks mental stimulation through being alone for 10 hours or more each day.
Fear	Fear of falling and of not being able to get up. Fear of further strokes.
Increase in weight	Because of lack of activity and eating as a substitute for living, she has gained nearly two stones.
Guilt	She feels she is restricting the life of her friend.
Dependency	She was previously very independent.

What are the problems besetting the friend?

Restrictions	A need to limit activities away from home.
Changes	She now has to fulfill her interest in walking alone, or not go at all.
Holidays	Country walking holidays are no longer possible; there is a need for expensive hotels with a lift and places to sit and look at a view rather than walk.

Trying not to look bored or restricted.
Alternating between understanding and irritation at the changes and the consequent guilt feelings.

What conclusions do these ladies draw? As professionals, they both have been involved with stroke patients and their families all of their working lives and have endeavoured to obtain gadgets for the patient's independence and "services" to fill the gaps of the essential creature needs. But, the physiotherapist writes, we now know that it is the psychological problems that are the permanent ones. Each household has to work these out for itself. It is not easy, if indeed it is possible, and whatever the degree of recovery, nothing is the same.

There are many other letters in a similar vein in which patients describe the frustrations and deprivations that are associated not with total disability but with taking longer and being clumsier at doing the things on which they had always prided themselves. Many detail peculiar difficulties such as finding one's way in familiar environments, of inhibiting uncalled-for tears, of recognising oneself in the mirror.

Here is a letter, full of spelling and typing errors, which sums it up neatly:

> I am a male of 68 years of age and I had my stroke on 27th August 1978 affecting my right side, not my speech. I can now walk of course with a severe limp and my arm is reasonably mobile but has little pressure. Of course I would like to walk properly again. According I am informed that I am lucky to have improved so much. I have seen so many people far worse than myself. What like to know if I can expect any further improvement. Further I would like to know if can get any further treatment. If so how am I to go about same? I would like know if there is any way that I can avoid a further stroke. I am taking daily walks as far my condition allows. I also take a matter of three weeks holiday per year. I do as much gardening as I am able to accomplish. I would also like to know if there is any occupation I could follow which help to pass the time—voluntary or otherwise. Finally would like to know if I am entitle to any benefits through the National Health such certain assistance in running a car. Any society I could join?

Please accept my apologies for the bad typing. I am not atall good with my left hand.

The six questions in Table 1 figure in that letter and in very many others. These are the questions our patients want to know and I fear that I seldom spend much time trying to answer them.

STROKE IN THE HEALTH SERVICE

Table 2 gives a few scraps of statistical information derived from the hospitals in the West Midlands. They show that nearly 90% of patients discharged alive from hospital after suffering a stroke spend less than 4 weeks in hospital. Ninety percent of all discharges were from medical wards. I was unable to obtain data on what proportion of these patients attended day hospitals or physiotherapy departments for continuing treatment; but in all cases, a point is reached where the patient has to be told that treatment is to be withdrawn. My letters tell me that this decision, though accepted as just and reasonable, is simultaneously resented as harsh and indelicate. The conviction that further treatment will lead to further improvement is an ever-present hope and perhaps a not entirely forlorn one, but one that our health care system cannot afford to sustain. Nonetheless, there are questions to be asked about this (see Table 3), and I am not at all sure how to answer them.

ACUTE OR CHRONIC

Stroke disguises its true nature from the health care system. It presents as an acute disease and in that guise, it enters hospital as an emergency. There is an assumption, that has almost the force of law, that illnesses of acute onset pursue

TABLE 1. *The stroke patient's questions*

1. Will I recover?
2. How long will it take?
3. What caused my stroke?
4. Will I have another?
5. What should I do to help myself?
6. What should I avoid to prevent another stroke?

TABLE 2. *Live discharges of stroke patients (ICD codes 431–434) from West Midlands hospitals*

	Number of patients discharged	Percentage discharged within 4 weeks	Percentage discharged after remaining more than 3 months
From medical wards	823	88	2
From geriatric wards	95	52	8
Both sources	918	85	3

Source: HAA West Midlands, 1979.

TABLE 3. *Withdrawal of treatment*

Who decides to withdraw treatment?
On what grounds?
How is this communicated?
How is the decision received?
What is provided to replace it?

an acute course—that victims die or recover almost as quickly as they take ill. This is true of fatal strokes—in the West Midlands, 80% of deaths in hospital from stroke occurred within 4 weeks of onset, which is true of some nonfatal strokes, too. However, a large proportion of stroke survivors remain disabled for a long period. Recognising this and fearing for the efficient use of their beds, many departments adopt the view that the criterion for discharge of stroke patients need not be complete functional recovery or maximum benefit from treatment, but rather, it could be ability of the family to manage at home. The decision to discharge early is often eagerly supported by the family, who seem deceived by the sudden onset of the illness into believing that it will suddenly go away once the patient is restored to his normal environment. After a series of predischarge procedures that in some overpressed and understaffed departments are in danger of becoming predischarge rituals, including the "OT (occupational therapy) assessment" and the "laying on of a home help"—the patient's wish is acceded to and he finds himself at home.

Optimism is soon dispelled and many patients write of a sense of abandonment, so often expressed in the sad little phrase "no one wants to know." Another complaint that frequently appears in the letters relating to this stage is that no one told them anything. This complaint hurts because we know it is not true. Most doctors tell me that they make a particular point of explaining carefully and clearly to patient and relative exactly what has happened and what they can expect in the future. Still, it seems that we tell them the wrong things, in the wrong way, at the wrong time, because the complaint is almost universal. The Chest, Heart and Stroke Association receives countless letters of appreciation for their little booklets answering twenty questions about stroke illness; always accompanied by the statement, "if only someone had told us this when he was in hospital." I accept that what we tell them is not enough. Patients and their relatives are quite unprepared to grasp the extent and nature of the disability and to come to terms with their feelings and experiences. Another correspondent reminded me that "paralysed limbs are painful to touch, to heat and to cold. Stroke patients get a lot of pain in the eye, nose, the mouth, and the neck of the affected side. A mouthwash is a necessary last thing at night to prevent choking on residual food in the weak side of the mouth." A hundred other unexpected behaviours and symptoms appear, yet there is no Doctor Spock to run to for an explanation of that behaviour. Many correspondents wrote to say what a relief it was, when they attended a stroke club, to find that others had observed similar behaviours to what they thought was unique to their own situation.

SOME SOLUTIONS

Stroke patients have extensive and continuing needs. So have all who suffer from chronic disabling diseases, and it would be wrong to make a special plea for the stroke victim. Yet the stroke patient dramatically typifies the failure of our health care system to identify and respond to continuing needs, as well as a certain lack of medical curiosity in studying the continuing changes in human behaviour and physiological function that follow from an assault on brain tissues. I favour three approaches: through the primary care team, the voluntary organisations, and the hospital services. Only the last is novel.

PRIMARY CARE

The family doctor is the standard target for the complaints of anyone who feels that his own special field of interest is failing to receive due attention. Our Glasgow study showed that general practitioners readily attended stroke victims to treat incidental illness, but offered little help for the stroke itself. When I asked general practitioners to comment on this finding, they admitted that they rarely visited stroke patients, but said, "What would you want us to do? All that most of them want is more physiotherapy or occupational therapy, and you know how difficult it is to get that for them; and anyway do you really think it would do them good?" They have a point, but I fear that these doctors may have too low an estimation of the regard in which they were held. Many patients only wanted an acknowledgment of their continued existence. Many had questions that they would like to ask—such questions as, "What should they do about sex and would it bring on another stroke?"—and who better than the family doctor to ask them of? My previous study took place 10 years ago, and the enlarged primary care team of today has much to offer stroke patients.

THE VOLUNTARY SECTOR

Stroke clubs and the Volunteers' Stroke Scheme, both initiated and stimulated by the Chest, Heart and Stroke Association, originated from the sense of rejection which patients felt when treatment was withdrawn. They thrive and multiply splendidly, renewing the faith of their members in their membership of the human race. Yet the Chest, Heart and Sroke Association tell us that the average interval between a stroke patient's discharge from hospital and his joining a stroke club is 3 years, and it is doubtful if as many as 10% of stroke victims attend clubs. Many don't want to go to a stroke club, but many more who would wish to do so are denied the opportunity, and not necessarily because there is no club in their region. Often it is just because no one has ever told them about it. Stroke clubs are not a panacea, but many stroke sufferers have written to the Chest, Heart and Stroke Association to say how their whole outlook on life has changed since they joined a club.

HOSPITAL

The hospital to which the patient was originally admitted does not normally play a continuing role in care after the patient's discharge, unless a technical problem persists like a high haematocrit necessitating frequent blood-letting, or unless he is on an anticoagulant or antiplatelet regime. Many of the 10% of hospital discharges who have been in geriatric units will continue attendance at the day hospital for a time and others may attend physiotherapy departments or occupational therapy or speech therapy departments or receive home treatment. However, sooner or later treatment must come to an end. The last thread is cut, and the patient is on his own.

I believe that a strong case can be made for what I call an "anniversary" clinic for stroke patients discharged from hospital (Table 4). They should attend routinely 6 months and 12 months after the stroke and annually thereafter. The anniversary clinic should be a multidisciplinary clinic attended by the patient and the relative, with evaluations from doctor, nurse, rehabilitation staff, and social worker. New symptoms should be sought, behavioural problems and functional difficulties identified, and advice on treatment given. The patients and relatives should have the opportunity of asking questions, and the professionals should submit themselves to the discipline of answering them honestly.

Multidisciplinary care is in favour, but the members of a multidisciplinary team tend to have multiple responsibilities, and it is no easy thing to bring them together at one time and place to focus on the needs of stroke patients. Only the conviction that there is a need and that good will accrue will act as a sufficient stimulus.

CONCLUSION

Stroke is a chronic illness with an acute onset, a vascular illness in neurological territory, a family illness with more than one victim, a challenging illness with much to teach about how the damaged brain regains function.

TABLE 4. *The anniversary assessment*

Medical	
Pathogenesis	Blood pressure
	Haematocrit
	Platelet function
	Cardiac rhythm
	Intracranial pathology
Diasability	Neuropsychiatric assessment
	Functional and social assessment
Health care	Diet, exercise, weight, feet
	Sweets, tobacco, alcohol
	Sleep, sex
Incidental	Unrelated disease
	Medication
Functional	
Environmental	
Psychological	
Interpersonal	
Social	

Medical care, preoccupied with hard data, may have overlooked the health care needs of long-term stroke survivors and the new information to be gathered systematically from listening to and observing these patients. There is no better stimulus to research than questions which patients ask and we cannot answer. I suspect that there is much truth to be found in the soft data that our stroke patients have committed to their letters.

ACKNOWLEDGMENTS

I would like to express my appreciation to the stroke patients and their relatives who wrote so feelingly to me, to Miss Hilda Walsh of the Chest, Heart and Stroke Association, and to the many doctors, physiotherapists, occupational therapists, speech therapists, social workers, stroke club organisers, and members who so kindly wrote to me.

REFERENCE

1. Isaacs, B., Neville, Y., and Rushford, A. (1976): The stricken: the social consequences of stroke. *Age Ageing*, 5:188–192.

Advances in Stroke Therapy, edited by
F. C. Rose. Raven Press, New York © 1982.

Psychosocial Aspects of Stroke Rehabilitation

R. Langton-Hewer

Consultant Neurologist, Frenchay Hospital, Bristol, England

The success or failure of rehabilitation programmes is usually measured in terms of the proportion of survivors who achieve independence in mobility and the activities of daily life. Indeed, the restoration of independence in these skills is a vital objective of rehabilitation. However, there is a growing awareness that stroke victims experience severe psychological and social problems that may be just as important as the mechanical ones caused by the obvious physical limitations of the hemiplegia. A recent paper (4) has suggested that a significant proportion of survivors manifest social disability despite complete, or near complete, physical restoration.

A stroke may be seen as a threat to the integrity of the family and is likely to have profound effects both on the patient and his close relatives. It raises many interrelated issues involving financial security, employment, ambition, future independence, the ability to drive a car, sexual activity, and social relationships. Common reactions occurring at different stages include shock, disbelief, guilt, feelings of rejection, anxiety, anger, unreasonable hope, hopelessness, and depression. The term "psychosocial" is currently used to describe the amalgam of psychological and social factors, and no worthwhile rehabilitation programme can afford to ignore this important dimension.

The nature and severity of psychosocial problems obviously will be influenced by many factors including the extent of the neurological deficit, whether or not the patient is admitted to hospital, his premorbid personality and the quality of his life, marital stability, and financial security. Although no two patients present precisely the same problems, nonetheless, certain patterns can be identified. Some of these are outlined in Tables 1 to 3 (2).

Psychological problems have been discussed by various workers including Epsmark (1) and Waite (8), the latter identifying three different phases: crisis, adjustment, and restoration. Our experiences (2) are similar and are described below.

THE FIRST TWO WEEKS

The patient himself is frequently in a state of shock and may not realise what is happening. The relatives, however, frequently react with extreme anxiety and some-

TABLE 1. *Psychological reactions—first 2 weeks*

High anxiety	
Patient	Relative
Shock	Shock
Frustration	Relief (that patient is alive)
Shame	Concern
	Anger

TABLE 2. *Psychological reactions—next 3 months*

Loss	
Patient	Relatives
Reactive depression	Financial worries
Unrealistic expectations or denial	Unrealistic expectations
Overidentification with remedial staff	Doubts about ability to cope

TABLE 3. *Psychological reactions—4 months onwards*

Adjustment	
Patient	Relatives
Confirmation of disability	Rejection
Rejection	
Frustration (work, driving, etc.)	Need for continued contact

times through anger and denial. At the same time, they may express relief that the patient has survived. The relatives are often unable to think rationally, and their emotions often appear illogical. The remedial staff have an important function in allaying anxiety by careful explanation and by helping with practical problems, particularly if the patient remains at home.

THE NEXT THREE MONTHS

As the patient's condition improves, he slowly becomes aware of his predicament and its implications, a process that may take several weeks, or even longer. Reactions at this time include anxiety, shame, and sometimes denial of what has happened. A stroke usually occurs suddenly, and many patients think that recovery will be equally quick, so that it is necessary to gently explain that recovery is likely to be slow, and will probably not be complete. Explanation can be difficult if there is significant dysphasia or intellectual deficit.

The patient who previously may have been the dominant member in the family, probably will be unable to take part in everyday decisions involving finance, his job, the children, and many other matters. The family may unconsciously expect him to adopt the role of a sick person, or even a child. As a result, many patients become depressed and are sometimes described as lacking motivation.

There is a tendency for patients and the family to become dependent upon the hospital, a phenomenon particularly liable to occur with patients who are kept in hospital for several weeks. It is easy for the relatives to come to feel that the handling of the patient can be undertaken only by professionals. As a result, they may invent all sorts of reasons why the patient cannot return home. Certainly, prolonged hospitalisation should be avoided, and relatives should be actively involved with remedial therapy from an early stage.

FOUR MONTHS ONWARDS—LONG-TERM ADJUSTMENT

Physical therapy is usually terminated after three or four months. At this point, the patient and family may react by becoming angry that so little has been achieved. Depression and feelings of rejection may occur in the patient and his family. Such a situation is only too likely to occur, and has been described by various workers (3,5).

The patient and his family remain highly vulnerable for many months following the stroke. Support should continue to be provided after physical therapy has stopped. In our experience, a follow-up period of 12 to 18 months is desirable. During this time, the patient must be helped to rebuild his life, and make the most of his residual capacities.

MANAGEMENT

In our experience, despite the fact that there is now a considerable literature on the subject, the management of psychosocial problems does not receive as much attention in practice as it appears to merit. Some of the reasons are:

1. The problems are complex and time consuming.
2. The benefits of involvement in this field are difficult to prove.
3. Data are not easily obtained and are difficult to present.
4. Few doctors and remedial therapists have received any appropriate training.
5. The social worker is the person most obviously involved. However, in the United Kingdom, social workers are not employees of the National Health Service. Experience over the last few years leads us to the conclusion that the Social Services Administration does not always understand the importance of experienced social work input in the field of severe physical incapacity.

We have been particularly fortunate in having an extremely experienced and able social worker who has been with us for 6 years, but not all units can expect to be so fortunate. However, it is obvious that the various psychosocial problems outlined above cannot be the sole responsibility of one person, and the importance of training for all members of the team is clear.

Because of the constraints of time, involvement probably is concentrated best at times of particular need (2), although remedial staff always should be available and willing to discuss problems. The three particular crises points are as follows:

1. When the stroke occurs. As mentioned above, the close relatives are likely to need support at this time.

2. The time of discharge from hospital.

3. At the time of discharge from active treatment (for example, when physiotherapy is stopped).

Many patients and relatives appear to benefit from individual counselling sessions. Group discussions for patients have been found to be helpful by some centres (7). Many centres run groups for relatives (6,9). The following matters are usually discussed:

1. Information about the stroke. Frequent questions include, What is a stroke? The cause of stroke? The risk of recurrence? The outlook? It may be helpful to distribute one or more simple booklets dealing with stroke illness.

2. Where can practical help be obtained? For example, provision of a commode, wheelchair, and services such as Meals on Wheels.

3. Financial advice—e.g. allowances and various entitlements.

4. How to handle a patient—emotionally and physically; for example, methods of transferring from bed to chair.

Many relatives need an opportunity to express their pent-up emotions (6). This can be done in groups and by individual counselling. Furthermore, many relatives find it helpful to share their experiences and feelings with others who are in a similar predicament. Some find it gratifying to realise that special attention is being given to their problem. It is certainly easy to neglect the family.

Following discharge from active treatment, the patient and his family ideally should be encouraged to remain in contact with the stroke unit. Advice always can be given by telephone, and we make it a practice to follow patients for at least 18 months. We also try to see the patient immediately if problems arise.

The Chest, Heart and Stroke Association has supported the development of stroke clubs throughout the United Kingdom. Over 260 are now in existence. In our own Health District, we have about 70 volunteers working with stroke families. Patients are encouraged to get out of the house at least once a week, and transport is provided for this. Various social gatherings are arranged. Hobbies of various sorts are encouraged, notably gardening. A special garden has been constructed for stroke patients, and this is proving a considerable success. All these activities are used to encourage social contact since social isolation is a significant cause of much long-term misery, and should, if possible, be avoided.

REFERENCES

1. Epsmark, S. (1973): Stroke before 50. A follow-up study of vocational and psychological adjustment. *Scand. J. Rehab. Med.*, Supplement 2.
2. Holbrook, M. (1981): *(personal communication)*.
3. Isaacs, B., Neville, Y., and Rushford, I. (1976): The stricken: the social consequences of stroke. *Age Ageing*, 5:188–192.
4. Labi, M. L. L., Philips, T. F., and Gresham, G. E. (1980): Psychosocial disability in physically restored long-term stroke survivors. *Arch. Phys. Med. Rehab.*, 61:561–565.

5. Mackay, A., and Nias, B. C. (1979): Strokes in the young and middle-aged: consequences to the family and to society. *J. R. Coll. Phys. Lond.*, 13:106–112.
6. Mykyta, C. J., Bowling, J. H., Nelson, D. A., and Lloyd, E. J. (1976): Caring for relatives of stroke patients. *Age Ageing*, 5:87–90.
7. Oradei, D. M., and Waite, N. (1974): Group psychotherapy with stroke patients during the immediate recovery phase. *J. Ortho. Psychiat.*, 44:386–395.
8. Waite, N. S. (1975): Social problems and the social work role. In: *Stroke and its Rehabilitation*, edited by S. Light, pp. 417–434. Waverly Press, Baltimore, Maryland.
9. Wells, R. (1974): Family stroke education. *Stroke*, 5:393–396.

Advances in Stroke Therapy, edited by
F. C. Rose. Raven Press, New York © 1982.

Lay Volunteers

Valerie Eaton Griffith

St. Martins, Grimm's Hill, Great Missenden, Bucks HP16 9BG, England

As an amateur, I spent 4 years working nearly every day with two severely dysphasic stroke patients. I started from a point of total ignorance as far as stroke was concerned. The result was a journey of discovery, and in a curious way, I believe that this is quite a solid way to learn—one's mind is so open that it is like a blank piece of paper. There are no preconceived ideas, and it gives one a rare chance to look at stroke patients both as they see themselves and as the families see them (3).

The philosophy that grew from this initial work has subsequently been reinforced and added to by the views of several thousand lay volunteers. These amateurs now work in the Volunteer Stroke Scheme, which has been sponsored by the Chest, Heart and Stroke Association (CHSA) since 1973. It is designed to put on a broader canvas the work that had been done by a team of amateurs with the original two stroke patients (1,2,4).

CHSA VOLUNTEER STROKE SCHEME

The scheme in each district is run by a lay supervisor and involves untrained volunteers helping stroke patients who have speech and associated problems. It also aims to help the patients regain their confidence and happiness, without which they are unlikely to attain maximum recovery. The scheme involves:

1. A small team of volunteers each visiting patients in their homes on a regular, weekly basis, to work with them on words of all sorts, numbers, money, telling the time, calendar, memory, shapes and so on, via games and activities. The visits are relaxed and neighbourly, with enjoyment as an essential ingredient.

2. A weekly club with transport arranged and occasional outings.

3. The most important function is to build a personal relationship with the stroke patient and his family, all of whom have been cruelly hard-hit.

The scheme works with the full support of the local health authorities and with the advice of doctors and speech therapists.

PATIENTS

The following points have emerged from working with the patients.

319

Before anything can be achieved, morale and confidence must be fostered. It is natural for a badly dysphasic stroke patient to be depressed, and it is important to allow him to show distress. The battle is to lift his morale and help him find some reason to fight back for his own recovery. It seems to us that both morale and confidence improve when the patient is occupied and working hard to help himself. However, he will need outside stimulation and plenty of human warmth to begin to achieve this. Volunteers find that any work designed to help particular problems is only of value if the way it is tackled is both relevant and of interest to their patient. This means that volunteers pay particular attention to the patient's personality, past work and hobbies, loves and hates, just as they would in any other social setting.

We have found that speech seems to come more easily when words are not consciously sought and the patient is at ease. It is important to try to create a situation where the patient has a prized bit of information to impart, when the thought itself helps to produce the words. Taking patients on "adventurous" outings can be one way of achieving this, when they are bursting to relate the events on their return (a coach breakdown can be a blessing in this respect). Another way to encourage a constructive atmosphere is for patient and volunteer to carry out some activity together which does not necessarily involve speech, for instance a game or a puzzle. This seems to help because silence is acceptable when there is action, whereas it causes stress when nothing else is happening.

Stress is however inevitable in a household where someone has had a bad stroke. It has many causes, not the least of which is that one partner has too much to do and one too little, with a consequent sense of guilt on both sides. Some stress caused by small irritants can be lessened, but to leave the patient out of the normal family ups and downs is likely to increase his frustration. Even the sharing of bad news helps avoid exclusion and is the lesser of two evils. To deny the patient the right to share trouble also takes from him the weapon of his own courage and his latent capacity to be the comforter.

It is wise to remember that will-power can become quenched as the result of a bad stroke, and the initiating spark must be provided by others. It is not always easy to see what will do this, and it is something that has to be searched for as each volunteer works with a patient. There is no doubt as we see it, that until confidence, morale, and self-respect have been restored to some degree, little progress will be made.

VOLUNTEERS

Because the volunteers are amateurs (which does not prevent them from observing and learning) their approach is simply that of good neighbours. They see the patient as a whole person—you or me in need of help. For this reason, we find it important that, albeit with a little guidance, the volunteers should be free to find their own best way of working at the various problems with their patient. This encourages the volunteers to continue because they themselves are involved and interested. It also has been noticed that volunteers as strangers are sometimes more effective than friends, since it can be a relief to the patient to be accepted as he is with no comparison with his former self.

In helping patients practise lost skills, taking them out and about or playing games, the volunteers help defeat the problems of boredom and frustration. The fact, too, that they are spending time with the patient because they want to rather than from a sense of duty helps to encourage the return of self-respect. It also helps the community to accept that stroke patients are normal people and not "out of their minds." Old friends, who had once felt too embarrassed and helpless, may start visiting again. All this will help towards the return of humour, the acceptance of lingering handicaps, and help to keep the hope of full recovery from gradually diminishing.

THE FAMILY

Perhaps one of the most important roles of a volunteer is as a support and confidante of the family, whose well-being is fundamental to a patient's progress. Clearly, support is essential. Perhaps the first and most important problem is that of overprotection, which may stem from the best of motives such as loving concern, but which is a destroyer. Overprotection leads to lack of self-respect in the patient and an ever increasing dependence, which in turn, lead to apathy and helplessness. Allowing the patient to take some risks (such as going to the shops alone) produces a fighting spirit and the will to go on and use what is still left to him.

Another problem the family may have to face is that man and wife so often have to reverse roles and this creates its own tension. In this connection, it is a sobering thought how well some patients manage who live alone.

REHABILITATION AND THE HOME

The majority of stroke patients will have had some rehabilitation before returning home. They will have painstakingly reacquired with professional help some physical and intellectual skills that they had lost. When they come home to take up the living of their own lives again, after a spell of abdication, as it were, they are doing so in a state of mourning for the whole person they once were.

This brings me to a troublesome point. So many patients do not continue to do at home those things which, with a professional by their side, they had shown themselves capable of doing, and neither do they always manage to make the most of what is left. I would like to suggest a few reasons that might contribute to this.

Possibly one of the worst things that happens to the seriously affected patients is a loss that is hard to describe, but what it amounts to is a loss of initiative, inventiveness, will-power, and imagination. This means that one action or thought fails to trigger off the next as is usual with you and me. I wonder whether this is given due regard in professional rehabilitation—whether everyone is worrying not only "can he do something?", but is he able to do it only when someone stands by his side and, as it were, winds up the clock? Should therefore a greater emphasis be placed on stimulation that might instill the kind of "do-it-yourself" spirit independent of someone else's initiative? If this is not possible because of the severity of brain damage, could not a routine be built up with a timetable for when the patient goes home? This could perhaps be handed to the families to help them plan the days.

Perhaps another reason why these patients do not always manage to reach their full potential when at home is because families do not have enough knowledge to understand both the problems and the possibilities. Volunteers are continually commenting on this point. Could not more time be spent on helping and advising families even at the expense, if necessary, of a few sessions for the patient? Because the family attitude affects the patient so strongly this will pay dividends for the patient himself. Another cause of bewilderment and aggrievement is that both patients and their families do not always understand why they see so little of their general practitioner. Perhaps this is because the dividing line between illness (when a doctor can help) and the after-effect (when there is little a doctor can do) is simply not appreciated. I believe it would help if this were gently explained.

Finally, important as it is for a stroke patient to go out into the world, his home is nevertheless the only place from which his life can be lived as fully as possible.

REFERENCES

1. Eaton Griffith, V. (1980): Observations on Patients Dysphasic after Stroke. *Br. Med. J.*, 281:1608–1609.
2. Eaton Griffith, V. (1975): Volunteer scheme for dysphasia and allied problems in stroke patients. *Br. Med. J.*, 3:633–635.
3. Eaton Griffith, V. (1970): *A Stroke in the Family*. Wildwood House, London.
4. Eaton Griffith, V., and Miller, C. L. (1980): Volunteer stroke scheme for dysphasic patients with stroke. *Br. Med. J.*, 281:1605–1607.

Subject Index

Subject Index

Stroke, *see also* Cerebrovascular
   disease
acute
   dexamethasone in, 54,59
   domiciliary care for, 299–303
   hematological tests, 21–22
   investigative aspects of, 21–25
   naftidrofuryl in, 74
   remedial therapy after, 231–234
acute or chronic, 308–309
categories of, in angiography, 164–
   165
as cause of death, 118–119
CBF and, 13
completed, management of, with
   dextran 40,55
continuing needs in, 305–312
descriptive epidemiology of, 101–
   103
early, glycerol in, 57
in elderly, dexamethasone in, 56
functional prognosis in, 119
functional recovery from, 201
gait assessment after, 213–222
geographical variation in,
   102–103
in the health service, 308
incidence of, 64,244–245
ischemic
   dextran 40 in, 57
   prostaglandins in, 63–68
long-term prognosis in, 119–124
medical/surgical management of,
   161–166
new postoperative, 174
ornithine alpha-ketoglutarate in,
   59
pathophysiology of, with positron
   emission tomography, 35–40
platelet behavior in, 130–131,
   134–135
prevention, *see also* European

   Stroke Prevention Study
   carotid surgery in, 169–176
   sulphinpyrazine in, 155–159
   after transient ischemic attacks,
      137–140
primary proliferative
   polycythemia and, 17–19
prognosis in, 200
racial and ethnic variations in, 103
recent, naftidrofuryl in, 58
recurrences of, 123–124
rehabilitation after, *see*
   Rehabilitation
seasonal variation in, 103
sex differences in, 102
threatened, antiaggregant drugs in,
   147–152
thrombotic tendency in, 129–135
treatable, 283
Stroke management, noninvasive
   techniques in, 27–33
Stroke presentation, 239
Stroke prevention study, *see*
   European Stroke Prevention
   Study
Stroke register, 258–259
Stroke trials, 53–61
Stroke unit, 237–254
   Avon, 275–280
   Bordeaux, 283–288
   Bristol, 275–280
   Dover, 257–261
   establishment of 263–267
   Greenwich, 269–273
   size of, 245
Subarachnoid hemorrhage (SAH),
   6–8,87–97
   aneurysmal, 87–97
   antifibrinolytic treatment in, 92–
      95
   in a community, 291–296
   incidence for, 292–293